# Science and Football VII

*Science and Football VII* showcases the very late [...] variety of sports known as 'football'. These inclu[...] (American football, Australian rules football and G[...] [...] rugby codes (union and league). Bridging the gap between th[...] [...] practice, this book is by far the most comprehensive collection of current research into football, presenting important new work in key areas such as:

- physiology of training
- performance analysis
- fitness assessment
- nutrition
- biomechanics
- injury and rehabilitation
- youth football
- environmental physiology
- psychology in football.

*Science and Football VII* is an essential resource for all sport scientists, trainers, coaches, physical therapists, physicians, psychologists, educational officers and professionals working across the football codes.

The papers contained within this volume were first presented at the Seventh World Congress on Science and Football, held in May 2011 in Nagoya, Japan. The meeting was held under the auspices of the International Steering Group on Science and Football, a representative member of the World Commission of Science and Sports.

**Hiroyuki (Hiro) Nunome** is Associate Professor in Biomechanics at Nagoya University, Japan. He is part of the International Steering Group on Science and Football and is the Vice President of the Japanese Society of Science and Football. He is well-known as a pioneer of biomechanics in soccer, particularly of kicking, with many advanced publications in the field.

**Barry Drust** is Reader in Applied Exercise Physiology at Liverpool John Moores University, UK. His main research interests are focused on the physiology of intermittent exercise. As well as his academic roles he has also provided sport science support to elite Premier League football teams and national associations.

**Brian Dawson** is Professor of Sport/Exercise Physiology in the School of Sport Science, Exercise and Health at the University of Western Australia. He is also Chair of the International Steering Group on Science and Football. He has published around 200 papers, many concerning physiology in football codes and other team sports.

# Science and Football VII

The Proceedings of the Seventh World Congress
on Science and Football

*Edited by*
**Hiroyuki Nunome, Barry Drust and
Brian Dawson**

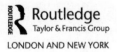 Routledge
Taylor & Francis Group

LONDON AND NEW YORK

First published 2013
by Routledge
2 Park Square, Milton Park, Abingdon, Oxfordshire OX14 4RN

Simultaneously published in the USA and Canada
by Routledge
711 Third Avenue, New York, NY 10017

First issued in paperback 2014

*Routledge is an imprint of the Taylor & Francis Group, an informa business*

*British Library Cataloguing in Publication Data*
A catalogue record for this book is available from the British Library

*Library of Congress Cataloging in Publication Data*
A catalog record for this book has been requested

ISBN 978-0-415-68991-5 (hbk)
ISBN 978-1-138-83772-0 (pbk)
ISBN 978-0-203-13187-9 (ebk)

Typeset in Times New Roman
by Zoe Miveld

# Contents

# Introduction

Dear Science and Football families,

It is our great pleasure to provide *Science and Football VII*. The current volume represents the latest scientific research covering all football codes published in the Seventh World Congress on Science and Football, concurrent with the Ninth Annual Conference of the Japanese Society of Science and Football. The event was held in Nagoya, Japan from 26–30 May 2011, hosted by Nagoya University. The series of Science and Football volumes providing a scientific record of these events have been milestones of the scientific activity geared towards bridging the gap between Science theory and Football practice. For the current volume, of 109 papers from the oral and poster materials submitted, 67 chapters were carefully chosen through twofold peer reviews. These were done by the International Steering Group on Science and Football and the Scientific Committee established for the meeting, with highly efficient administrative help provided by Zoe Miveld at the office of the Research Institute of Sport and Exercise Sciences at Liverpool John Moores University. The book covers every key aspect, including:

- biomechanics
- exercise physiology
- match analysis
- motor behaviour
- performance profiling
- sports medicine
- training science, coaching and psychology.

Sports scientists, trainers, coaches, physiotherapists, medical doctors, psychologists, educational officers and professionals working in the range of football codes will welcome this in-depth, comprehensive, essential and up to date resource.

The World Congress of Science and Football has proud traditions: initiated by the late Professor Tom Reilly at Liverpool in 1987, later followed by meetings at Eindhoven in 1991, Cardiff in 1995, Sydney in 1999, Lisbon in 2003 and Antalya in 2007. The Nagoya Congress continued the line and tradition of these previous conferences under the kindly endorsement and guidance of the International Steering Group on Science and Football, being one of a number of member groups affiliated to the World Commission of Science and Sports, charged by the International Council for Sports Science and Physical Education (ICSSPE).

The Seventh World Congress was officially supported by the Japan Football Association, Japan Rugby Football Union, Japan American Football Association, Nagoya University and Japanese Society of Science and Football, and also benefited from the support of congress partners, exhibitors, drink and meal partners, advertisement partners and presentation partners. With effective support and advice from the International Steering Group, the Congress had an abundant program including: 12 symposia, one keynote, one seminar, one round table session, 19 podium sessions and two poster sessions. Background support for the meeting was ably provided by the staff of JTB Global Marketing & Travel, our academic colleagues and student volunteers from Nagoya University, Chukyo University, Yamagata University and Liverpool John Moores University. A special thanks goes to Koh Sasaki for coordinating the link with the Japan Rugby Football Union.

The Book of Abstracts for the Congress was published in a special supplement of *Football Science*, an international journal published by the Japanese Society of Science and Football. The volume is available at: http://www.shobix.co.jp/jssf/index.cfm.

The Congress award tradition was continued and given a new name: the 'Tom Reilly New Investigator Award'. The winners for oral presentations were: 1st Vanessa Martinez-Lagunas, 2nd Diminic Orth and 3rd Daniel Barreira. The winners for posters were: 1st Hironari Shinkai, 2nd Yusuke Tabei and 3rd Tomas Maly. Also, the Australian Football League Best Paper award went to Johann Bilsborough.

The host of the next Congress was decided after formal presentations by pre-selected candidates. After careful discussion, Copenhagen, Denmark was chosen as the site of the Eighth World Congress on Science and Football in 2015. As with previous Congresses, it is hoped that this Congress will stimulate further research into Science and Football and encourage the participants to implement theory into practice.

**Editors: Hiroyuki Nunome, Barry Drust and Brian Dawson**

# Part I

# Biomechanics

# CHAPTER ONE

# Aerodynamic characteristics
# of new soccer balls

T. Asai

University of Tsukuba, Japan

## 1. INTRODUCTION

Many studies have been conducted on the aerodynamics of sports balls, for example, golf balls (Bearman and Harvey, 1976; Smits and Ogg, 2004), cricket balls (Mehta *et al.*, 1983), tennis balls (Haake *et al.*, 2000; Mehta and Pallis, 2001), baseballs (Watts and Ferrer, 1987), rugby balls (Seo *et al.*, 2004), volleyballs (Wei *et al.*, 1988; Cairns, 2004), and soccer balls (Asai *et al.*, 2007). Mehta (1985) conducted the first proper review of sports ball aerodynamics by investigating the performance of cricket balls, golf balls, and baseballs in detail and demonstrated that the drag on a ball is largely determined by the size and deflection of its wake. However, few such studies have been conducted on new soccer balls. Specifications for soccer balls are determined by Fédération Internationale de Football Association (FIFA), and new soccer balls that meet these specifications are routinely manufactured and used in competitive and recreational sports around the world. However, the aerodynamic characteristics of such newly manufactured soccer balls have not been clarified.

In this study, we have aimed to compare the basic aerodynamic characteristics of conventional and new soccer balls by using wind tunnel tests.

## 2. METHODS

### 2.1 Wind tunnel test

We measured the aerodynamic forces acting on different types of balls in a low-speed wind tunnel having a 0.7 m × 0.7 m rectangular cross-section (turbulence level ≤ 1%). Two full-size official FIFA soccer balls were tested: one conventional ball Adidas Teamgeist II (relatively flat with 14 panels; Figure 1a) and one newly designed ball Adidas Jabulani (small ridges or protrusions with 8 panels; Figure 1b).

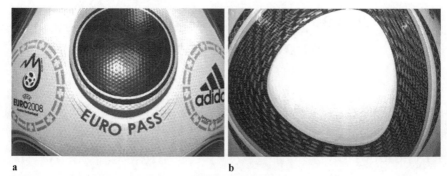

a                                    b

**Figure 1** Surfaces of (a) a conventional ball Adidas Teamgeist II (smooth with 14 panels) and (b) newly designed ball Adidas Jabulani (ridged with 8 panels).

The soccer ball was attached to a stainless steel rod, as shown in Figure 2. Data were acquired by using a three-component strut-type balance (LMC-3531-50NS; Nissho Electric Works) for 8.192 s and recorded on a personal computer using an A/D converter board (sampling rate: 1000 per second).

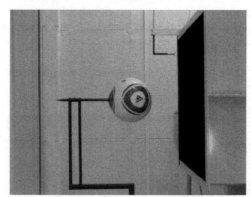

**Figure 2** Setup for wind tunnel test.

Aerodynamic force data were collected at wind speeds $U$ ranging from 6–30 m/s. The force acting in the direction opposite to the direction of the wind, drag ($D$), and the force acting sideways on the basis of frontal views ($L$) were calculated from the experimental data collected under a range of conditions. The aerodynamic forces measured in the experiment were then used to calculate the drag coefficient ($C_d$) and lift coefficient ($C_l$) using the following equations:

$$C_d = \frac{D}{\frac{1}{2}\rho U^2 A} \quad (1)$$

$$C_l = \frac{L}{\frac{1}{2}\rho U^2 A} \quad (2)$$

Here, $\rho$ is the density of air (1.2 kg/m$^3$); $U$, the flow velocity (m/s); and $A$, the projected area (m$^2$) of the soccer ball. Moreover, we calculated the power spectra of an unsteady lift force in order to analyze the characteristics of lift force fluctuations using fast Fourier transform (FFT).

## 3. RESULTS AND DISCUSSION

### 3.1 Drag coefficient

In the experiments, the critical Reynolds number (Re) for a conventional soccer ball (Adidas Teamgeist II) was approximately $2.8 \times 10^5$, while, interestingly, that for the new ridge type ball (Adidas Jabulani) was slightly higher at approximately $3.2 \times 10^5$ (Figure 3). Moreover, $C_d$ for the new ball was less than that for the old ball at high Re values.

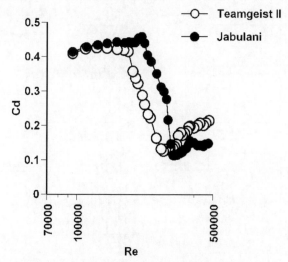

**Figure 3** Drag coefficient ($C_d$) versus Reynolds number (Re) of conventional ball (Teamgeist II; 14 panels) and new ball (Jabulani; 8 panels).

In the supercritical regime, the drag coefficient for the new ball (ridge type) (0.11) was smaller than that for the conventional ball (0.13) and vice versa in the subcritical regime. These results suggest that the aerodynamic drag coefficient of a newly designed soccer ball is closer to that of a smooth sphere than the drag coefficient of a conventional ball. The lift coefficient for both the conventional and ridge type balls showed significant instability at certain speed ranges, but the average lift coefficient did not exhibit any consistent trends.

## 3.2 Lift force fluctuation

The lift force applied to the conventional and new balls used in this experiment was approximately 0 N on an average, but investigations into the time sequence of changes revealed oscillations in the force waveform (Figure 4). For both the conventional and new balls, the magnitude of the oscillations increased when the wind speed was increased from 9 to 16 to 25 and finally to 30 m/s; further, the conventional and new balls did not exhibit large differences in the magnitudes. From the power spectrum of the lift force calculated by the FFT, both the conventional and new balls showed large amplitudes in a low-frequency range below ~6 Hz (Figure 5). The amplitude of the power spectrum increased as the wind speed increased from 9 to 16 to 25 m/s. Figure 6 shows a comparison of the relationship between the maximum amplitudes in the power spectrum and wind speed for the conventional and new balls. Large differences were not observed, but the maximum amplitude was slightly smaller in the new ball at higher speeds (Re = 3.0 × 10$^5$ to 4.5 × 10$^5$). This is probably due to the small ridges on the surface of the new ball; we aim to investigate this in detail in a future study.

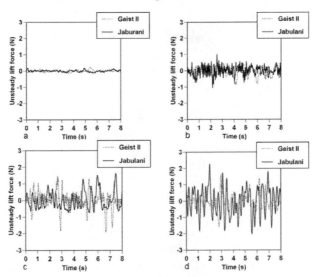

**Figure 4** Unsteady lift force of the conventional ball and new ball at flow speeds of (a) 9 m/s, (b) 16 m/s, (c) 25 m/s, and (d) 30 m/s.

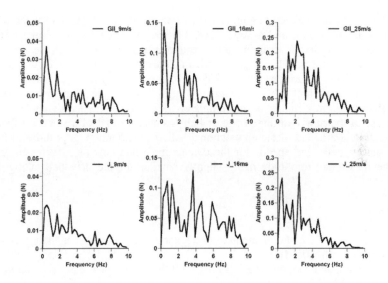

**Figure 5** Power spectrum of the lift force calculated for the conventional ball and new ball by fast Fourier transform (FFT) at flow speeds of 9 m/s, 16 m/s, and 25 m/s.

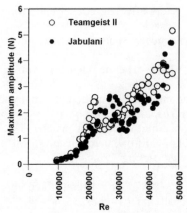

**Figure 6** Relationship between the maximum amplitude of the power spectrum and wind speed for the conventional ball and new ball.

## 4. CONCLUSIONS

In this study, we have aimed to compare the basic aerodynamic characteristics of a conventional soccer ball and a new soccer ball by employing wind tunnel tests. Furthermore, in order to examine the aerodynamic instability near the critical Reynolds regime (Re = ~3.0 × $10^5$), we calculated the power spectra of an unsteady lift force using fast Fourier transform (FFT). The critical Reynolds number for the conventional soccer ball was approximately 2.8 × $10^5$, whereas that for the ridge type ball was slightly higher at approximately 3.2 × $10^5$. The aerodynamic drag coefficient of the newly designed soccer ball is closer to that of a smooth sphere than the drag coefficient of the conventional ball. The maximum amplitudes of the power spectra and wind speeds for the conventional and new balls were similar, with the maximum amplitude being slightly smaller for the new ball at higher speeds.

## References

Asai, T. *et al.*, 2007, Fundamental aerodynamics of the soccer ball. *Sports Engineering*, **10**, 101–109.

Bearman, P.W. and Harvey, J.K., 1976, Golf ball aerodynamics. *Aeronautical Quarterly*, **27**, 112–122.

Cairns, T.W., 2004, Modeling the lift and drag forces on a volleyball. In Hubbard *et al.*, (eds) *The Engineering of Sport 5*, Vol. 1, Sheffield: The International Sports Engineering Association, pp. 97–103.

Haake, S.J. *et al.*, 2000, Engineering tennis–slowing the game down. *Sports Engineering*, **3**, 131–143.

Mehta, R.D. *et al.*, 1983, Factors affecting cricket ball swing. *Nature*, **303**, 787–788.

Mehta, R.D., 1985, Aerodynamics of sports balls, *Ann Rev Fluid Mech*, **17**, 151–189.

Mehta, R. and Pallis, J., 2001, The aerodynamics of a tennis ball, *Sports Engineering*, **4**, 177–189.

Seo, K. *et al.*, 2004, Regular and irregular motion of a rugby football during flight. In Hubbard *et al.* (eds) *The Engineering of Sport 5*, Vol. 1, Sheffield: The International Sports Engineering Association, pp. 567–573.

Smits, A.J. and Ogg, S., 2004, Golf ball aerodynamics. In Hung, G.K. and Pallis, J.M. (eds) *Biomedical Engineering Principles in Sports*, New York: Kluwer Academic, pp. 333–364.

Watts, R.G. and Ferrer, R., 1987, The lateral force on a spinning sphere: Aerodynamics of a curveball. *Am J Physics*, **55**, 40–44.

Wei, Q. *et al.*, 1988, Vortex-induced dynamics loads on a non-spinning volleyball. *Fluid Dynamics Research*, **3**, 231–237.

# CHAPTER TWO

# Injury occurrence and footwear performance on artificial soccer turf

T. Sterzing

Li Ning Sports Science Research Center, Beijing, P.R. China

## 1. ARTIFICIAL SOCCER TURF

Artificial soccer turf has been controversially discussed in relation to game characteristics, injuries, and footwear throughout its developmental stages. The first generation of artificial turf was originally directed towards American football and dates back to the 1960s. One of the first installations was at the Astrodome in Houston, TX, USA (Levy *et al.*, 1990). It solely consisted of a concrete bottom layer covered by a short and dense artificial fiber carpet. The second generation was developed in the 1980s, featuring an elastic bottom layer covered by a carpet of longer and less dense artificial fibers with a sand infill. The third generation was developed in the 1990s, keeping the elastic bottom layer but featuring a more elaborated fiber carpet having a combined sand and rubber infill. This general structure represents the gold standard of artificial soccer turfs today with further developmental efforts ongoing by numerous manufacturers. Due to the different manufacturers, exact specifications of the different components as wells as manufacturing and installment processes of artificial soccer turf may vary.

FIFA ensures the standard of artificial soccer turf pitches by providing 1-star or 2-star certificates after inspection of the installed surface, comparing it to high quality natural grass pitch characteristics (FIFA, 2011b). The number of FIFA certified artificial soccer turf installations is rapidly increasing. Globally, certified installations doubled within one year from 357 in 2010 to 719 in 2011 (FIFA, 2011a). In 2004 2-star artificial soccer turf was included in the FIFA rules of the game as an official playing surface. Since then, soccer match play on artificial turf has been taken place during national regular season competitions in various countries. Also international competitions like the U17 World Cup in Peru and the U20 World Cup in Canada were held on artificial turf.

The breakthrough for artificial soccer turf as the official match play surface was made possible by an improvement of game characteristics and the reduction of injury occurrence. Whereas earlier generations of artificial turf showed considerably different ball bounce and ball roll, subsequently causing different playing behavior (Lees and Lake, 2003), the third generation showed only minor differences compared to natural grass. Here, sliding tackling represents a noteworthy exception, as on artificial soccer turf considerably less sliding tackling occurs compared to natural grass. Whereas injury occurrence was increased for earlier generations of artificial soccer turf (Arnason *et al.*, 1996), prospective studies on injury occurrence on third generation artificial soccer turf compared to natural grass generally revealed no increased injury frequencies. Interestingly, a discrepancy between the objective playing characteristics and the respective subjective perception by players was observed, indicating some bias of players towards artificial soccer turf.

## 2. INJURY OCCURRENCE

Increased injury occurrence in game and practice used to be a major problem of the earlier generations of artificial soccer turf. For currently used artificial soccer turfs, prospective injury surveys consistently show that the overall number of injuries that were sustained during match and training activities is similar to the number of injuries observed on natural grass (Ekstrand *et al.*, 2006; Fuller *et al.*, 2007a, 2007b; Steffen *et al.*, 2007). However, types of injury may slightly differ. Ekstrand *et al.* (2006) reported that more ankle sprains on artificial soccer turf were observed, which has also been shown in a subgroup analysis of young female soccer players (Steffen *et al.*, 2007). Additionally, the injury risk for away team players, potentially being less familiarized with artificial soccer turf was shown to be higher in competitive match settings (Ekstrand *et al.*, 2006). Currently, there is a lack of knowledge about the role of general climatic as well as temporary weather conditions as potential confounding factors for the quantity and type of injuries on artificial soccer turf.

## 3. FOOTWEAR INFLUENCE

Stud configuration of soccer footwear considerably influences agility running performance and respective player's perception (Sterzing *et al.*, 2009). With the implementation of artificial soccer turf players faced playing on a "new" artificial turf but using footwear that was originally designed for playing on natural grass. Thus, a three phase research project was carried out to establish manufacturing guidelines for traction outsoles well suited for playing on artificial turf (Sterzing *et al.*, 2010). The research project included a status quo evaluation (phase I), knowledge based prototype testing (phase II), and a market comparison (phase III). During all phases, a comprehensive footwear evaluation approach was applied consisting of mechanical, biomechanical, athletic performance, and perception testing procedures. This approach is commonly accepted among footwear scientists (Sterzing and Brauner, 2010).

It was found that a functionally designed artificial soccer turf outsole enables players to run faster and receives better subjective perception in comparison to firm and soft ground footwear when used during soccer specific agility running. Higher biomechanical traction ratios were observed in those shoes in which players ran faster, suggesting that breaking and propulsion efforts were more effective during cutting movements. In contrast, mechanical traction characteristics were observed to be highest for a traditional soft ground outsole configuration in which players ran slowest. This displays a noteworthy discrepancy between the suitability of mechanical versus biomechanical traction characteristics for actual usage during play. Alongside, key aspects for a functional traction concept were derived (Figure 1), underlining that purely mechanical traction testing does not provide sufficient insight for the suitability of different shoe surface interfaces. The general concept of mechanically available versus biomechanically utilized traction during shoe ground interaction illustrates the importance of sensory motor skills that allow athletes to adapt their sport specific movement patterns according to varying circumstances.

| Mechanical Availability | Biomechanical Utilization |
|---|---|
| – Material | – Anthropometrics |
| – Geometry | – Body Composition |
| – Interface Angle | – Motor Performance Skills |
| – Loading | – Training Status |

**Figure 1** Functional traction concept.

In further course of the research project, the findings of phase I were used to build knowledge based prototypes for testing of phase II. In phase III, the final artificial soccer turf prototype was compared to three high quality commercially available soccer shoes of top brands that were assigned for artificial soccer turf. The market comparison showed that the final artificial soccer turf prototype outperformed these three shoes models.

Whereas the above addressed research predominantly focused on performance aspects, the following study examined loading aspects of the lower extremities loading due to different footwear conditions on artificial turf (Müller *et al.*, 2010a). Four footwear conditions were analyzed during an active 135° turning movement. Shoe conditions included the final artificial soccer turf prototype shoe of the study referred to above (AT), a firm ground (FG), a soft ground (SG), and a custom made non-studded outsole configuration (AT_0). Touch down angles between shoe and surface in sagittal and frontal planes did not differ among the studded soccer shoes. The non-studded outsole showed reduced touch down angles in both planes to compensate for the removed geometrical traction elements. Additional findings displayed the characteristic relationship between medio-lateral horizontal foot translation and internal ankle eversion moment (Figure 2). Lower traction properties resulted in increased foot translation and coincided with reduced ankle loading. Higher traction properties resulted in reduced foot translation and coincided with increased ankle loading.

It has been shown that athletic footwear function highly depends on the respective surface it is used on. Hence, the implementation of artificial soccer turf pushed the athletic footwear companies to initiate corresponding research. Innovative, reasonably designed artificial soccer turf shoes were shown to provide superior biomechanical and athletic performance characteristics also matching players' perception. Moreover, such type of footwear also decreased internal ankle eversion joint moments during turning movements in comparison to firm and soft ground shoes. Based on these findings, general guidelines for artificial soccer turf footwear were derived. It is suggested that artificial soccer turf footwear should use a rather high number of relatively low stud elements.

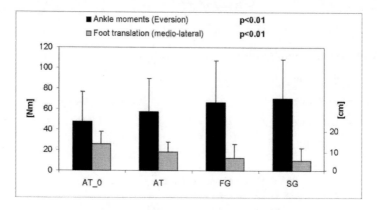

**Figure 2** Medio-lateral foot translation and ankle eversion moments for a 135° turning movement in different soccer shoe conditions on third generation artificial soccer turf (AT_0: no studs, AT: artificial turf, FG: firm ground, SG: soft ground (Müller *et al.*, 2010a).

## 4. CONCLUSION AND PERSPECTIVE

Although artificial soccer turf was included in the rules of the game in 2004, manufacturers have not sufficiently addressed this topic with regard to respective soccer footwear. Initial guidelines for artificial soccer turf shoes have been established, suggesting multiple rather short stud elements to be well suited for playing on artificial soccer turf (Sterzing *et al.*, 2010). However, continued research is mandatory on the topic as the various FIFA licensed manufacturers provide different types of artificial turf constructions. Thus, it needs to be analyzed whether the provided artificial soccer shoe guidelines are suited for all artificial soccer turf types or only for selected ones. Furthermore, the ongoing development efforts of artificial soccer turf should be watched carefully and potentially necessary adaptations to soccer shoe outsole configurations should be made. When playing on natural grass, players use different stud types in response to changing weather and surface conditions. The concept of hard ground, firm ground, and soft ground studs as well as the screw-in stud concept, enabling players to use different stud lengths, has long been established as the gold standard. In contrast, little is known about the influence of varying climatic and temporarily changing weather conditions on the shoe surface interface characteristics of artificial turf. As there is a lack of scientific knowledge, scientific research should be assigned in order to address this relevant and important topic.

A general functional traction concept for soccer footwear was derived. It was shown that mechanically available traction of a shoe surface interface is not identical with the biomechanically utilized traction soccer, which players encounter during breaking and propulsion efforts. Therefore, well suited traction properties of soccer shoes are rather an optimization function of mechanical traction properties instead of a maximization function (Sterzing *et al.*, 2008; Müller *et al.*, 2010b). It should be noted that the general concept of mechanical availability of traction and respective biomechanical utilization is not soccer specific but was applied previously in the context of walking locomotion (Fong *et al.*, 2009).

A comprehensive view of the information provided points towards a potential link between current generation of artificial soccer turf, type of footwear used, and related injury risk. Some injury surveys carefully indicate an increased number of ankle sprains on artificial turf (Ekstrand *et al.*, 2006; Steffen *et al.*, 2007). The analysis of footwear influence on lower extremity loading identified relatively high loads, especially ankle eversion moments, for firm ground soccer shoes compared to the artificial soccer turf prototype shoe on artificial turf (Müller *et al.*, 2010a). As currently the majority of players still use firm ground stud designs when playing on artificial turf, a potential relationship between these findings should be carefully considered. It may be assumed that players put themselves at a slightly increased risk of sustaining ankle sprains by picking less appropriate types of footwear. Performance evaluation of soccer shoes on artificial turf showed that specific artificial turf outsole configurations allow even better agility running performance. Therefore, undertaking such risk is not justified as no beneficial performance margin can be obtained (Sterzing *et al.*, 2010). It needs to be acknowledged that solid scientific evidence for these considerations is missing. Unfortunately, published injury surveys did not include the type of footwear worn by subjects during playing on artificial and natural surfaces when sustaining injuries. This important piece of information is strongly recommended to be included in future injury surveys.

The injury survey by Ekstrand *et al.* (2006) showed also greater injury risk for away team players during match play. The implications of this finding are important as in coming years an increased number of "mixed" national leagues may be present. These leagues feature a number of teams playing on natural grass and a number of teams playing on artificial turf as their home turf. Specific practice units should be developed and also executed in order to ensure timely and sufficient familiarization with the artificial turf prior to match day. It needs to be addressed that with further increase of artificial turf installations, national leagues may encounter a reversed situation with natural grass pitches maybe becoming relatively unusual to some of the players. Therefore, precautions should be taken to allow players to become familiarized when switching playing surfaces in general.

## References

Arnason, A. *et al.*, 1996, Soccer injuries in Iceland. *Scand J Med Sci Sports*, **6**, 40–45.

Ekstrand, J. *et al.*, 2006, Risk of injury in elite football played on artificial turf versus natural grass: a prospective two-cohort study. *Brit J Sports Med*, **40**, 975–980.

FIFA, 2011a, *www.fifa.com* (accessed 12.06.2011).

FIFA, 2011b, FIFA quality concept for artificial turf – handbook of test methods. Zurich, *www.fifa.com* (accessed 12.06.2011).

Fong, D. *et al.*, 2009, Human walks carefully when the ground dynamic coefficient of friction drops below 0.41. *Safety Science*, **47**, 1429–1433.

Fuller, C.W. *et al.*, 2007a, Comparison of the incidence, nature and cause of injuries sustained on grass and new generation artificial turf by male and female football players. Part 1: match injuries. *Brit J Sports Med*, **41**, 20–26.

Fuller, C.W. *et al.*, 2007b, Comparison of the incidence, nature and cause of injuries sustained on grass and new generation artificial turf by male and female football players. *Brit J Sport Med*, **41**, 27–32.

Lees, A. and Lake, M., 2003, The biomechanics of soccer surfaces and equipment. In *Science and Football II* , pp. 120–135.

Levy, M. *et al.*, 1990, Living with artificial grass: a knowledge update Part 1: Basic science. *Am J Sports Med*, **18**, 406–412.

Müller, C. *et al.*, 2010a, Different stud configurations cause movement adaptations during a soccer turning movement. *Footwear Science*, **2**, 21–28.

Müller, C. *et al.*, 2010b, Comprehensive evaluation of player-surface interaction on artificial soccer turf. *Sports Biomechanics*, **9**, 193–205.

Steffen, K. *et al.*, 2007, Risk of injury on artificial turf and natural grass in young female football players. *Brit J Sports Med*, **41**, 33–37.

Sterzing, T. and Brauner, T., 2010, Untersuchungsverfahren in der Sport- und Fußballschuhforschung. *Orthopädieschuhtechnik*, **6**, 43–49.

Sterzing, T. *et al.*, 2008, Discrepancies between mechanical and biomechanical measurements of soccer shoe traction on artificial turf. In *Proceedings 26: Symposium of the International Society of Biomechanics in Sports*, Seoul, Korea, pp. 339–342.

Sterzing, T. *et al.*, 2009, Actual and perceived running performance in soccer shoes: a series of eight studies. *Footwear Science*, **1**, 5–17.

Sterzing, T. *et al.*, 2010, Traction on artificial turf: development of a soccer shoe outsole. *Footwear Science*, **2**, 37–49.

# CHAPTER THREE

# The influence of footwear on ball handling in soccer

T. Sterzing, C. Müller and T. Wächtler

Institute of Sport Science, Chemnitz University of Technology, Germany

## 1. INTRODUCTION

The specific interaction between foot and ball is the defining component of soccer. To date, related research has mainly focused on standardized kicking scenarios of stationary balls (Barfield, 1998; Kellis and Katis, 2007; Lees et al., 2010). Ball velocity as well as ball accuracy also depend on kicking technique (Levanon and Dapena, 1998; Nunome et al., 2002; Kristensen et al., 2005; Neilson and Jones, 2005; Sterzing et al., 2009a). Ball velocity of full instep kicks (Sterzing and Hennig, 2008) as well as ball accuracy of inner instep kicks (Hennig and Sterzing, 2010) were shown to be influenced by soccer footwear. These studies indicated that barefoot compared to shod kicking increased ball velocity but reduced ball accuracy.

However, ball handling comprises more actions than only kicking. In a survey about the importance of ball handling skills in eleven soccer specific situations, players regarded them to be important in most situations that require foot to ball interaction (Sterzing et al., 2011). Also, shoes and balls were reported to play a fairly important role for good ball handling. For this research, we defined ball handling as "player to ball interaction aiming to control or transfer the ball with the foot". Recently, a soccer specific ball handling test battery was introduced by Sterzing et al. (2010). In contrast to more comprehensive soccer performance test protocols (Roesch et al., 2000), the newly introduced protocol consisted of testing situations exclusively requiring foot and ball interaction, evaluating dribbling, juggling, lofted passing of a stationary ball, one touch passing of a rolling ball, passing from aerial, and receiving from aerial.

The goal of this research was to investigate the influence of four different footwear conditions on actual and perceived ball handling performance of soccer players. It was hypothesized that wearing soccer shoes allows better ball handling compared to wearing non-soccer specific footwear or playing barefoot.

## 2. METHODS

Nineteen male soccer players participated in this study (age: $24.0 \pm 3.6$ yrs, height: $178.3 \pm 1.9$ cm, mass: $72.1 \pm 3.1$ kg). Average soccer experience was $15.6 \pm 4.5$

yrs and 6.4 ± 3.0 hrs/wk. Skill level was heterogeneous and ranged from fourth to tenth in the German league. Two soccer shoe models, a non-soccer specific indoor court shoe, and a barefoot condition were included in the study: Puma King® (S-PK), Puma V1.10® (S-V1), Puma Vibrant 5 Trix® (C-VT), barefoot (BAR). All shoes were UK size 8. The two soccer shoe models were highly different to each other (S-PK: leather, wide and long (Brannock D, 262 mm), open lacing with fold over, 320 grams; S-V1: TPU finemold, narrow and short (Brannock C, 254 mm), covered lacing, 237 grams). The indoor court shoe served to question the generally assumed superiority of soccer shoes over non-soccer specific footwear for ball handling tasks (C-VT: Polyester mesh with injected TPU trimmings, very wide and short (Brannock E, 254 mm), open lacing, 333 grams). The barefoot condition provided no artificial interface between the foot and the ball. Footwear conditions were tested in randomized order between subjects and performance tasks. The ball used in this study was an official Puma King® size 5 soccer ball with an inflation pressure of 1 bar. All procedures of this study were approved by the ethics committee of Chemnitz University of Technology for subject testing. Prior to testing all subjects gave written informed consent.

Perception testing was performed as a sequence of dribbling, one touch passes of rolling balls, lofted passes, passes from aerial, and juggling. It incorporated all components of the objective testing performed thereafter. Players rated ball handling suitability of each footwear condition on a 100 mm visual analogue scale, labelled *very good* (0) at the left end and *very bad* (10) at the right end. Respective pain was rated on a 100 mm visual analogue scale, labelled *very low* (0) at the left end and *very high* (10) at the right end. The objective testing protocol included five ball handling tasks explained as follows.

Dribbling (a): Players went through a narrow dribbling course including multiple turns three times each in the respective shoe conditions. Variables were running time [sec] captured by double light barriers (*TAG Heuer HL 2-31, Marin-Epagnier*, Switzerland) and ball contacts [number] captured with a hand counter (*Tally Counter, Sport Thieme*, Germany). Lower running times were associated with better ball handling. Since traction is important for soccer agility running courses (Sterzing *et al.*, 2009a), only the two soccer shoe conditions were included in this task. Potentially small traction differences of the soccer shoes were assumed no confounding variables as running speed for this dribbling task was submaximal.

Juggling (b): Players juggled the ball as often as possible for 20 seconds two times each in the respective testing conditions. Only ball contacts with the foot [number] were counted as performance variable (*Tally Counter, Sport Thieme*, Germany). More ball contacts indicated better ball handling performance.

Lofted pass of stationary ball (c): Players performed five lofted passes of a stationary ball towards a target point located 20 m away. The distance [cm] between the target point and the point where the ball hit the ground first served as the performance variable. The tester identified the exact location of ball bounce, marked it with a chip and measured the respective distance with a tape measure. Smaller deviations to the target point were associated with better ball handling.

One touch pass of rolling ball (d): Players performed five low, one touch passes of balls that were rolling towards them. The task was to pass the ball beyond a "goal line" located 10 m away and direct it as close as possible to a target point located right in the middle of it. The rolling approach of the ball was standardized by usage of a custom made mechanical ball rolling apparatus (Sterzing *et al.*, 2011). The distance [cm] between the target point and the location where the ball actually crossed the "goal line" served as the performance variable. It was read immediately from a laid out tape measure by the tester. Smaller distances between "goal line crossing point" and target point indicated better ball handling.

One touch pass from aerial (e): Players performed five high, one touch passes of balls flying towards them. The task was to pass the ball towards a target point located 8 m away. The flying approach of the ball was standardized by a custom made mechanical ball throwing apparatus (Sterzing *et al.*, 2011). The distance [cm] between the target point and the point where the ball hit the ground first served as the performance variable. The tester identified the exact location of ball bounce, marked it with a chip and measured the respective distance with a tape measure. Smaller deviations from the target point indicated better ball handling.

For statistical evaluation the repetitive trials of each ball handling task were averaged. Means and standard deviations were calculated for each footwear condition across all subjects. Student's t-tests ($p < 0.05$) or repeated measures ANOVA ($p < 0.05$), followed by Bonferroni post-hoc tests ($p < 0.05$), were applied. Subjective variables were contrasted with objective variables to evaluate whether players' perception of ball handling suitability matched their actual ball handling performance.

## 3. RESULTS

As expected, pain perception during ball handling was considerably higher in the barefoot condition compared to all three shod conditions ($p < 0.01$). Ball handling suitability was perceived worse for the indoor court shoe compared to the two soccer shoes and barefoot ($p < 0.01$). Although not statistically significant, there was a trend towards attributing better ball handling suitability to the S-V1 condition compared to S-PK and BAR (Figure 1).

Table 1 summarizes the objective ball handling performance results. The S-V1 evoked faster dribbling times compared to the S-PK ($p < 0.05$). This performance benefit was achieved while maintaining a homogenous number of ball contacts. During juggling, the soccer shoe models allowed most ball contacts. However, this was significant only compared to barefoot ($p < 0.01$). Between the shod conditions no differences in ball contacts were observed.

No statistically significant differences were found between testing conditions for those ball handling tasks that allowed only one touch ball contact (lofted pass of stationary ball, one touch pass of rolling ball, one touch pass from aerial). However, for aerial ball passes a strong trend ($p = 0.06$) pointed towards better ball handling performance of the soccer shoes compared to the non-soccer specific indoor court shoe and barefoot.

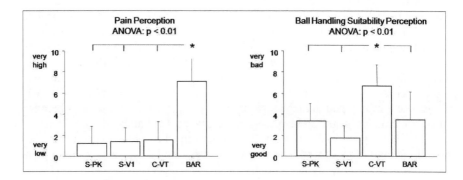

**Figure 1** Subjective perception variables VAS (pain: 0 - very low, 10 - very high; ball handling suitability: 0 - very good, 10 - very bad).

**Table 1** Objective performance variables.

| Task | Unit | S-PK | S-V1 | C-VT | BAR | p-Value |
|------|------|------|------|------|-----|---------|
| (a) | [s] | 7.31 ± 0.63 | 7.07 ± 0.69 | - | - | p < 0.05 |
| | [contacts] | 14.1 ± 1.1 | 13.6 ± 1.3 | - | - | p = 0.13 |
| (b) | [contacts] | 44.2 ± 10.8 | 44.4 ± 10.6 | 42.6 ± 7.7 | 40.8 ± 8.8 | p < 0.01 |
| (c) | [cm] | 208.3 ± 60.6 | 188.1 ± 62.4 | 199.0 ± 56.3 | 224.9 ± 78.0 | p = 0.20 |
| (d) | [cm] | 59.9 ± 28.5 | 64.8 ± 40.3 | 64.7 ± 36.6 | 78.4 ± 33.9 | p = 0.22 |
| (e) | [cm] | 171.4 ± 61.7 | 182.6 ± 81.9 | 226.6 ± 114.2 | 218.2 ± 107.0 | p = 0.06 |

## 4. DISCUSSION

Ball handling perception displayed less trust in non-soccer specific footwear compared to soccer specific footwear and barefoot. The comparison of the two soccer shoe models, although not significant, suggests that, subjectively, players might prefer the narrower, shorter, and lighter shoe properties of the S-V1 for ball handling tasks. In contrast, the leather upper of the S-PK compared to the TPU upper of the S-V1 was not preferred.

Objective performance measurements revealed statistically discriminative potential only in those tasks that required multiple ball contacts (dribbling and juggling). A summed effect of multiple, rather small performance benefits during each ball contact may be the reason for this. No statistical differences were observed for one touch ball handling tasks, suggesting performance was not influenced by the different footwear used. However, in all one touch ball handling tasks shod conditions showed a similar trend to better performance compared to barefoot. Earlier research has shown inner instep kicking for barefoot to be less accurate than for shod kicking (Hennig *et al.*, 2009). This was suggested to be due to less even characteristics of the uncovered anatomical structures of the barefoot compared to the shod foot (Hennig and Sterzing, 2010). In the present research, barefoot ball handling tended to be less accurate than respective shod performance, being in line with those earlier observations.

Among the three shod conditions the non-soccer specific indoor court shoe was clearly perceived worst with respect to ball handling suitability, although objective data did not show solid statistical differences for the respective performance values. This means that subjective and objective data did not reflect each other in the present research. Therefore, human sensory as well as psychological mechanisms during the perception of footwear performance in ball handling tasks are not necessarily related to actual motor performance.

The absence of more solid objective performance differences among the footwear conditions may have various reasons. As the subject group's skill level was quite heterogeneous, it might be worth looking at a more homogenous pool of elite soccer players. It also needs to be taken into consideration that there simply is no bigger measurable influence of the footwear used in this study. Also, as the tested footwear differed in multiple features, the various single shoe features may have cancelled out with respect to objective ball handling performance.

## 5. CONCLUSION

This study showed that soccer footwear contributes to performance of ball handling in some cases and generally contributes to respective perception in soccer. Ball handling performance was perceived differently by players when wearing different footwear. Actual ball handling performance was shown to be different in some but not in all performance tasks of this study. Better discrimination potential for objective ball handling quality of different shoe conditions seem to be present in those tasks requiring multiple ball contacts and potentially during those that are more difficult.

Future research should aim to investigate the influence of specific, isolated shoe properties on ball handling performance and their respective perception, such as dimension (size, fit), upper material (type, thickness), upper geometry (shape, profile) and shoe flexibility. Also, for a better understanding of the underlying mechanisms of soccer ball handling related to footwear, the application of biomechanical and mechanical testing procedures is recommended.

### Acknowledgements

Research was supported by Puma® Inc., Germany. A more comprehensive paper on the presented content was published earlier (Sterzing *et al.*, 2011).

## References

Barfield, W.R., 1998, The biomechanics of kicking in soccer. *Clinics in Sports Medicine*, **17**, 711–728.

Hennig, E.M. *et al.*, 2009, Soccer footwear and ball kicking accuracy. *Footwear Science*, **1**, 85–87.

Hennig, E.M. and Sterzing, T., 2010, The influence of soccer shoe design on playing performance - a series of biomechanical studies. *Footwear Science*, **2**, 3–11.

Kellis, E. and Katis, A., 2007, Biomechanical characteristics and determinants of instep soccer kick. *J Sports Sci Med*, **6**, 154–165.

Kristensen, L.B. *et al.*, 2005, Comparison of precision in the toe and instep kick in soccer at high kicking velocities. In *Science and Football V*, pp. 70–72.

Levanon, J. and Dapena, J., 1998, Comparison of the kinematics of the full-instep and pass kicks in soccer. *Med Sci Sport Exer*, **30**, 917–927.

Lees, A. *et al.*, 2010, The biomechanics of kicking: A review. *J Sport Sci*, **28**, 805–817.

Neilson, P.J. and Jones, R., 2005, Dynamic soccer ball performance measurement. In *Science and Football V*, pp. 21–27.

Nunome, H. *et al.*, 2002, Three-dimensional kinetic analysis of side-foot and instep soccer kicks. *Med Sci Sports Exerc*, **34**, 2028–2036.

Roesch, D. *et al.*, 2000, Assessment and evaluation of football performance. *Am J Sports Med*, **28**, pp. S29–S39.

Sterzing, T. and Hennig, E.M., 2008, The influence of soccer shoes on kicking velocity in full instep soccer kicks. *Exerc Sport Sci Rev*, **36**, 91–97.

Sterzing, T. *et al.*, 2009a, Velocity and accuracy as performance criteria for three different soccer kicking techniques. In *Proceedings of the 27th International Conference on Biomechanics in Sports*, Limerick, Ireland, pp. 243–246.

Sterzing, T. *et al.*, 2009b, Actual and perceived running performance in soccer shoes: A series of eight studies. *Footwear Science*, **1**, 5–17.

Sterzing, T. *et al.*, 2010, Bewertung der Ballbehandlung im Fußball. In *Proceedings of the 7th dvs-Sportspiel-Symposium*, Münster, Germany, pp. 9–15.

Sterzing, T. *et al.*, 2011, Shoe influence on actual and perceived ball handling performance in soccer. *Footwear Science*, **3**, 97–105.

# CHAPTER FOUR

# Unanticipated compared to preplanned turning movements increase lower extremity loads in football players

C. Müller, T. Sterzing and T. L. Milani

Institute of Sport Science, Chemnitz University of Technology, Germany

## 1. INTRODUCTION

Football is characterized by short, abrupt and dynamic, non-cyclic movements like accelerations, decelerations and changes of directions (Ekblom, 1986). FIFA (2009) reported that general changes of running velocity and running directions occur every 4–6 seconds during a football game. Changes of direction can be categorized as cutting movements (0–90° relative to original running direction) or turning movements (90–180° relative to original running direction). Dynamic changes of directions are very common in football and occur in numerous game situations. Unanticipated turning movements (UA) especially occur during rapid transitions from offensive to defensive playing situations, when reacting to opponent's movement paths as well as when reacting to sudden or unexpected ball passes. Preplanned turning movements (PP) are predominantly used for feints within or without ball. Generally, all actions during a football game are either preplanned or unanticipated movements. Thereby preplanned movements mark active actions of a player based on his personal performance plan. Unanticipated movements mark reactive actions triggered by the specific performance of opponents or other elements of the game situation like passes or turnovers. Thus, a large percentage of all defensive actions can be described as unanticipated movements.

Football is a sport with a very high injury rate. Thereby, more than 70% of the injuries occur at the lower extremities (Ekstrand and Gillquist, 1983; Dvorak and Junge, 2000). Non-contact injuries primarily occur during rapid changes of direction (Besier et al., 2001). A main reason for non-contact injuries is the relative fixation of the foot to the surface in combination with a rotational component initiated by body segments proximal to the foot. This specific interface scenario is predominantly observed during rapid turning movements. The general mechanism of turning movements can be subdivided into three phases (Andrews et al., 1977). In phase one, the upper body of the player is decelerated by the stance leg. In phase two, the trunk and pelvis rotate around the stance leg towards the new running direction. In phase three, the stance leg itself rotates towards the new running direction and initiates the propulsion of the player. In all three phases considerably high loads act on the player's lower extremities.

The majority of biomechanical cutting and turning studies only focused on preplanned type of movements, although it already has been pointed out that these do not reflect all games situations (Stacoff *et al.*, 1996; Sell *et al.*, 2006). In recent years, more studies, specifically focusing on unanticipated movement types, were carried out (Ford *et al.*, 2005; Landry *et al.*, 2007). In summary, these studies observed higher knee moments during unanticipated compared to preplanned movements as well as gender specific movement patterns during unanticipated movements. So far, all these findings are based on research designs using non-football footwear and therefore dealing with non-football specific shoe ground interfaces.

The general sequence of mechanisms for preplanned movements is characterized by initially self-selected action, foot strike orientation in the new running direction, and specific muscle activation for the stabilization of joints to reduce joint moments. In contrast, unanticipated movements are characterized by initial temporal restrictions, a subsequent less well prepared foot strike, and unspecific muscle activation resulting in increased joint moments (Abernethy 1996; Besier *et al.*, 2001, 2003; Cuisinier *et al.*, 2005; Brown *et al.*, 2009). The objective of this study was to investigate the kinematics and kinetics of the lower extremities during preplanned and unanticipated football turning movements while wearing football shoes. It was hypothesized that lower extremity loadings were increased during unanticipated turning movements.

## 2. METHODS

Twenty-three experienced football players (age: 24.3 ± 2.6 years, height: 178.3 ± 3.7cm, weight: 71.8 ± 6.3kg, exposure: 6.3 ± 2.2 hrs/wk) participated in this study. All procedures adhered to the general guidelines for subject testing at Chemnitz University of Technology, Germany. Subjects were required to give informed consent prior to testing.

The study took place on third generation artificial football turf (*Liga Turf 240 22/4 RPU, Polytan, Burgheim, Germany*) in a laboratory environment. Two shoe conditions were used in this study, an artificial turf prototype shoe, which was positively evaluated in previous research (Sterzing *et al.*, 2010) and a firm ground shoe type, which is commonly used on artificial football turf. For preplanned turning movements, subjects performed a 135° turn relative to their original approach direction. For unanticipated turning movements subjects performed either a 135° turning movement or straight ahead running due to a randomized light signal indication, provided 150–200ms before contacting the force plate area. Ground reaction force data were collected by a Kistler force plate (9287BA, 900x600mm, 960Hz), lower extremity kinematics by a 12-camera Vicon motion analysis system (MX-3, 240Hz). For the latter, 25 reflective anatomical and tracking markers were placed on the lower extremities. The lower extremity segments (thigh, shank, foot) were reconstructed from the medial and lateral anatomical markers, which allow defining the dimensions and the local coordinate system. Kinematic (Low pass, Butterworth, 30Hz) and kinetic (Low pass, Butterworth, 200Hz) data were filtered and further processed in Visual 3D (C-Motion Inc., Rockville, MD, USA). Ankle and knee joints were assigned six degrees of freedom; the coordination reference frame used for each segment was the Cardan sequence XYZ with the X-axis medio-lateral oriented, the Y-axis anterior-posterior, and the Z-axis proximal-distal (Kadaba *et al.*, 1990). The inverse dynamics is based on the method of global optimization by Lu and O'Connor (1999). The subjects performed five repetitive trials for each type of turning movement.

Investigated variables were ground contact time, horizontal foot translation, defined as the relative motion of the foot on the surface during ground contact (Müller *et al.*, 2010), foot and leg alignment during the turning movements, including foot strike adduction angle, ankle angles and knee angles, as well as net internal joint moments for ankle and knee. For all these variables means and standard deviations were calculated and analyzed by two-way (type of movement, shoe condition) repeated measures ANOVA. Post-hoc tests were applied according to Bonferroni ($p<0.05$).

## 3. RESULTS AND DISCUSSION

In general, all variables turned out to be shoe independent. Therefore, means were calculated over both shoe conditions for results. Ground contact time was significantly increased for unanticipated movements compared to preplanned movements (Table 1). For horizontal foot translation no differences were observed among both turning movements.

**Table 1** Ground contact time (GCT) and horizontal foot translation (HFT) for preplanned (PP) and unanticipated turning movements (UA).

| Variable | Unit | PP | UA | p-value |
|---|---|---|---|---|
| GCT | [s] | $0.50 \pm 0.31$ | $0.55 \pm 0.38$ | $< 0.01$ |
| HFT (medio-lateral) | [cm] | $5.41 \pm 5.30$ | $7.03 \pm 5.17$ | $= 0.18$ |
| HFT (anterior-posterior) | [cm] | $5.28 \pm 5.73$ | $4.35 \pm 6.05$ | $= 0.23$ |

At initial ground contact, subjects showed a decreased foot adduction angle and decreased tibial rotation towards the new running direction for the unanticipated movement (Table 2). Thus, kinematic differences were observed, suggesting that foot and leg alignment was less well prepared at initial ground contact for unanticipated turning movements.

**Table 2** Foot angles, ankle angles and knee angles at touchdown (TD) and toe-off (TO) in degree ($^\circ$).

| Variable | Phase | PP | UA | p-value |
|---|---|---|---|---|
| Foot plantarflexion | TD | 28.2 ± 7.4 | 30.4 ± 7.0 | = 0.38 |
| Foot inversion | TD | 10.1 ± 9.2 | 9.3 ± 10.7 | = 0.41 |
| Foot adduction | TD | 55.0 ± 16.3 | 49.7 ± 19.6 | < 0.01 |
| Ankle eversion | TD | 6.4 ± 4.3 | 4.2 ± 3.6 | = 0.08 |
| Ankle eversion | TO | 21.0 ± 6.3 | 23.4 ± 7.1 | = 0.06 |
| Knee flexion | TD | 16.8 ± 6.3 | 17.4 ± 9.0 | = 0.30 |
| Tibial rotation | TD | 25.8 ± 8.7 | 20.1 ± 11.9 | < 0.05 |

Additionally, ankle eversion angle was slightly decreased for unanticipated movements at initial ground contact. In contrast, at final ground contact, ankle eversion angle was slightly increased for the unanticipated compared to the preplanned movements. Subsequently, related ankle eversion magnitude (PP: 15° ± 7, UA: 19° ± 7) was significantly increased for unanticipated movements during ground contact (p<0.01).

Ankle moments as well as knee moments were significantly increased for unanticipated movements. Knee flexion (PP: 231Nm ± 84, UA: 256Nm ± 82, p<0.05) and ankle eversion moments (PP: 60Nm ± 12, UA: 68Nm ± 10, p<0.01) were more than 10% increased. Furthermore, knee rotation (PP: 56Nm ± 22, UA: 61Nm ± 23, p<0.05) and ankle plantarflexion moments (PP: 222Nm ± 38, UA: 241Nm ± 46, p<0.05) were increased up to 8% for unanticipated movements compared to preplanned movements. Figure 1 illustrates the ankle eversion moment for both types of movements.

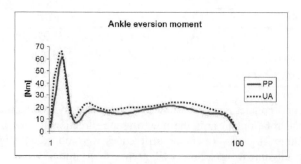

**Figure 1** Ankle eversion moment for preplanned (PP) and unanticipated movements (UA), normalized to 100 data points (1 - touchdown to 100 - toe-off).

Distinct movement adaptations were observed for unanticipated turning movements compared to preplanned movements. These adaptations describe a mechanism chain featuring a less suitable foot and leg alignment towards the new running direction at foot strike, resulting in increased joint moments of the lower extremities. The less well prepared foot strike was based on the temporal restrictions induced. Subjects primarily compensated for that by an increased ankle eversion amplitude during the turning movement. In combination with a higher ankle eversion moment, this indicates higher loads on the distal part of the lower extremities during unanticipated movements.

## 4. CONCLUSION

This research showed that an unanticipated, 135° turning movement while wearing football shoes showed similar mechanisms present in related studies investigating unanticipated movements while wearing non-studded athletic footwear. Unanticipated movements may be a potential risk factor for football injuries. Primarily the distal part of the lower extremities was shown to be highly loaded during unanticipated movements. A potentially higher injury risk during unanticipated turning movements is based on higher joint moments in combination with a similar amount of foot translation compared to preplanned turning movements. Additionally, it was shown that obvious varying motion sequences overshadowed traction properties of football footwear. In this case, artificial turf prototype condition and firm ground condition provoked marginal influences on the movement behavior between unanticipated and preplanned movements.

In future studies, the effect of different reaction times for unanticipated movements should be analyzed. It is hypothesized that shorter reaction time periods change the kinematics and kinetics even more severely, whereas longer reaction time periods diminish those movement adaptations between unanticipated and preplanned movements. Additionally, different football specific movements, like cutting and jumping, should be investigated with regard to preplanned and unanticipated movements.

## Acknowledgement

This research was supported by Puma Inc., Germany.

## References

Abernethy, B., 1996, Training the visual-perceptual skills of athletes: Insight from the study of motor expertise. *Am J Sport Med*, **24**, 89–92.
Andrews, J.R. *et al.*, 1977, The cutting mechanism. *Am J Sport Med*, **5**, 111–121.
Besier, T.F. *et al.*, 2001, Anticipatory effects on knee joint loading during running and cutting maneuvres. *J Med Sci Sports Exerc*, **33**, 1176–1181.

Besier, T.F. *et al.*, 2003, Muscle activation strategies at the knee during running and cutting maneuvers. *J Med Sci Sports Exerc*, **35**, 119–127.

Brown, T.N. *et al.*, 2009, Differences between sexes and limbs in hip and knee kinematics and kinetics during anticipated and unanticipated jump landings: Implications for ACL injury. *Brit J Sport Med*, **43**, 1049–1056.

Cuisinier, R. *et al.*, 2005, Effects of foreperiod duration on anticipatory postural adjustments: Determination of an optimal preparation in standing and sitting for a raising arm movement. *Brain Res Bull*, **66**, 163–170.

Dvorak, J. and Junge, A., 2000, Football injuries and physical symptoms: A review of the literature. *Am J Sports Med* **28**, 3–9.

Ekblom, B., 1986, Applied physiology of soccer. *J Sport Med*, **3**, 50–60.

Ekstrand, J. and Gillquist, J., 1983, The avoidability of soccer injuries. *Int J Sport Med*, **4**, 124–128.

FIFA, 2009, Health checks in football. www.fifa.com (26.6.2009).

Ford, K.R. *et al.*, 2005, Gender differences in kinematics of unanticipated cutting in young athletes. *J Med Sci Sport Exerc*, **37**, 124–129.

Kadaba, M.P. *et al.*, 1990, Measurement of lower extremity kinematics during level walking. *J Orthop Res*, **8**, 383–392.

Landry, S.C. *et al.*, 2007, Neuromuscular and lower limb biomechanical differences exist between male and female elite adolescent soccer players during an unanticipated side-cut maneuver. *Am J Sports Med*, **35**, 1888–1900.

Lu, T.W. and O'Connor, J.J., 1999, Bone position estimation from skin marker coordinates using global optimization with joint constraints. *Journal of Biomechanics*, **32**, 129–134.

Müller, C. *et al.*, 2010, Different stud configurations cause movement adaptations during a soccer turning movement. *Footwear Science*, **2**, 21–28.

Sell, T.C. *et al.*, 2006, The effect of direction and reaction on the neuromuscular and biomechanical characteristics of the knee during tasks that simulate the noncontact anterior cruciate ligament injury mechanism. *Am J Sport Med*, **34**, 43–54.

Stacoff, A. *et al.*, 1996, Lateral stability in sideward cutting movements. *J Med Sci Sports Exerc*, **28**, 350–358.

Sterzing, T. *et al.*, 2010, Traction on artificial turf: development of a soccer shoe outsole. *Footwear Science*, **2**, 37–49.

# CHAPTER FIVE

# Cross-sectional change of ball impact in instep kicks from junior to professional footballers

H. Shinkai[1], H. Nunome[2], H. Suito[3], K. Inoue[2] and Y. Ikegami[2]

[1]Faculty of Education, Art and Science, Yamagata University, Japan
[2]Research Centre of Health, Physical Fitness and Sports, Nagoya University, Japan
[3]Faculty of Psychological and Physical Science, Aichi Gakuin University, Japan

## 1. INTRODUCTION

Along with the forward swing of the kicking leg, ball impact is one of the most important factors for fast ball kicking in soccer. Ball impact is a phase during which the players transfer the momentum of their kicking limb to the ball. Through daily training, the players acquire ways to impart the leg and foot momentum into the ball effectively. In most instep kicking, rapid passive motion of the kicking foot occurs due to large ball reaction force during ball contact (Asai *et al.*, 2002; Nunome *et al.*, 2006; Shinkai *et al.*, 2009). To enhance the ball impact efficiency, it has been considered that the magnitude of the foot deformation needs to be minimized by ankle rigidity at ball contact (Asami and Nolte, 1983; Rodano and Tavana, 1993; Lees and Nolan, 1998).

To date, there have been several studies to describe the maturity process of ball kicking technique in soccer. With regard to the forward swing of the kicking leg, it has been reported that the maximum angular velocity of the shank or the values at ball contact increased with age (Bloomfield *et al.*, 1979; Luhtanen, 1988). On the other hand, the kicking foot motion during ball impact phase and those changes from childhood to adolescent soccer players have never been systematically investigated.

The aim of this study was to investigate the change of ball impact characteristics in instep kicking with physical growth of the soccer players by the cross-sectional method.

## 2. METHODS

Fifty-one skilled male soccer players from 8 to 24 years old, including six professionals, participated in this study. All players belonged to a Japanese professional football club or its youth academy.

After an adequate warm-up, subjects performed several maximal instep kicks using their dominant leg with a free approach run. The target (0.88 m square) was set 5 m ahead and just above ground level. Success and failure of hitting the target was measured by the high-speed video image (250 Hz) recording around the target. Moreover, rough impact position of the foot with the ball was checked visually by ultra-high-speed video images. One successful shot, when the player impacted the ball around the centre of instep and the ball hit the target, was selected from each subject for analysis.

FIFA approved soccer ball of size four (mass = 0.374 kg, inflation = 700 g/cm$^2$) or size five (mass = 0.42 kg, inflation = 900 g/cm$^2$) was used for subjects between 8 and 12 years old and over 13 years old, respectively. All subjects wore the same type of soccer shoes for outdoor practice to minimize the influence of type of shoe on the interaction between foot and ball during ball contact. Two electrically synchronized ultra-high-speed video cameras (Photron Ltd., FASTCAM-512 PCI) were set up on the kicking leg side and backward. The sampling rate of the cameras was set at 2000 Hz to capture adequately the instantaneous foot and ball motion during ball contact. White markers were securely fixed onto the ball and several anatomical landmarks on the lateral side of the kicking limb: head of fibula, lateral malleolus, lateral side of calcaneus, fifth metatarsal base and fifth metatarsal head.

Three-dimensional coordinates of each marker were obtained by the direct linear transformation (DLT) method. Tri-axial angular foot motion of (plantar/dorsal flexion, abduction/adduction, inversion/eversion) was calculated using the shank segment vector (pointing from lateral malleolus towards the head of fibula) and foot segment vector (pointing from the lateral side of calcaneus toward the fifth metatarsal head). Angular displacements during ball contact, whose criterion value was the angle of the foot at the instant of the initial ball contact, were also calculated. All angular data were digitally filtered by a fourth-order Butterworth low-pass filter at 200 Hz.

The contact time between the foot and the ball was measured from the lateral side video image by counting the number of frames. The foot velocity (fifth metatarsal base) just before ball impact and the resultant ball velocity (centre of the ball) were calculated. The ball-foot velocity ratio provided an index of efficiency of ball impact and was represented by the ratio of ball velocity to foot velocity. To quantify how much the mass was imparted for the collision, effective striking mass of the kicking limb was estimated from the equation of conservation of momentum using the mass of the ball, foot velocities just before and after ball impact, and ball velocity (Plagenhoef, 1971). For comparison of this parameter, the mass of the player's foot was also estimated using coefficient for segment mass proportions

(Jensen, 1989). The foot mass of the players over 21 years old was calculated regarding as 20 years old player.

## 3. RESULTS AND DISCUSSION

Body mass (range from 23 to 76.4 kg), foot velocity before ball impact (range from 14.5 to 24.2 m/s), ball velocity (range from 14.5 to 34.1 m/s), and ball-foot velocity ratio (range from 0.98 to 1.53) increased systematically with player's age. Luhtanen (1988) published the only study that reported the ball velocity of instep kicking of skilled young soccer players from 9 to 18 years old. The resultant ball velocity of this study showed distinctively higher values than those reported by him in all age groups. The ball velocity was strongly correlated with the player's body mass (r = 0.94, $P < 0.01$) and the foot velocity (r = 0.94, $P < 0.01$). On the other hand, the average contact time between foot and ball was 8.9 ± 0.4 ms and was consistent for all age groups.

The kicking foot was forced into plantar flexion (5.9 ± 4.6 deg), abduction (6.2 ± 4.3 deg), and eversion (2.2 ± 2.8 deg) during ball contact. These passive foot motions were commonly observed in most trials regardless of age. The magnitude of passive foot motions except for abduction and changes of foot angles during ball contact were similar to those of Shinkai *et al.* (2009) also reported for skilled adult players. Figure 1 shows the relationship between angular displacement of passive plantar flexion during ball contact and ball-foot velocity ratio. To date, it has been suggested by several studies (Asami and Nolte, 1983; Rodano and Tavana, 1993; Lees and Nolan, 1998) that the state of rigidity of the foot is a vital factor for good foot-ball impact. Therefore, these angular displacements of the foot during ball impact have been considered the index of maturity of ball impact technique. However, in this study, ball-foot velocity ratio which is an index of ball impact efficiency was correlated weakly with foot angular displacement for all directions (abduction/adduction, r = -0.09; inversion/eversion, r = 0.13). These results show that the ball impact technique of skilled younger players of this study was mostly completed.

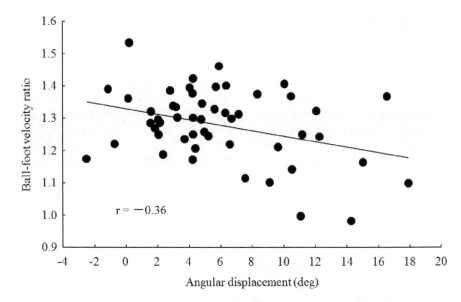

**Figure 1** Relationship between angular displacement of plantar (+) / dorsal (-) flexion
during ball contact and ball-foot velocity ratio.

The effective striking mass of the kicking limb (ranged from 0.69 to 2.36 kg) was strongly correlated with the estimated foot mass of the players (range from 0.48 to 1.37 kg, r = 0.91) and ball-foot velocity ratio (see Figure 2). Moreover, the sum of the mass of foot and shoe (ranged from 0.68 to 1.69 kg) corresponded to 84.0 ± 9.6 % of the effective striking mass of the kicking limb (Figure 3). Lees and Nolan (1998) speculated that if the ankle becomes more rigid at the ball impact, the effective striking mass would increase by adding some part of the shank mass on the foot mass. However, our results suggested that if the foot hit the ball with adequate position (i.e. around the location of its centre of mass), the ball impact is most likely assumed to be a collision between the shod foot and ball.

To enhance the striking mass, increasing the mass of the foot is essential for the players having good enough ball impact technique. Therefore, it can be considered that the mass of the foot (as a proportion of the body mass) of the players has great influence on the ball impact efficiency.

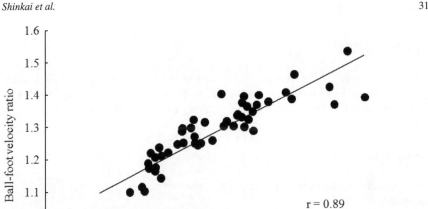

**Figure 2** Relationship between effective striking mass of the kicking limb and ball-foot velocity ratio.

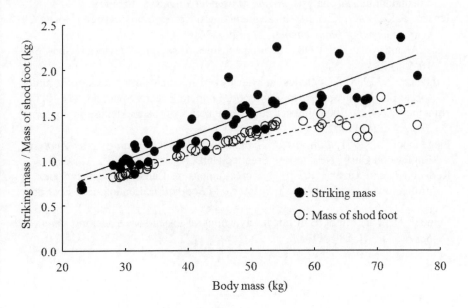

**Figure 3** Comparison of the effective striking mass of the kicking limb and
the sum of the mass of foot and shoe.

## 4. CONCLUSION

The physical size of the soccer players has great influence on the ball impact efficiency. Therefore, due to the small mass of the foot, younger players have some disadvantage in kicking the fast ball effectively even if their kicking technique is skilful.

### Acknowledgements

This research was partially supported by a grant from Yamaha Motor Foundation for Sports.

### References

Asai, T. *et al.*, 2002, The curve kick of a football I: Impact with the foot. *Sports Engineering*, **5**, 183–192.

Asami, T. and Nolte, V., 1983, Analysis of powerful ball kicking. In H. Matsui and K. Kobayashi (eds) *Biomechanics VIII-B*, Champaign, Illinois: Human Kinetics Publishers, pp. 695–700.

Bloomfield, J. *et al.*, C.M., 1979, Development of the soccer kick: A cinematographical analysis. *J Hum Movement Studies*, **5**, 152–159.

Jensen, R.K., 1989, Changes in segment inertia proportions between 4 and 20 years. *Journal of Biomechanics*, **22**, 529–536.

Lees, A. and Nolan, L., 1998, The biomechanics of soccer: A review. *J Sport Sci*, **16**, 211–234.

Luhtanen, P., 1988, Kinematics and kinetics of maximal instep kicking in junior soccer players. In *Science and Football*, London: E & FN Spon, pp. 441–448.

Nunome, H. *et al.*, 2006, Impact phase kinematics of instep kicking in soccer. *J Sport Sci*, **24**, 11–22.

Plagenhoef, S., 1971, *Patterns of Human Motion: A Cinematographic Analysis*, Englewood Cliffs, New Jersey: Prentice-Hall.

Rodano, R. and Tavana, R., 1993, Three-dimensional analysis of instep kick in professional soccer players. In *Science and Football II*, London: E & FN Spon, pp. 357–363.

Shinkai, H. *et al.*, 2009, Ball impact dynamics of instep soccer kicking. *Med Sci Sport Exer*, **41**, 889–897.

# CHAPTER SIX

# The validity of the Shadowbox™ magnetic and inertial tracking system for measuring soccer-specific movements

T. R. Flanagan[1] and L. A. Thompson[2]

[1] US Ski & Snowboard Association, Park City, USA
[2] RMIT University, Bundoora, Australia

## 1. INTRODUCTION

Previous match analysis studies on soccer (Hennig and Briehle, 2000) and Australian rules football (Edgecomb and Norton, 2006) have successfully used a Global Positioning System (GPS) to track the general locomotion and movement patterns of players around the field. However, many sport specific actions such as kicking, tackling and passing were not captured and quantified in these studies. For a complete movement analysis, all movements made by players including locomotion and sport specific actions should theoretically be measured. Current match analysis technologies used by researchers, however, are not sensitive enough to measure both global movements on the field and to capture sports specific actions made by players.

One possible solution to solve this problem is the use of a wearable magnetic and inertial tracking system during match play to capture the motion of limbs and relative displacement of the player around the field. This system uses motion sensors (accelerometers, gyroscopes and magnetometers) to continuously measure the position, orientation, direction and speed of movement without the need for external references. This technology has recently incorporated more powerful sensor components, is miniature and has been trialled in sports biomechanics research as a motion tracking solution in ski racing (Brodie *et al.*, 2008).

The Shadowbox™ (Shadowbox, Park City, USA) is a commercially available miniature magnetic and inertial navigation system. It was originally designed for detecting the movements of wake boarders and has very high capacity sensors. To date, the validity of such technology to accurately detect the 3D motion of a soccer player's limb remains unclear, particularly the accuracy of the triaxial inertial and magnetic sensors. The purpose of this study, therefore, was to evaluate the validity of the 3D displacement data derived by a portable magnetic and inertial motion tracking system, the Shadowbox™, against a criterion camera-based 3D motion capture system, the Vicon MX™ (Vicon Motion Systems Ltd, Oxford, UK), during a series of soccer-specific actions.

## 2. METHODS

One healthy male competitive soccer player (age = 26 yrs; mass = 78 kg; stature = 181 cm) volunteered and consented to act as a subject in this study. The subject's task was to perform a kick (drive) of a ball, a one-touch pass of a ball and a slide tackle while his motion was tracked simultaneously by the Shadowbox™ and the calibrated Vicon MX™ motion analysis system.

The Shadowbox™ (dimensions: 9 x 6 x 2 cm, mass: 132 g) was securely attached to the right ankle of the subject using adhesive tape. The Shadowbox™ contained a triaxial accelerometer, gyroscope and magnetometer. Raw data from these sensors were collected at a sample rate of 100 Hz. Reflective markers were placed on the subject using the Vicon plug-in-gait method (Riley *et al.*, 2007). The 'ankle' reflective marker was placed on the Shadowbox™ to track its actual location in the data collection space using the camera-based Vicon MX™ motion analysis system (Figure 1). Vicon MX™ cameras were placed around the data collection space (7 m x 4 m). The Vicon MX™ system included 6 x MX-T20 cameras (2.0 megapixel resolution/500 frames per second) and 4MX-T40 cameras (4.0 megapixel resolution/370 frames per second). The cameras also included 10 near infrared high power surface strobes for detecting the reflective markers placed on the body. Vicon data was averaged over time and exported as 100 Hz data.

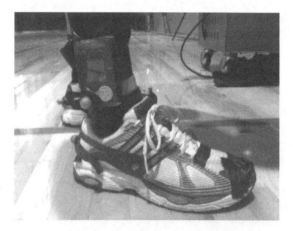

**Figure 1** The Shadowbox™ magnetic and inertial navigation system.

Raw data from the Shadowbox™ sensors was downloaded via USB interface and imported into MATLAB software for data processing. A quaternion-based extended Kalman filter was used to combine the raw sensor data to generate an estimate of the Shadowbox™ position, velocity and attitude using the methods of van der Merwe and Wan (2004) and Bachmann *et al.* (2001). Figure 2 illustrates a block diagram of the Kalman Filter procedure used to derive the displacement of the Shadowbox™. A Pearson product-moment correlation was then calculated between the 3D displacement data for the Shadowbox™ and the Vicon MX™ for each action to determine the dependence between the two methods.

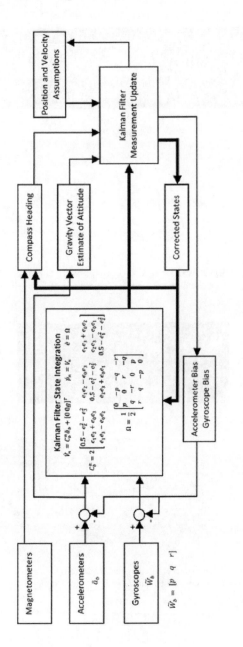

**Figure 2** Block diagram of the quaternion-based extended Kalman filter method.

## 3. RESULTS

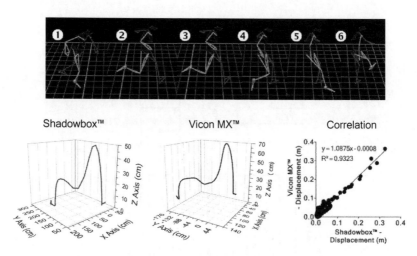

**Figure 3** Ankle 3D displacement data measured by the Shadowbox™ versus
the Vicon MX™ during a kick (from toe-off then kick to until end-of-follow-through) of a soccer ball.

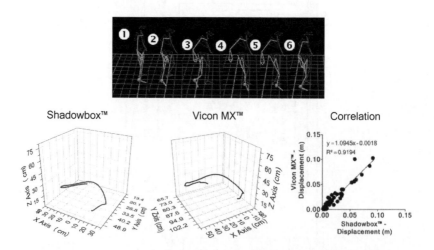

**Figure 4** Ankle 3D displacement data measured by the Shadowbox™ versus the Vicon MX™ during a
one-touch pass (from toe-off then kick to end-of-follow-through) of a soccer ball.

When attached to the ankle, the Shadowbox™ tracking system was proven to have high validity against the criterion Vicon MX™ motion tracking system during a series of soccer specific acitons ($R^2$=0.93 for kicking a ball, $R^2$=0.92 for one-touch pass of a ball and $R^2$=0.95 for slide tackle). The comparative ankle 3D displacement data and correlations between the two sensor systems for each action are illustrated in Figures 3, 4 and 5.

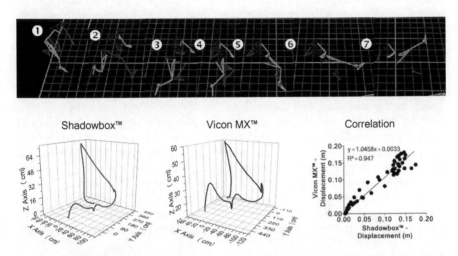

**Figure 5** Ankle 3D displacement data measured by the Shadowbox™ versus the Vicon MX™ during a slide tackle (2 steps, then leg swing to end of follow-through).

## 4. DISCUSSION

This experiment demonstrated that the Shadowbox™ was able to precisely track the limb of a soccer player during sport specific actions. Data from both motion analysis systems tracked similar pathways and the 3D displacement estimated by both systems was very strongly correlated. The Vicon MX™ was selected as a criterion method due to its high resolution and has previously been used by various researchers as a criterion to evaluate new motion analysis technologies (Webster, *et al.*, 2005; Duffield *et al.*, 2010). The Shadowbox™ system, therefore, was sensitive enough to remotely track the subtle limb movements of a soccer player. However, further testing on more subjects with a variety of different brand inertial sensors is recommended for future research.

A quaternion-based extended Kalman filter was used, primarily using the methods of van der Merwe and Wan (2004), because it has been proven as an effective method for real-time estimation of rigid body motion to calculate limb displacement. The use of quaternions reduces the chance of singularity errors known as "gimball lock" and the extended Kalman filter reduces the computational requirements, making it possible for real-time estimates of attitude.

Inertial sensors have recently become more sensitive with improved dynamic ranges. However, they are still susceptible to sensor drift over time. The incorporation of GPS sensors as an external reference with inertial sensors has been one effective method of correcting the drift (Brodie *et al.,* 2008). While the Shadowbox™ is relatively miniature and lightweight, it is still not small enough for use during an actual soccer match. However, the sensor components are very small and flat. Future modification of this technology into the sole of a shoe, for example, would make the sensors undetectable to the player. The storage and real-time transmission of raw data could also be achieved by the incorporation of onboard flash memory and patch antenna technology.

Despite the need for miniaturization and incorporation into a shoe or shin guard, the concept of using a magnetic and inertial navigation system as a suitable tracking device to measure limb movements looks promising. The suitability of this technology will continue to improve as the sensors become more precise and the post-processing that was done in this research becomes incorporated into commercial software systems. Future research could also focus on measuring sport specific parameters over extended periods of play. This type of motion analysis system could lead to real-time performance analysis during matches, improved knowledge of the decline in physical performance and improved understanding of the physical performance requirements of elite soccer match play.

## 5. CONCLUSION

The Shadowbox™ motion tracking system had high validity against the criterion method, the Vicon MX™ motion tracking system, during a series of soccer specific movements made by a soccer player.

### Acknowledgements

The authors would like to acknowledge the technical advice from Joe van Niekerk.

### References

Brodie, M. *et al.*, 2008, Fusion motion capture: A prototype system using inertial measurement units and GPS for the biomechanical analysis of ski racing. *Sports Technology*, **1**, 17–28.

Bachman, E. *et al.*, 2001, Inertial and magnetic posture tracking for inserting humans into networked virtual environments. In *Proceedings of the ACM Symposium on Virtual Reality Software and Technology*, Banff, pp. 9–16.

Duffield, R. *et al.*, 2010, Accuracy and reliability of GPS devices for measurement of movement patterns in confined spaces for court-based sports. *J Sci Med Sport*, **13**, 523–525.

Edgecomb, S.J. and Norton, K.I., 2006, Comparison of global positioning and computer-based tracking systems for measuring player movement distance during Australian football. *J Sci Med Sport*, **9**, 25–32.

Hennig, E.M. and Briehle, R., 2000, Game analysis by GPS satellite tracking of soccer players. *Arch Physiol Biochem*, **108**, 44.

Riley, P.O. *et al.*, 2007, A kinematic and kinetic comparison of overground and treadmill walking in health subjects. *Gait & Posture*, **26**, 17–24.

van der Merwe, R. and Wan, E.A., 2004, Sigma-point Kalman filters for integrated navigation. In *Proceedings of the 60^{th} Annual Meeting, Institute of Navigation*, Dayton, OH, pp. 641–654.

Webster, K.E. *et al.*, 2005, Validity of the GAITRite® walkway system for the measurement of averaged and individual step parameters of gait. *Gait & Posture*, **22**, 317–321.

# CHAPTER SEVEN

# Biomechanics of punt kicking

K. Ball

Institute of Sport Exercise and Active Living (ISEAL) and School of Sport and Exercise Science, Victoria University, Melbourne, Australia

## 1. INTRODUCTION

The punt kick is a feature of all the football codes. It involves starting with the ball held in the hands with the body moving towards the target. In the last two steps, the ball is released such that it falls to a position where the kick foot can strike it. The ball is then forcefully contacted by the foot near the ground to be propelled through the air to the target. It is used as the primary means of disposal in Australian and Gaelic football, tactically in the rugby codes and American football and by association football goalkeepers when kicking out.

While the association football kick has developed a strong research base, the punt kick is substantially less studied. Importantly, the kick has two features that stand it apart from association football; for most punt-kick sports, the ball is ovoid rather than round and the ball is dropped before the kick rather than on the ground. These two key features mean that independent kicking studies are essential. At the previous Science and Football conference in 2007, Professor Brian Dawson noted this kick needs to be researched more thoroughly, particularly in Australian Football (AF). This paper reviews the work done and presents new data in research at Victoria University examining the biomechanics of the punt kick.

## 2. KICKING FOR DISTANCE

The ability to kick the ball further is an important attribute for all the kicking sports. Ball (2008a) examined technical aspects of the punt kick in AF. Twenty-eight elite AF players kicked for maximum distance on their regular training ground. High speed video (2D, 500Hz) was digitized to obtain technical factors and regression analyses were used to examine their relationship with kick distance. Larger foot speed, greater shank angular velocity and a higher ball position at ball contact, as well as a larger last step, were all significantly correlated with distance. In regression analyses, foot speed and shank angular velocity, as well as the distance between the support foot and the ball in the horizontal direction explained 67% of the variance in distance. Ball (2008a) recommended increasing foot speed, shank angular velocity and increasing the last step distance to improve distance kicking. Ball (2008a) also noted the importance of ball position at the point of impact but suggested this is more likely an optimisable rather than maximisable factor.

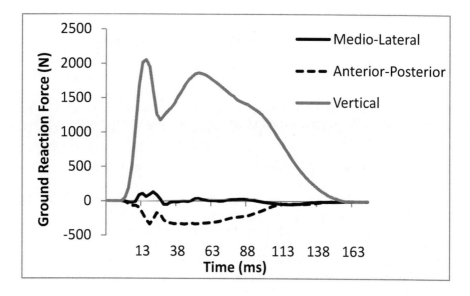

**Figure 1** Example GRF pattern from support foot landing until toe off after ball contact
(note anterior-posterior forces always negative or braking).

An important finding within this study was the identification of a continuum of styles. At one end of the continuum (termed 'knee-strategy') players produced very large knee angular velocities at ball contact and relatively low thigh angular velocity (in many cases none at all). At the other end of the continuum (termed 'thigh-strategy') players produced a relatively larger thigh angular velocity and relatively lower knee angular velocity at ball contact. Ball (2008a) reported that while no performance difference existed between the ends of the continuum (i.e. similar distances kicked) knee-strategy kickers exhibited significantly larger knee flexion in forward swing while thigh-strategy kickers showed greater hip angular velocity at ball contact.

Ground reaction force data and support leg kinematics have also been shown to play a role in producing greater foot speed at ball contact. Pilot work in the Victoria University laboratory examined the relationship between ground reaction forces, support leg kinematics and performance in elite AF players. Ground reaction forces (GRF) under the support leg were collected using an AMTI LG6-4 force plate for maximal and sub-maximal drop punt kicks. Optotrak Certus operating at 100 Hz also collected support leg kinematics from support foot landing until toe off after ball contact. Similar to soccer kicking (e.g. Lees *et al.*, 2010), braking forces only existed during the support leg stance phase before the kick, with no propulsive forces evident (see Figure 1 for an example GRF curve). Foot speed at ball contact was found to correlate with peak forces in Fz (vertical force, $r = 0.69$, $p = 0.02$) and Fy (braking force, $r = 0.68$, $p = 0.04$). Foot speed also correlated with a more extended support leg at initial foot contact (r = -0.73, p = 0.004) and at maximum flexion (r = -0.71, p = 0.006). This differed to the findings of Dicheria *et al.* (2006) who found a more flexed support leg knee was associated with more accurate kicking. While the study might have been influenced by the testing environment (the laboratory had a low ceiling and the kick distance was very short, 15 m), these contrasting results need to be evaluated in future studies as they might indicate a difference in optimal performance technique for distance compared to accuracy kicking.

A similar mechanism was proposed to explain the relationship between centre of mass (CM) motion and foot speed in the punt kick. Ball (2011a) examined five elite AF players performing maximal and sub-maximal kicks specifically looking at CM motion in the last step. Optotrak Certus operating at 100 Hz collected full body kinematics from kick foot toe off until ball contact. Ball (2011a) found that maximal kicks exhibited larger CM approach speeds (3.7 v 3.3 m/s) and larger reduction in CM velocity from support foot landing until ball contact (1.5 v 1.2 m/s) compared to sub-maximal kicks. Further, a large effect existed between foot speed and reduction in CM velocity during stance (r = 0.77) indicating greater deceleration was associated with greater foot speeds. A similar finding was reported by Potthast *et al.* (2010) for soccer kicking where greater CM deceleration was associated with greater ball speeds. Ball (2011a) also reported that while maximal kicks produced a greater approach speed compared to sub-maximal kicks, correlation analysis within the maximal kicks indicated a negative relationship (i.e. greater approach speed associated with smaller foot speed, r = -0.95). This did not support the findings of Ball (2008a) who found approach speed was associated with kick distance. Ball (2011a) noted that with only five players tested, more research with larger numbers of subjects is needed to better define the relationship between GRF, support leg kinematics, CM motion and performance in punt kicking.

## 3. IMPACT

Ball (2008a) noted that variance in distance was still left unexplained by kinematic analyses and suggested the nature of impact is also likely to influence the kick. A number of studies have been performed examining impact in AF and rugby league kicks providing a sound research platform and a good database for future work. Ball (2008b) analysed ball to foot interaction of elite AF players performing 30 m and 50 m kicks using 1000 Hz video. Two dimensional video analysis indicated that the ball stays in contact with the boot for between 9 and 12 ms and moves approximately 0.2 m during this time. Foot to ball speed ratios lay between 1.1 and 1.3 and as reported for soccer (e.g. Tsaousidis and Zatsiorsky, 1996), work is performed on the ball, with significantly more work performed in the 50 m kick compared to the 30 m kick (271 v 198 J). It is a very forceful activity, with the average force applied to the ball by the foot lying between 900 and 1100 N.

Impact in different rugby league kicks has been the focus of one study. Ball (2010) used 6000 Hz video to evaluate impact characteristics of the rugby league drop punt (45 m kick), bomb (kick for maximal height), drop kick (ball strikes the ground before being contacted by the foot) and grubber (ball kicked along the ground) as well as the goalkick. Ball to foot contact times were lower (6–8 ms) and work on the ball higher (290–342 J) compared to values reported by Ball (2008b), Smith *et al.* (2009) for AF kicks. Ball (2010) suggested this might be influenced by the lighter rugby league ball (400 v 450 g) or potentially the coefficient of restitution differences between the AF and rugby league ball. Ball (2010) also noted differences existed between the kicks within rugby league. For example, foot trajectory at ball contact varied from horizontal (0 degrees) for the grubber, 7 degrees for the 45 m kick and 24 degrees for the bomb. Impact factors also exhibited a range of values with foot to ball speed ratios ranging from 1.22–1.30, work ranging from 290 J to 342 J and ball displacement from 0.12 m (grubber), to 0.20 m (45 m kick) and 0.23 m (drop kick). Ball (2010) highlighted that these differences emphasised the need to evaluate the different kicks within any sport separately, identifying this as a limitation of both punt kick and soccer kicking research.

Differences in impact characteristics have been found between preferred and non-preferred leg kicks. Smith *et al.* (2009) compared elite AF players kicking for maximal distance using 6000 Hz video of impact. Smith *et al.* (2009) found the preferred leg produced significantly larger foot and ball speeds, change in shank angle while the ball was in contact with the foot and work done on the ball compared to the non-preferred leg. However, of interest, the ratio between foot and ball speed has tended not to differ significantly between kick legs, suggesting foot speed is the major determinant. Nunome *et al.* (2006) found a similar result in soccer kicking, with no difference in foot to ball speed ratios between the preferred (1.35) and non-prefered (1.32) leg kicks. However, Ball (2010) noted that mis-kicks were not evaluated by Smith *et al.* (2009) and these might be expected to exhibit a lower foot to ball speed ratio.

Senior and junior kickers have also been compared and important practical findings have been reported. Ball (2010) found that foot and ball speeds were considerably slower in juniors (foot speed: 26.5 v 21.3 m/s, ball speed: 32.6 v 24.7 m/s). Juniors also applied significantly less work on the ball, a combination of being able to apply less force to the ball during impact (1023 v 679 N) and applying it over a shorter distance (0.22 v 0.20 m). Interestingly foot to ball speed ratio did not differ statistically, although Ball (2010) noted the difference (1.16 for juniors, 1.23 for seniors) still held practical significance. Further foot speed once again did not explain all the variance in ball speed meaning impact factors were still influential. Ball (2010) recommended that while increasing foot speed should be a focus, impact factors should not be ignored. Also important, ankle plantar flexion during impact was greater for junior players (senior = 4°, junior = 6°, p < 0.003). This finding suggests that training to reduce plantar flexion during impact through kicking drills and conditioning of the ankle musculature might be beneficial to improving kick distance for juniors.

## 4. COORDINATION

Another important area of study is examining coordination in kicking. Hancock and Ball (2008) tested five elite AF players perfoming kicks with the preferred and non-preferred legs. Three dimensional data were collected at 200 Hz using Optotrak Certus and knee angle-knee angular velocity phase plane diagrams were examined. Hancock and Ball (2008) found differences between kick legs were range of motion (ROM) and speed rather than timing and cordination based.

Falloon *et al.* (2010) and Ball (2011b) expanded this evaluation to include the hip and pelvis. Falloon *et al.* (2010) examined five elite AF players kicking a 45 m pass with both legs. Once again, differences seemed to be range of motion and speed based. However an interesting difference in movement pattern was identified. The preferred leg exhibited greater knee and pelvis ROM and knee angular velocity at ball contact. Conversely the non-preferred leg produced greater hip angle ROM and hip angular velocity at ball contact. Ball (2011b) suggested this might be due to three reasons. First it could be a locking of degrees of freedom, as described by Bernstein (1967) for a less trained skill. It could also be indicating a less efficient sequencing of the movement where momentum developed in the hip and thigh is not transferred as well to the shank and foot. Finally it could be due to control at the hip allowing for lateral adjustment of the leg to execute the kick successfully as typically the non-preferred side balldrop is more variable. Interestingly this pattern was also evident in junior kickers (9–11 years old) indicating this movement pattern is established very early (Farrow and Ball, 2011).

## 5. CONCLUSION

In summary, important technical factors have been identified for performance in the punt kick. Greater kick distances have been associated with larger foot speed, shank angular velocity, a larger last step before the kick and ball position at ball contact. A knee and a thigh strategy exists among punt kickers in AF. Greater foot speeds have been associated with greater braking forces, a more extended support leg and a greater deceleration of the CM in the last step before ball contact. Impact factors are important to the kick and differ between kick legs and between senior and junior kickers. Finally an interesting difference exists between the preferred and non-preferred legs with the preferred leg using the knee and pelvis more while the non-preferred leg uses the hip more in kicking.

A number of important future directions exist for the evaluation of punt kicking. Linking the important kinematic factors identified in previous studies with kinetic factors is essential to better understand the underlying mechanics of the punt kick. Within this study, different kick types need to be evaluated separately as has been highlighted in rugby league kick research. Further this work needs to include more evaluation of trunk and upper body mechanics to evaluate posture and the influence of trunk axial rotation on punt kicks. Evaluation of distance and accuracy kicks, in particular examining the role of the support leg is an area of potential conflict in the literature and needs to be resolved. Finally, and perhaps most importantly given it is the distinctive aspect of the punt kick compared to other kicks, the technique of controlling and dropping the ball optimally and the interceptive task of striking it with the foot need to be assessed.

## References

Ball, K., 2008a, Biomechanical considerations of distance kicking in Australian Rules football. *Sports Biomechanics*, **7**, 10–23.

Ball, K., 2008b, Foot interaction during kicking in Australian Rules Football. In *Science and Football VI*, London: Routledge, pp. 36–40.

Ball, K., 2010, Foot to ball interaction for different kicks in rugby league. In Jensen, R. *et al.* (eds) *Proceedings of the 28ᵗʰ International Conference on Biomechanics in Sports*, Northern Michigan University: USA, pp. 458–461.

Ball, K., 2011a, Centre of mass motion in punt kicking. *Port J Sport Sci*, **11**, 45–48.

Ball, K., 2011b, Kinematic comparison of the preferred and non-preferred foot punt kick, *J Sport Sci*, **29**, 1545–1552.

Bernstein, N., 1967, *The Coordination and Regulation of Movements*. London: Pergamon.

Dichiera, A. *et al.*, 2006, Kinematic patterns associated with accuracy of the drop punt kick in Australian Football. *J Sci Med Sport*, **9**, 292–298.

Falloon, J. *et al.*, 2010, Coordination profiles of preferred and non-preferred foot kicking in Australian Football. In Jensen, R. *et al.* (eds) *Proceedings of the 28ᵗʰ ISBS Conference*, Northern Michigan University: USA, pp 466–469.

Farrow, D. and Ball, K., 2011, Preferred and non-preferred leg kicking in junior players. Technical report for the AFL research board, Melbourne, Australia.

Hancock, A. and Ball, K., 2008, Comparison of preferred and non-preferred foot kicking in Australian Football. In Burnett, A. (ed) *Proceedings of the ESSA Conference*, Australian Catholic University: Melbourne, pp. 45.

Lees, A. *et al.*, 2010, The biomechanics of kicking in soccer: A review, *J Sports Sci*, **28**, 805–817.

Nunome, H. *et al.*, 2006, Impact phase kinematics of instep kicking in soccer. *J Sport Sci*, **24**, 11–22.

Potthast, W. *et al.*, 2010, The success of a soccer kick depends on run-up deceleration. In Jensen, R. *et al.* (eds) *Proceedings of the 28ᵗʰ ISBS Conference*, Northern Michigan University: USA, pp. 462–465.

Smith, J. *et al.*, C., 2009, Foot to ball interaction in preferred and non-preferred leg Australian Rules kicking. In Anderson, R. *et al.* (eds), *Proceedings of 27ᵗʰ ISBS Conference*, Limerick University: Ireland, pp. 650–653.

Tsaousidis, N. and Zatsiorsky, V., 1996, Two types of ball-effector interaction and their relative contribution to soccer kicking. *Human Movement Science*, **15**, 861–876.

# CHAPTER EIGHT

# Biomechanics of goal-kicking in rugby league

K. Ball, D. Talbert and S. Taylor

Institute of Sport Exercise and Active Living (ISEAL) and School of Sport and Exercise Science, Victoria University, Melbourne, Australia

## 1. INTRODUCTION

Goal-kicking in rugby league and union is an important component of winning games. Goal-kicks are taken after a penalty has been awarded to the attacking team or after a try has been scored and are taken from different distances and angles from the goal. The goal-kick is performed by placing the ball on a tee and attempting to kick the ball over the crossbar and between the upright posts on the full. It comprises approximately 30% of total points scored in rugby league games (2007 Australian National Rugby League season) and is often the difference between teams. In rugby, Ortega et al. (2009) reported finding winning teams kicked more penalty goals compared to losing teams. Importantly, the same number of penalty kicks were awarded to winning and losing teams but winning teams kicked more penalty goals (2.76 compared to 1.76 goals, $p = 0.001$) highlighting the importance of accurate kicking.

In spite of the importance of goal-kicking, there is little scientific work examining goal-kicks. In the only technical analysis of either rugby code, Bezodis *et al.* (2007) examined five university first team rugby kickers performing kicks for accuracy and distance. Three dimensional data were collected for the full body during each kick (VICON, 120Hz). The authors reported angular momentum of the non-kick side arm was greater in the more accurate kickers in the anterior-posterior axis (axis direction in the kick direction) and about the longitudinal axis (i.e. vertical line through the trunk). The authors suggested that this was due to better control of whole body momentum and for altered trunk positioning. Bezodis *et al.* (2007) also reported more skilled kickers adopted a ball contact position where the trunk leaned towards the kick side while less skilled kickers leaned away from the kick.

In the only technical analysis of technique in rugby league goal-kicking Ball (2010) examined ball to foot interaction and launch characteristics for four elite National Rugby League goal-kickers using 6000 Hz video. Ball (2010) reported a number of technical elements important to impact including foot to ball speed ratios of 1:2, distance the ball travels while in contact with the boot (0.22 m) and the average work applied to the ball by the foot (306 J). This related to an average force of 1391 N indicating the rugby league goal-kick is a very forceful task (calculated from data in the Ball 2010 study using work divided by distance). Of note, Ball (2010) reported the ball moved through a relatively large change in orientation angle while on the boot (17°) which was substantially larger than other rugby league kicks (5 ° or less for long kicks) and the junior kicker in this group was also the most variable.

There is currently no work evaluating full body technical aspects of the rugby league kick. This work is needed to establish an evidence-base to define the technical elements that are associated with successful kicking for use in development programmes. The examination of elite performers and differences between successful and unsuccessful shots within this group is the most appropriate focus to begin this work. Further, the evaluation of current coaching cues is an appropriate feature to evaluate in this analysis of goal-kicking. This approach can identify important information immediately useable by coaches. Three coaching cues commonly used in rugby league kicking are 'stay upright' (typically communicated after missed kicks as 'leaned off the kick'), 'square to the target' and 'momentum through the kick'. 'Square' refers to adopting a trunk position in which the line of the shoulders and hips as viewed from above are perpendicular to the line of shot (i.e. the chest faces towards the goal). 'Momentum' refers to full-body motion during the kick with the aim to move closer to the goal during and after ball contact. The usefulness of these cues needs to be evaluated. The aims of this study were to describe the technique of rugby league goal-kicking and to examine differences between successful and unsuccessful kicks. In particular, these coaching points were evaluated.

## 2. METHODS

Four elite goal-kickers (age $24 \pm 3$ years) participated in this study. All players had kicked in the national rugby league (NRL) and/or for their country in international rugby league senior games. This represented an unusual and important cohort as within a single club there are typically only one or two kickers for this analysis to be performed. Eighteen reflective markers were placed on each arm (wrist, elbow, shoulder), leg (hip, knee, ankle), foot (head of the $5^{th}$ metatarsal) and pelvis (right and left anterior superior iliac spine, ASIS, and posterior superior iliac spine, PSIS). Players then performed between five and 15 goal-kicks on their usual training ground from 40m in front of the goalposts. This was another important feature of this work, with kicks taken on the playing arena and in a familiar environment for participants. Each trial was filmed by three Basler A602FC-2 cameras (100 Hz) and video was digitized in VICON MOTUS from kick foot toe off until ball contact. Data were smoothed using a fourth order Butterworth digital filter (10 Hz cut-off) and used to calculate technical parameters. Centre of mass was calculated using anthropometric data from Clauser *et al.* (1969). All calculations were performed within VICON MOTUS (X = direction of kick, Y = vertical, Z = perpendicular to the line of kick).

The kick was described qualitatively from video observation and by quantifying key technical parameters. Body lean or 'staying upright' was evaluated by measuring trunk angle at ball contact (defined by a line between the hips and shoulders viewed in the XY plane, or side on to the line of the kick). 'Squaring' to the target was evaluated by the hip (left and right ASIS) and shoulder angle about the vertical axis. Centre of mass (CM) velocity in the direction of the kick at ball contact was used to determine if players kicked 'through the ball'.

## 3. RESULTS

Table 1 reports technical parameters for the goal-kicking group. All players leaned away from the ball, moved their CM towards the target at and through ball contact. Pelvis and shoulder angles were non-zero (the value that would indicate the kicker is square at contact).

**Table 1** Technical parameters for the league goal-kick (approach angle and velocity calculated at kick foot toe off in the last step before kick. All other parameters at ball contact).

| Parameter | Mean | sd |
|---|---|---|
| Foot speed (m/s) | 21 | 1 |
| Ball speed (m/s) | 27 | 3 |
| Foot:Ball speed ratio | 1:26 | 0:16 |
| Knee angle (°) | 145 | 14 |
| Knee angular velocity (°/s) | 1044 | 361 |
| Trunk angle (YZ plane or front view, °) | 28 | 7 |
| Pelvis angle (XZ plane or overhead view, °) | 21 | 7 |
| Shoulder angle (XZ plane or overhead view, °) | 28 | 7 |
| CM velocity (m/s) | 2.6 | 0.4 |
| Support foot ankle to centre of ball (m) | | |
|     Forwards/backwards | 0.14 | 0.10 |
|     Lateral | 0.29 | 0.08 |
| Approach velocity (m/s) | 3.0 | 0.8 |
| Approach angle (°) | 31 | 12 |

Table 2 reports success for each kicker as well as selected parameters for comparison. Coach rankings aligned with both success in games and in testing. Trunk angles at BC indicated no player was upright or leaning towards the ball but the best kicker did produce the most upright trunk posture. No clear pattern existed for the kick foot to non-kick-side arm. Player 2 produced a low success rate (25%) although one kick hit the upright.

**Table 2** Success, coach rating and selected technical parameters for individual players (1–4).

|   | Success (%) | Coach rank | Game success (%) | Approach steps | Approach angle |
|---|---|---|---|---|---|
| 1 | 80 | 2 | Not available | 5 | 22 |
| 2 | 25 | 4 | 67 | 8 | 20 |
| 3 | 60 | 3 | 75 | 5 | 44 |
| 4 | 100 | 1 | 81 | 3 | 38 |

## 4. DISCUSSION

All goal-kickers started the kick by placing the ball on the tee, tilting it forward (30–40 $^\circ$) with its long axis pointed towards the goal. All players aligned the seam and/or long axis of the ball with the intended direction of ball flight. For the three right foot kickers, this position was slightly to the right of centre as they reported having a curved kick through the air. Each goal-kicker then used measured steps to move back to the top of their run-up. This varied from three steps back and two across to five steps back and four across. After pausing for 5–10 seconds, two of the four kickers began their approach by taking a step backwards before moving towards the ball, one took two steps backwards and one kicker moved forward with the first step. Approach velocity increased during the run-up with the last step into the kick being the largest. During this last step, the kick leg lagged behind the body achieving a greater stretch at the front of the hip. The support foot landed beside the ball with the toe approximately pointing towards the goal. At this point the pelvis was rapidly posteriorly tilted and rotated towards the ball with a counterbalancing motion of the support side arm rotating downwards and across the body in the opposite direction. The knee continued to flex during the initial stage of the forward swing as the thigh began extending. Near mid forward swing, the thigh slowed and the knee rapidly extended to ball contact. At ball contact the lower body adopted an angled position as viewed from the front while the trunk was approximately upright. All players struck the ball close to its point on the instep of the foot. The ball deformed while on the boot such that it contacted from approximately where the laces on the boot began to just above the top of the boot. Motion after ball contact tended to be a skip of the support foot with the whole body either moving directly towards or to the non-kick side.

Ball speeds (27 m/s) were similar to the 26.44 m/s reported by Holmes *et al.* (2006) and 23–25 m/s reported by Bezodis *et al.* (2007) for rugby goal-kicking. Knee angular velocity at impact (1044 $^\circ$/s) lay within the ranges for instep soccer kicking of 860–1720 °/s (Nunome *et al.,* 2002). Approach speed (3 m/s) was also similar to soccer kicking (3–4 m/s, Kellis and Katis, 2007) but approach angle (31°) was considerably straighter than the 43° reported by Egan *et al.* (2007).

Elite rugby league kickers do 'kick through the ball'. The group centre of mass velocity of 2.6 m/s towards the ball indicated that the body was continuing to move forward through ball contact. This was supported on an individual basis, with all players and all kicks producing a positive CM velocity at ball contact. Importantly, the pelvis was also moving forward at the time of contact for all players highlighting that the CM motion was not simply produced by the kick leg moving rapidly angularly forward. This is significant from an applied point of view in light of the 'snap' technique evident in many kickers where the support leg remains on the ground after ball contact with players either remaining on the spot of falling to the side. This style of kick was evident for two of the kickers tested here but clearly the body continues to move forward during ball contact. The vector of CM through the kick is an important next step in this work to determine if this influences successful and unsuccessful kicks.

Previous work identified more accurate rugby kickers exhibited a trunk angle tilted towards rather than away from the ball (Bezodis *et al.,* 2007). While no kickers produced a trunk angle that tilted towards the ball in this study, the kicker considered the most accurate (kicker 4 who did not miss during testing) exhibited the most upright trunk angle (20° compared to 21–38°). Further, the remaining three kickers produced greater trunk angles (i.e. leaned off more) in missed kicks compared to their successful kicks (Table 3). While more work is needed to explore this finding, a more upright trunk might allow for a leg swing plane more aligned with the intended path of the ball, a more balanced body and head position or might position the hip and pelvis joints more optimally for an accuracy task. This finding supported the error identified as 'leaning off the ball' as accurate and adopting a more upright trunk position would seem to be a good technical cue.

**Table 3** Trunk lean (viewed from the front, zero = upright, positive value = leaning away from the ball).

|          | Goal (°) | Miss (°) |
|----------|----------|----------|
| Player 1 | 21       | 32       |
| Player 2 | 23       | 27       |
| Player 3 | 34       | 38       |

Elite kickers do not 'square to the target'. Group mean values for shoulders (28°) and pelvis (21°) indicated that the trunk was facing slightly to the left of the goals (or to the right for the left foot kickers). As such, this coaching cue would seem to be incorrect. However, post-hoc analysis of kick accuracy showed that for two kickers, a 'squarer' trunk position was evident for successful kicks. So the use of this cue might be appropriate for some players in becoming 'more square' rather than 'square'. This is worth further exploration in future studies.

Other technical parameters differed between successful and unsuccessful kicks and between players but these showed an individual-specific nature. Support foot position relative to the ball and qualitative observation of position of the ball on the foot at ball contact (from high speed video) both showed differences but no clear pattern emerged between kickers. Similarly, the support side arm showed differences in motion between kickers and between successful and unsuccessful kicks. This was found to be important by Bezodis *et al.* (2007) in rugby kicking and is also an important area for evaluation in future rugby leage goal-kicking research.

Individual differences were particularly evident in the preparation, run-up and approach angle. Among this group, preparation time varied from 5–10 seconds, the run-up varied from 3–8 steps, approach angle varied from 20–41°. Sampling 12 NRL kickers during the 2011 season, ten stepped backwards before coming forwards, approach steps ranged from two to seven and approach angles varied from relatively straight (evident in one kicker who took four steps backwards and one step to the side to position the start of the run-up) to very angled (evident in a three step back and five step sideways to the top of the run-up position). Based on these different aproaches and the individual differences evident in successful kicks for different individuals, it is clearly important to coach this skill on an individual basis rather than applying a theoretical 'perfect kick' model.

## CONCLUSION

Players kicked through the ball by moving their whole body through impact but did not exhibit the 'square at contact' coaching cue. A more upright trunk at ball contact seems to be linked to better performance.

### References

Ball, K., 2010, Foot to ball interaction for different kicks in rugby league. In Jensen, R. *et al.* (Eds), *Proceedings of the 28th International Conference in Biomechanics in Sports*, Northern Michigan University: USA, pp. 458–461.

Bezodis, N. *et al.*, 2007, Contributions of the non-kicking-side arm to rugby place-kicking technique. *Sport Biomechanics*, **6**, 171–186.

Clauser, C.E. *et al.*, 1969, *Weight, Volume and Centre of Mass of Segments of the Human Body*. AMRL Technical Report 69□–70, Wright-Patterson Air Force Base, Ohio.

Egan, C.D. *et al.*, 2007, Effects of experience on the coordination of internally and externally timed soccer kicks. *J Motor Behav*, **39**, 423–432.

Holmes, C. *et al.*, 2006, Ball launch characteristics for elite rugby union players. In *Engineering of Sport 6*, pp. 211–216.

Kellis, E. and Katis, A., 2007, Biomechanical characteristics and determinants of instep soccer kick. *J Sport Sci Med*, **6**, 154–165.

Nunome, H. *et al.*, 2002, Three dimensional kinetic analysis of side-foot and instep kicks. *Med Sci Sport Exer*, **34**, 2028–2036.

Ortega, E. *et al.*, 2009, Differences in game statistics between winning and losing rugby teams in the Six Nations Tournament. *J Sport Sci Med*, **8**, 523–527.

# CHAPTER NINE

# The role of the axial skeleton during rugby union punt kicking

M. Sayers and J. Morris

School of Sport and Health Sciences, University of the Sunshine Coast, Australia

## 1. INTRODUCTION

There are approximately 60 kicks per game of international level rugby union (IRB, 2010), with the majority of these involving the ball being dropped from the hands and kicked (punted) before it strikes the ground. Punt kicking is a fundamental skill for many of the football codes and yet it has been subject to limited scientific investigation. Previous biomechanical research on punt kicking has been completed primarily on Australian Football (AFL) players (Ball, 2008; Cameron and Adams, 2003; Dichiera et al., 2006). Typically, this research has concentrated on the two dimensional (2D) sagittal plane kinematics of the lower limbs and has not examined the skill in three dimensions (3D), or the contribution of other segments to performance. The absence of 3D data on punt kicking is particularly surprising given that research on soccer kicking has indicated that segmental movements in all three planes contribute to ball velocity for kicks off the ground (Lees and Nolan, 2002; Lees et al., 2009).

The majority of studies on kicking kinematics have focused on the lower limbs, with limited research on the role that the axial skeleton plays in determining kicking proficiency. This is surprising as there is potential for the trunk and pelvis to assist in generating higher foot speeds during kicking activities, as these movements have been reported previously to have a key role in other sports skills where distal end-point velocity is developed as a result of whole body movements (Elliott, 2006; Hume et al., 2005; Welch et al., 1995). Research on kicking a ball from the ground has reported that the pelvis moves from being tilted anteriorly 25 deg at the start of the kick to having 20 deg of posterior tilt at ball contact (Lees et al., 2009). This research also indicated that approximately 13 deg of rotation occurs at the pelvis about the segment's anterior-posterior axis during the kick, with the pelvis lifted on the kicking side to allow greater knee extension during the swing phase. In addition, rotational trunk movements have been shown to be a significant contributor to the change in knee extension moments (58%) when kicking a soccer ball from the ground (Naito et al., 2010).

Research on the role of the axial skeleton in punt kicking is limited. In a study on AFL punt kicking Dichiera et al. (2006) reported that accurate AFL kickers had greater anterior pelvic tilt during the backswing phase than inaccurate kickers.

However, participants in this project were instructed to kick for maximum accuracy and so the relationships between pelvic movements and punt kicking ball velocity remain unreported. Similarly, Ball (2008) suggested pelvic rotation about a vertical axis may be an important contributor to punt kicking performance, but to date only coaching observations on pelvic rotation have been reported. Accordingly, the aim of this study was to examine the 3D movements of the pelvis and thorax during a punt kick to determine their influence on ball velocity.

## 2. METHODS

Thirteen semi professional (S-Pro) male Rugby players (age 23.5 y ± 4.9, weight 91.7 kg ± 12.3, height 1.79 m ± 0.06) and 17 male recreational (Rec) kicking sport athletes (age 23.7 y ± 7.9, weight 80.9 kg ± 12.2, height 1.81 m ± 0.05) volunteered to participate in this study. This research was approved by the University of the Sunshine Coast Human Research Ethics Committee.

Retro-reflective markers were located on key thorax and pelvis landmarks. Pelvis markers were attached bilaterally on the anterior and posterior superior iliac spines with a single marker positioned over the spinous process of S2. Thorax markers were attached over the suprasternal notch, xiphoid process and the spinous processes of C7 and T10 (Wu *et al.*, 2005). Three additional markers were also placed on a standard rugby ball (Gilbert Barbarian, size 5). Following a structured warm-up, participants were then instructed to perform six punt kicks for maximum velocity. To reduce the effects of fatigue, there was a 4 min rest between each kick.

Data were collected at 500 Hz using a seven camera motion capture system (Qualisys AB, Gothenburg, Sweden). These data were then modelled in 3D using standard biomechanical software (Visual3D, C-Motion, Inc., USA) to construct a two segment rigid body model of the thorax and pelvis (Wu *et al.* 2005). A global reference system was established with the positive y-axis in the intended direction of ball travel, the x-axis perpendicular to the intended direction of ball travel (positive direction to the right) and the positive z-axis pointing vertically. Thorax and pelvis kinematics were calculated relative to the global reference system with anterior–posterior tilt, lateral tilt and axial rotations defined using Euler angle calculations as angular rotation about each segment's x, y and z-axes. The orientation of the thorax relative to the pelvis was also recorded as a relative measure of trunk flexion, trunk lateral flexion and trunk rotation. All rotations were defined using the right hand orthogonal rule. A time frequency algorithm adapted from Nunome *et al.* (2006) was used to smooth the data prior to it being processed to compute linear and angular velocities for each segment.

The differences between the participant groups were determined using one-way ANOVA. Pearson Product Moment correlation coefficients were used to determine the relationships between ball velocity and pelvis, thorax and trunk displacements, range of motion (ROM) and maximum angular velocities. Statistical analysis of the data was be performed using the statistics package SPSS for Windows (version 19), with an alpha level of $p < 0.05$.

## 3. RESULTS

The S-Pro group had significantly faster foot speeds at ball contact (22.95 ± 2.01 m/s) than the Rec kickers (16.11 ± 2.77 m/s, p<0.001). This group also had significantly greater ROM in the pelvic orientation about the z-axis (22 ± 10 deg) than the Rec kickers (12 ± 14 deg, p=0.031). There were no other significant differences in the orientation of the pelvis during the key phases of the kick. Both groups performed the kick with the pelvis tilted up laterally on the kicking leg side with limited variation in this position (ROM S-Pro 5 ± 4 deg, Rec 7 ± 5 deg). The S-Pro participants had significantly greater ROM in trunk flexion (33 ± 5 deg) than the Rec kickers (18 ± 21 deg, p=0.023), with the trunk being more flexed at both the start of the swing phase (p=0.02) and at ball contact (p=0.013). There were no other significant differences in thorax or trunk ROM about the other axes of rotation, or the 3D orientation of these segments during the key phases of the kick. Comparison of the maximum velocities of the segments in the three planes of motion indicated that the S-Pro kickers had greater maximum trunk flexion (p<0.001) and pelvic posterior tilt velocities (p=0.002) than the Rec kickers. Similarly, the S-Pro kickers also recorded significantly greater pelvic axial rotation velocities (259 ± 57 deg/s) than the Rec kickers (165 ± 93 deg/s, p=0.004). There was no difference in the rate of trunk axial rotation between groups (S-Pro -165 ± 52 deg/s, Rec -133 ± 65 deg/s, p=0.157). Representative pelvis and trunk data from a participant from each group has been included in Figure 1. Typically, the peak posterior pelvic tilt velocity occurred prior to the peak in pelvic axial rotation velocity for the S-Pro group.

Overall, significant moderate correlations were recorded between ball velocity and maximum velocity of posterior pelvic tilt (r=0.76, p<0.001), maximum axial pelvic axial rotation velocity (r=0.51, p=0.004) and the maximum trunk flexion velocity (r=0.66, p<0.001). However, within the recreational group the only kinematic variable that correlated with ball velocity was the maximum velocity of posterior pelvic tilt (r=0.81, p<0.001). In the semi-professional group significant correlations were recorded between ball velocity and both maximum axial pelvic axial rotation velocity (r=0.72, p=0.005) and the maximum trunk flexion velocity (r=0.63, p=0.021).

## 4. DISCUSSION

The purpose of this study was to determine whether differences exist in the 3D kinematics of the pelvis and thorax during rugby punt kicking between semi-professional and recreational punt kickers. The relationships between ball velocity and 3D rotation velocities of the pelvis and thorax were examined with the aim of providing a greater understanding of the role that these segments have in punt kicking performance.

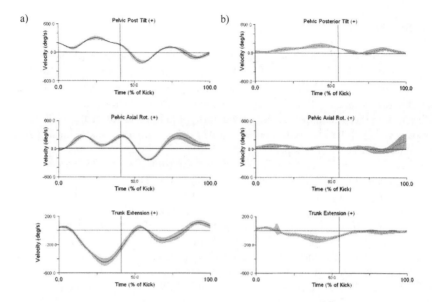

**Figure 1** Pelvic anterior-posterior tilt, axial rotation and trunk extension data for a S-Pro (a) and Rec (b) kicker. Data starts at the plant of the non-kicking leg (0%) and ends at the point of maximum hip flexion (100%). The vertical line represents ball contact.

The values for ball velocity at ball contact reported for the S-Pro group in this study are slower than those reported previously for professional AFL players (26.4 m/s) (Ball, 2008). These differences may have been influenced by the skill levels of the participants, as punt kicking in AFL is a more important part of the game than it is in rugby. Whether this difference is typical for athletes from these sports is not yet known and is open for further investigation.

The pattern of pelvic lateral tilting reported here was similar to research on soccer kicking that indicated the pelvis is raised on the kicking leg side by 10 deg at ball contact (Lees *et al.*, 2009). These researchers suggested that this action enabled greater knee extension throughout the swing and therefore increased ball speed. However, the small absolute pelvic lateral tilt values reported in this study are less than those for kicking a ball from the ground (Lees *et al.*, 2009), which coupled with the relatively small ROM values, indicates that the pelvis is held in a relatively stable position about the y-axis throughout the punt kick. Lees *et al.* (2010) suggested that a more stable pelvis in the frontal plane allowed for greater precision of foot position at ball contact.

A key finding of this project concerned differences in the anterior/posterior and axial pelvic movements between the groups. The ROM in axial pelvic rotation values reported for the S-Pro group were similar to those by Lees *et al.* (2009) for kicking a soccer ball from the ground (between 30 to 36 deg). This action no doubt contributed to the high pelvic axial rotation velocities obtained by the S-Pro group and was a key predictor of ball velocity. Although no differences existed in the rate of trunk axial rotation between groups, the counter rotation between the pelvis and trunk has been reported in rugby place kicking (Bezodis *et al.*, 2007). These results could indicate that the trunk was undergoing a stretch-shorten cycle as a means to generate faster ball speeds, a characteristic common to other sports that utilise pelvic and thorax rotations to develop high distal segment velocities (Hume *et al.*, 2005). The use of the stretch shorten cycle in kicking a soccer ball from the ground has been thought to account for 43% of the difference in ball speeds between novice and elite players (Shan and Westerhoff, 2005). In addition, the S-Pro kickers also recorded greater rates of posterior pelvic tilt than the Rec kickers (Figure 1). This action has been suggested to have an important role in generating a stretch-shorten cycle on the front of the hip and hence increase the rate of hip flexion during the kick (Ball, 2008; Lees *et al.*, 2009). Although not able to generate the same rate of posterior tilt velocity as the S-Pro group, the Rec kickers relied heavily on this action to develop ball velocity.

It was hypothesised that the differences in the pelvic movement strategies adopted by the S-Pro and Rec groups were representative of skill level, with the S-Pro group utilising a more complex multi-planar movement pattern as a means of developing greater ball velocities. Conversely, the Rec group utilised a simple movement strategy that relied on movements in the sagittal plane to develop ball velocity. Interestingly, research on AFL punt kicking has suggested that the rapid pelvic axial rotation can lead to large shear forces applied through pelvis. When considered in light of the findings from this project, it would appear that the rapid multi-planar movements of the pelvis that appear vital to punt kicking performance may also be contributing factors for several of the common pelvic and hip injuries that plague athletes from kicking sports (Orchard *et al.*, 1999; Williams, 1978).

## 5. CONCLUSION

This is the first study to report the complex 3D movements of the pelvis and thorax during punt kicking. The S-Pro kickers presented with a more complex movement strategy at the pelvis and thorax than the less capable Rec kickers. The increased axial rotation and posterior tilt velocity of the pelvis were key determinants of the high punt kicking ball velocities developed by the S-Pro group. Conversely, less skilled punt kickers place greater emphasis on simple flexion/extension movement patterns through the axial skeleton, a strategy that appears to limit punt kicking ball velocity. Further investigations using segmental interaction methods are needed to quantify the relative roles of the axial skeleton in generating ball velocity during Rugby punt kicking.

## References

Ball, K., 2008, Biomechanical considerations of distance kicking in Australian Rules Football. *Sports Biomechanics*, **7**, 10–23.

Bezodis, N. *et al.*, 2007, Contributions of the non-kicking-side arm to rugby place-kicking technique. *Sport Biomech*, **6**, 171–186.

Cameron, M. and Adams, R., 2003, Kicking footedness and movement discrimination by elite Australian Rules footballers. *J Sci Med Sport*, **6**, 266–274.

Dichiera, A. *et al.*, 2006, Kinematic patterns associated with accuracy of the drop punt kick in Australian Football. *J Sci Med Sport*, **9**, 292–298.

Elliott, B., 2006, Biomechanics and tennis. *Brit J Sport Med*, **40**, 392–396.

Hume, P.A. *et al.*, 2005, The role of biomechanics in maximising distance and accuracy of golf shots. *Sports Med*, **35**, 429–449.

IRB, 2010, *Statistical Review and Match Analysis: Six Nations 2010*. Dublin: International Rugby Board.

Lees, A. and Nolan, L., 2002. Three dimensional kinematic analysis of the instep kick under speed and accuracy conditions. In *Science and Football IV*, London: Routledge, pp. 16–21.

Lees, A. *et al.*, 2009, Understanding lower limb function in the performance of the maximal instep kick in soccer. In *Proceedings of the 6th International Conference on Sport, Leisure and Ergonomics*, London: Routledge, pp. 149–160.

Lees, A. *et al.*, 2010, The biomechanics of kicking in soccer: A review. *J Sports Sci*, **28**, 805–817.

Naito, K. *et al.*, 2010, Multijoint kinetic chain analysis of knee extension during the soccer instep kick. *Human Mov Sci*, **29**, 259–276.

Nunome, H. *et al.*, 2006, Impact phase kinematics of instep kicking in soccer. *J Sport Sci*, **24**, 11–22.

Orchard, J. *et al.*, 1999, Muscle activity during the drop punt kick. *J Sport Sci*, **17**, 837–838.

Shan, G. and Westerhoff, P., 2005, Full-body kinematic characteristics of the maximal instep soccer kick by male soccer players and parameters related to kick quality. *Sports Biomechanics*, **4**, 59–72.

Welch, C.M. *et al.*, 1995, Hitting a baseball: A biomechanical description. *J Orth Sports Phys Ther*, **22**, 193–201.

Williams, J.G., 1978, Limitation of hip joint movement as a factor in traumatic osteitis pubis. *Brit J Sport Med*, **12**, 129–133.

Wu, G. *et al.*, 2005, ISB recommendation on definitions of joint coordinate systems of various joints for the reporting of human joint motion – Part II: Shoulder, elbow, wrist and hand. *Journal of Biomechanics*, **38**, 981–992.

# CHAPTER TEN

# A biomechanical analysis of the knuckling shot in football

S. Hong[1], C. Chung[2], K. Sakamoto[1], R. Nagahara[1] and T. Asai[1]

[1] University of Tsukuba, Japan,[2] Seoul University, Korea

## 1. INTRODUCTION

In recent times, ball impact techniques have improved, and various ball impact point with the foot, swing motions, and more complicated curving kicks are being performed by football players. For example, top professional athletes who use the instep while kicking curve shots are often able to apply topspin in addition to sidespin. Such an intentional application of topspin to a ball is an extremely specialised technique that results in shots that drop more than conventional curve shots. A few top-level football players (e.g. C. Ronaldo) are also capable of kicking the knuckling shot, in which a ball is intentionally kicked with very low or no spin; due to the effects of random turbulence, such balls have an unpredictable wobble. Moreover, as a result of the excitation of an irregular vortex oscillation in the ball wake, the knuckleball results in the ball wavering or dropping unpredictably (Asai *et al.*, 2008).

Several studies on the non-spinning knuckleball have measured the steady aerodynamic forces in a wind tunnel (Carré *et al.*, 2004) and have investigated the reasons for irregular variations in the ball flight path using fluid mechanics (Asai *et al.*, 2006; Hong *et al.*, 2010). However, there are virtually no knuckleball studies on the kicking motions or ball impact characteristics; as a result, the mechanisms of this shot have not been elucidated, possibly because this phenomenon occurs at extremely high speeds. Moreover, there are relatively few football players who can intentionally perform the knuckling shot, and even among them, most have low success rates. In this study, we have used a system of four high-speed video cameras to investigate the swing characteristics of the kicking leg while kicking the knuckling shot. And then, we have tried to elucidate the impact process of the kicking foot at ball impact and the technical mechanisms of the knuckling shot through the comparison with the motion of curve and straight shots.

## 2. METHODS

Five adult male football players (mean height: 1.76 m ± 0.03; mean weight: 67.2 kg ± 4.2; mean age: 21.6 years ± 1.3) from the Tsukuba University soccer team, without any history of major lower limb injuries or diseases, volunteered to participate in this study; informed consent was obtained from them. All the participants had been playing regularly for the university team and were capable of kicking the knuckling shot. Each player kicked either non-spinning or low-spinning soccer balls towards the centre of the goal a total of 20 times. The results of these kicks were judged by three instructors each with an experience of more than 10 years in soccer instruction. The analysis was subject to 10 instances where the kicked ball reached the goalpost with a knuckle effect being observed at a significant level. Furthermore, 10 straight and 10 curve shots kicked with instep and curve kicks, respectively, were also analyzed for comparison with the knuckling shot.

Two high-speed cameras (Fastcam, Photron Inc., Tokyo, Japan; 1000 fps, 1024 × 1024 pixels) were set up 2 m from the site of impact with a line of sight perpendicular to the kicking leg side. In addition, two semi-high-speed cameras (EX-F1, Casio Computer Co., Ltd., Tokyo, Japan; 300 fps; 720 × 480 pixels) were positioned at the rear and on the kicking leg sides (Figure 1a).

To calibrate the performance area, a calibration frame (2.0 × 2.0 × 2.0 m) with 27 control points was recorded before the trials. A digitizing system (Frame DIAS IV, DKH Inc., Tokyo, Japan) was employed to manually digitize the anatomical body landmarks. The direct linear transformation (DLT) method (Abdel-Azis and Karara, 1971) was used to obtain three-dimensional (3D) coordinates of each landmark. The performance area (2.0 × 2.0 × 2.0 m) was calibrated with a net root mean square error of 5 mm. The 3D coordinates were expressed as a right-handed orthogonal reference frame fixed on the ground (X-axis: the horizontal forward direction from the ball set point; Y-axis: the horizontal left direction; Z-axis: the vertical direction).

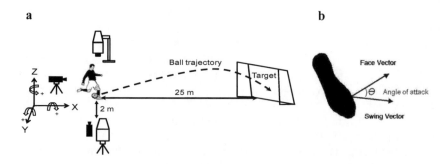

**Figure 1** Diagram of experimental setup (a), orientation of face and swing vectors (b).
Modified from Hong *et al.* (2012), with permission.

The face vector at impact was defined as a normal vector of the line from the toe point to the heel point (Miura and Sato, 1999). The swing vector at impact was defined as the average velocity vector of the toe and heel points. The angle of attack was defined as the angle between the face and swing vectors (Figure 1b). The obtained data was analyzed statistically using analysis of variance followed by Post-hoc Tukey's test for multiple comparisons between variables. The variables used between the three testing sessions were joint torque and angle of attack. All the statistical procedures were performed using statistical software (SPSS Japan, Inc., Tokyo, Japan). Statistical significance was set as $p < 0.05$.

## 3. RESULTS AND DISCUSSION

### 3.1. Ball–foot impact

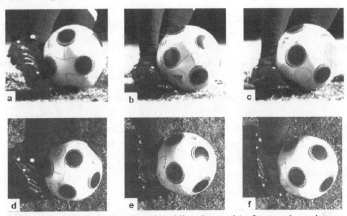

**Figure 2** (a, d) Straight shot; (b, e) knuckling shot; and (c, f) curve shot at impact (a, b, c: side view; d, e, f: top view).

Figure 2 depicts sample images of the straight shot, knuckling shot, and curve shot at the ball impact. In contrast to the comparatively extended position of the ankle joint in the straight shot (a, d), in the curve shot, an L-shaped flexion of the ankle joint at the impact (c, f) can be observed (Asai *et al.*, 1998). Further, the ankle joint at the impact in the knuckling shot (b, e) was flexed in an approximate L-shape that is similar to that of the curve shot. In other words, the ankle joint posture when impacting the ball was closer to that of the curve shot than that of the straight shot. Although similar trends were observed in the other subjects as well, some individual differences were noticed in the ankle joint angle at ball impact; it is possible that the same knuckling shot could be performed using impact methods other than those measured in this study.

### 3.2 Impact process

Figure 3 depicts the top view and side view of a sample travel path for the ankle during the ball impact process. In the top view, although the direction of motion of the displacement in the straight shot and that in the knuckling shot are somewhat bent towards the inside of the swing and are nearly identical, the direction of motion of the displacement is significantly directed towards the outside in the curve shot. Moreover, this displacement was considerably greater in the curve shot (50 mm) than in the straight shot and knuckling shot (4 mm and 0.6 mm, respectively). In the side view, the straight shot moved downwards whereas both the knuckling shot and curve shot moved somewhat upwards.

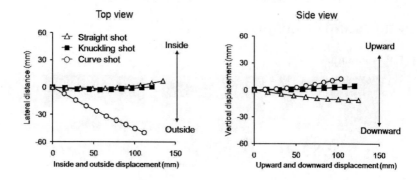

**Figure 3** Ankle joint displacement during ball impact.
Modified from Hong *et al.* (2012), with permission.

### 3.3. Angle of attack

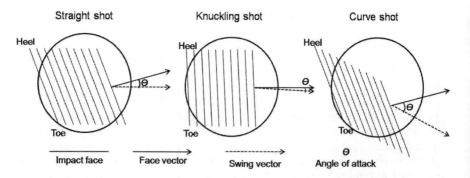

**Figure 4** Face and swing vectors during ball impact. The angle formed by the face and swing vectors during impact (angle of attack) increases progressively.

Figure 4 shows the face and swing vectors as well as their angles of attack for the straight shot, knuckling shot, and curve shot, respectively. The angle of attack (the initial contact) for the knuckling shot was approximately 4°, which was smaller than those for the straight and curve shots, approximately 19° and 35° respectively. These angles of attack are believed to correlate with the production of rotational forces at the surface of ball contact (Asai *et al.*, 2005). Moreover, the average values of the angle of attack formed by the face and swing vectors at the instant of impact (the first frame of the impact process) were 19.7° ($SD = 3.5°$), 3.8° ($SD = 1.5°$), and 32.6° ($SD = 3.9°$) for the straight shot, knuckling shot, and curve shot, respectively. A statistically significant difference was noted. From these results, it can be considered that the lower angle of attack for the knuckling shot in comparison with that for the other shots is the reason for the low rotational frequency of the ball.

### 3.4. Torques of knee joint and hip external rotation

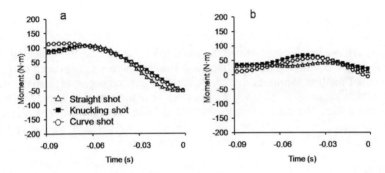

**Figure 5** (a) An example of knee extension and (b) hip external rotation from leg cocking to impact in the straight, knuckling, and curve shots.

The peak values for the knee extension in the straight shot, knuckling shot, and curve shot in Figure 5a were 108.0 N·m, 106.2 N·m, and 114.9 N·m, respectively. Table 1 lists the peak torques of the knee joint and hip external rotations (mean ± *SD*). The mean peak torque values of the knee extensions were 110.0 N·m (*SD* = 8.4 N·m), 106.1 N·m (*SD* = 8.5 N·m), and 116.7 N·m (*SD* = 9.4 N·m) for the straight shot, knuckling shot, and curve shot, respectively. The patterns of the knee extension for all the three shots were clearly similar. In addition, the values were within the range of peak values (83–122 N·m) of previous researches on knee extensions (Luhtahnen, 1988; Nunome *et al.*, 2002).

From Figure 5b, the peak values of hip external rotation for the knuckling shot (67.0 N·m) was higher than that for the straight shot (41.2 N·m) and curve shot (58.1 N·m). Moreover, the mean peak values of the hip external rotation were 39.1 N·m (*SD* = 3.4 N·m), 67.2 N·m (*SD* = 6.0 N·m), and 53.1 N·m (*SD* = 5.8 N·m) for the straight shot, knuckling shot, and curve shot, respectively. A statistically significant difference was noted (Table 1). Nunome *et al.* (2002) have reported hip external rotation peak values of 56 N·m (*SD* = 12 N·m) for a side-foot kick and 33 N·m (*SD* = 8.0 N·m) for an instep kick. Their instep kick results are similar to the hip external rotation values for the straight shot in this study; in addition, their results for the side-foot kick have greater similarity with the result of the knuckling shot in this study than their instep kick results. From these results, it can be considered that compared to the other shots, the knuckling shot exerts a greater external rotation torque on the hip during leg forward swing phase and has a tendency to push the heel forward and impact with the inside of the foot (Figure 2b and 2e).

**Table 1** Peak torque of knee extension and hip external rotation (mean ± SD).

|  | Straight shot | Knuckling shot | Curve shot | P |
|---|---|---|---|---|
| Maximal knee extension (N·m) | 110.0±8.4 | 106.1±8.5* | 116.7±9.4* | <0.05 |
| Maximal hip external rotation (N·m) | 39.1±3.4* | 67.2±6.0* | 53.1±5.8* | <0.05 |

## 4. CONCLUSIONS

In this study, we have demonstrated the ankle joint at impact in the knuckling shot to be flexed in an approximate L-shape in a similar manner to the curve shot. The hip external rotation torque in the knuckling shot exerted a greater than the other shots, which suggests a tendency to push the heel forward and impact with the inside of the foot. The angle of attack in the knuckling shot was smaller than that in the other shots and its smallness was believed to be a factor in soccer kicks generating the balls with smaller rotational frequencies.

## References

Abdel-Aziz, Y.I., 1971, Direct linear transformation from comparator coordinates into object space coordinates in close-range photogrammetry. In *Proceedings of the ASP/UI Symposium Photogrammetry*, Falls Church, VA, pp. 1–18.

Asai, T. *et al.*, 1998, The physics of football. *Physics World*, **11**, 25–27.

Asai, T. *et al.*, 2005, Computer simulation of ball kicking using the finite element skeletal foot model. In *Science and Football V*, London: Routledge, pp. 77–82.

Asai, T. *et al.*, 2006, Flow visualization on a real flight non-spinning and spinning soccer ball. In *The Engineering of Sport 6*, Munich: Springer, pp. 327–332.

Asai, T. *et al.*, 2008, A study of knuckle effect in football. In *Science and Football VI*, London: Routledge, pp. 64–69.

Carré, M.J. *et al.*, 2004, Understanding the aerodynamics of a spinning soccer ball. In Hubbard M., *The Engineering of Sport 5 Vol 1*, California: USA, pp. 70–76.

Hong, S. *et al.*, 2010, Unsteady aerodynamic force on a knuckleball in soccer, In *The Engineering of Sport 8*, Wien: Elsevier, pp. 2455–2460.

Hong, S. *et al.*, 2012, Ball impact dynamics of knuckling shot in soccer. *Procedia Engineering*, **34**, 200–205.

Luhtanen, P., 1988, Kinematics and kinetics of maximal instep kicking in junior soccer players. In *Science and Football*, London: E & FN Spon, pp. 449–455.

Miura, K. and Sato, F., 1998, The initial trajectory plane after ball impact. *Science and Golf III*, Human Kinetics, pp. 535–542.

Nunome, H. *et al.*, 2002, Three-dimensional kinetic analysis of side-foot and instep soccer kicks. *Med Sci Sports Exerc*, **34**, 2028–2036.

# CHAPTER ELEVEN

# Ideal dive technique in high one-handed soccer saves: top hand versus bottom hand

N. Smith and R. Shay

Chichester Centre for Applied Sport and Exercise Sciences, Chichester, UK

## 1. INTRODUCTION

The game of soccer comprises of ten outfield players and only one goalkeeper. Subsequently, the goalkeeper can be regarded as the most specialised position on the soccer field. Recent advances in player training and equipment have led to new breed of athletic goalkeepers, who utilise different techniques to those seen previously. Such techniques will enable goalkeepers to deal with the modern game and ball, and thus leaving current coaching manuals out of date. Referring to the manuals supplied by the English FA (Wade, 1981), the most significant omission from the goalkeeping literature is the coaching of 'diving saves' to the modern keeper.

Goalkeeping manuals suggest diving should focus on the facilitation of a learner's ability to attack the ball with both hands (Coles, 2003). Yet, when diving at full stretch it will not be possible to attack the ball with both hands as this will shorten the distance that the goalkeeper can reach (Welsh, 1999) by using a combination of spinal lateral flexion and shoulder elevation. These saves are termed aerial saves (Kostelis, 2007), and are the focus of the current study as they do not appear in current coaching literature.

Observation of elite goalkeepers shows a variation in the performance of aerial saves. The 'bottom hand technique' (BHT) is the more traditional technique where the goalkeeper leads with the hand of the direction in which they are diving (Figure 1). The 'top hand technique' (THT) entails the use of the hand initially on the side opposite to where the ball is travelling. The arm abducts, often in combination with greater rotation of the hips and trunk, to reach above and around the head to make the save. The absence of these techniques from coaching literature creates difficulties for coaches who attempt to instruct performers in the principles behind each technique, and as to when they should be used.

Previous work by Suzuki *et al.* (1988) calculated the path of the goalkeeper's Centre of Mass (COM) whilst diving to save balls suspended in a laboratory. Data showed that higher level keepers dived more directly, and with greater velocity than novice keepers. As a result, the expert's COM vertical displacements were lower than their novice counterparts. Further work by Spratford *et al.* (2009)

investigated dives to keeper's preferred and non-preferred side, and concluded those to the non-preferred side reduced the ability to dive directly towards the ball, and also induced a greater amount of pelvic and torso rotation. Ecological validity was compromised in these studies, however, by the use of suspended balls in a laboratory setting.

The current authors postulate that the incorrect selection of either BHT or THT for a particular save has led to many goalkeeping errors at elite level. The aim of the current study was to investigate which areas of the goal would be best covered using either the BHT or THT to inform goalkeepers and coaches how to improve the number of shots saved. It was hypothesised that due to the top hand arm position, keepers must displace their COM further to save with THT.

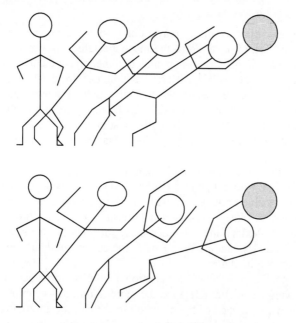

**Figure 1** Graphics of two saving techniques: Bottom Hand Technique (top) and Top Hand Technique (bottom).

## 2. METHODS

### Pre-testing

A hand notation system was used to analyse selected games between 1992–2010 seasons from elite level English, European and International competitions. The goal was divided into four zones representing the ball destination during high, one handed saves. Twenty saves were analysed using BHT, and 20 using THT. Results showed an even distribution of saves using BHT (50%) and THT (50%) to the Top Outer (TO) portion of the goal, and saves with THT predominantly (85%) occurred in the Top Middle (TM) zone.

## Participants

Eight male participants volunteered for the study (age 22±4 years). Goalkeepers had mass 88.04kg (±19.88) and height 183.88cm (±7.85). All goalkeepers had a minimum of one year's playing experience at English semi-professional level. Subjects provided informed consent after clearance was provided by the University Ethics committee. Participants wore their own goalkeeping attire yet were instructed to wear tight fitting clothing for anatomical landmark identification. Body markers were not used due to the high impact nature of the testing.

## Equipment

Outdoors on a natural turf surface, an association football goal was covered by a 'goal division sheet' (Tildenet, Bristol) identifying the four target areas, each of 108 x 103cm. A marker was placed in the centre of the goal, two yards in front of the goal-line. A further two disks were placed 12 yards from the goal-line in front of the goalkeeping areas to be tested, between which the server would strike the football (Mitre Ultimatch, Mitre Sports International, London ) toward the goal.

Two 50 Hz video cameras (Sony Handycam, Japan) were used. Camera 1 in the frontal plane was placed in the centre of the goal, 20m from the goal line. A view perpendicular to ball flight was recorded to assess ball velocity. Footage was manually digitised using Vicon Motus 9 software (Vicon, Oxford, UK).

## Procedure

Upon a verbal cue, the goalkeeper made a 'game related movement'; laterally, anticlockwise, around the outside and in front of the disk, whilst the server struck a ball to the goalkeeper's left, at the tested Goal Area (GA). The four GA were measured from the dimensions stated above to provide two areas in the Top Outer, Top Middle, Bottom Outer and Bottom Middle sections of the left hand side of the goal. Each trial was aimed to a GA in a randomised order. Only one side of the goal was analysed once experimenters were satisfied that subjects could adequately perform both techniques to each side of the goal. Each trial was noted for the quality of serve, the GA in which the save was made and the technique used. The goalkeeper completed two successful saves from each goal section for both THT and BHT.

## Data analysis

The authors judged that participants performed saves not natural to them by using the THT in the bottom GA, therefore these GA were disregarded prior to analysis, leaving the top middle and outer GA.

Trials selected for subsequent analysis were required to have a consistent ball serve velocity (18 m/s±10%). Body segment parameters obtained from DeLeva (1996) were applied to an 18 point full body model and raw data was smoothed using a generalised, cross-validated quintic spline. Key variables extracted were; time of save from toe-off to ball contact, peak velocity of COM, max COM height, time of max COM height, COM height at toe-off, COM height at ball contact and COM displacement at toe-off, and hand displacement at ball contact. Paired sample t-tests were performed for key variables between BHT and THT in SPPS 16.0 for windows. Statistical significance was set at $P<0.05$.

## 3. RESULTS

Key variables objectifying a shot destined for goal were the vertical and horizontal distance of the ball away from the take-off foot. To move the body towards this position the Centre of Mass (COM) must also be moved vertically and horizontally. From this position of COM, when the ball reaches the goal-line the success of a save will then depend on the distance that the goalkeeper can extend either their top or bottom hand to make contact with the ball.

### Top middle goal area

Differences on the top middle goal area show there were differences in the distances from the centre of mass to the hand at the point of the save. The BHT displayed greater reach in the horizontal direction, whilst the THT displayed greater reach in the vertical direction. Results showed the BHT also gave a greater horizontal distance from the point of toe-off to the saving position.

**Table 1** Significant differences between BHT and THT in the top middle goal area (values in metres).

|                          | bottom hand | top hand | p-Value |
|--------------------------|-------------|----------|---------|
| COM-hand horizontal      | 0.552       | 0.387    | <0.001  |
| COM-hand vertical        | 0.722       | 0.914    | 0.03    |
| Horizontal hand position | 1.012       | 0.882    | 0.03    |

## Top outer goal area

**Table 2** Significant differences between BHT and THT in the top outer goal area (values in metres).

|                          | bottom hand | top hand | p-Value |
|--------------------------|-------------|----------|---------|
| COM-hand horizontal      | 0.589       | 0.419    | <0.001  |
| Horizontal hand position | 1.337       | 1.015    | 0.003   |
| COM horiz displacement   | 0.748       | 0.596    | 0.03    |
| COM-hand vertical        | 0.705       | 0.839    | <0.001  |
| Vertical hand position   | 1.874       | 2.017    | 0.01    |

Differences in the top outer goal area show greater horizontal distances achieved using the BHT in overall distance of the hand, distance travelled by the COM and distance of the hand from the COM at ball contact. When using the THT in this top outer corner of the goal saves showed greater vertical hand position, and vertical distance between the COM at the hand at the point of ball contact. The hypothesis that goalkeepers would have to displace their COM further to save with the THT was subsequently rejected.

## 4. DISCUSSION

The study aimed to show which areas of the goal would be best covered by BHT or THT, with the hypothesis that when using THT a goalkeeper would have to displace their COM further to make the save, as horizontal reach would be limited using THT, and vertical position of the COM may be higher for the same save when using THT compared to BHT. The hypothesis was rejected yet recommendations for dive technique were interpreted from the data.

When using BHT for the most challenging saves in the top outer area, there were strong (non-significant) trends for the COM to have greater horizontal displacement (BHT 0.33m; THT 0.26m) and vertical displacement (BHT 0.11m; THT 0.07m) when using BHT. Such results agree with Suzuki *et al.* (1988) who claimed elite goalkeepers dive more directly at the ball, and would suggest that BHT technique would therefore be more consistent with the principles of good dive technique. We state the BHT is more consistent with the principles of good diving technique of diving directly at the ball, and creates more of an opportunity to get both hands behind the ball (Coles, 2003) yet this does not exclude the selection of THT in game situations. For example, the goalkeeper may not achieve both the height and distance needed to make the save using the BHT (with the most direct COM path), as it may require an additional energy expenditure that is not possible. So the ability to make a save with a lower COM path (i.e. using the THT) could allow the goalkeeper to save shots otherwise not energetically possible. Such situations may also arise when the goalkeeper has misjudged the flight of the ball and has set off too early (so COM is falling at the point of the save). In addition, the increasing popularity of free kicks where the ball is struck with minimal spin a 'knuckleball' effect may also increase the unpredictability of ball flight, and the requirement to use THT once the dive has been initiated.

Spratford *et al.* (2009) found dives made towards the weaker side displayed an additional hip and trunk rotation around the vertical axis towards the ball, and also an inability to move the COM directly to the ball. Similarities between the dive technique of the weaker side and our THT dives suggest there may be a link. Moreover, COM results obtained from the present study would suggest the THT displays a COM path less direct to the ball than the BHT. This infers a THT could be a result of diving to the goalkeeper's weaker side. Whilst a plausible explanation to the movement pattern observed, our performers were still able to produce both techniques diving to just one side during the current study. Future work would require a systematic study of THT and BHT in conjunction with preferred handedness to solidify this proposed relationship. Such work would not only help explain goalkeepers choice of saving technique for a given save, but also indicate if it is preferable for coaches to instil symmetry in coaching over reliance on preferred handedness.

The current study showed that ball velocities were consistent at a mean of 17.8ms$^{-1}$, yet this is considerably slower than maximal instep kick velocities taken from other studies with professional subjects of 29.5ms$^{-1}$ (Smith *et al.*, 2008) due to the need for an accuracy constraint. The effect of this ecological ball feed also meant greater variability in ball placement which meant that for each goal area, the balls saved with THT and BHT were not in exactly the same place. If such ecological validity is to be maintained in future studies, however, the current authors would suggest that trials where the shot was not saved, yet the goalkeeper had a large displacement and were deemed to be making maximal effort should be analysed, as opposed to only the trails where a successful save had occurred.

## 5. CONCLUSIONS

The current study concludes that the use of BHT provides a more direct line to the ball in line with traditional coaching technique (Suzuki *et al.*, 1988; Coles, 2003). In addition to a trend of increased COM velocity using BHT, greater horizontal displacement was also possible. The authors would therefore recommend the coaching and use of the BHT where possible. Whilst THT showed greater vertical displacements of the hand were possible, this technique would only be recommended for the top middle goal areas, or for situations where the initial dive parameters determined the dive to have occurred either too low, or too early to intercept the ball, or when late adjustments are required due to an alteration in ball trajectory. Due to the increasing frequency of these saves in the modern game we propose that both BHT and THT saves are included within governing body run on coaching literature. It is proposed that to fully understand the selection of these techniques further work is required into the three dimensional nature of the saves and the relationship between preferred and non-preferred limbs.

### References

Coles, D., 2003, In *Goalkeeping, The Specialist*. Marlborough: The Crowood Press.

De Leva, P., 1996, Joint centre longitudinal positions computed from a selected subset of Chandler's data. *J Biomech*, **29**, 1231–1233.

Kostelis, G., 2007, What a save! *Soccer Journal*, **52**, 20–23.

Smith, N. *et al.*, 2008, The power flow through the swinging limb during an instep kick in soccer. In *Proceedings of the International Society for Biomechanics in Sports*, p. 541.

Spratford, W. *et al.*, 2009, The influence of dive direction on the movement characteristics for elite football goalkeepers. *Sports Biomechanics*, **8**, 235–245.

Suzuki, S. *et al.*, 1988, Analysis of the goalkeeper's diving motion. In *Science and Football*, London: E. & F.N. Spon, pp.468–475.

Wade, A., 1981, In *The FA Guide to Teaching Football*. Published on Behalf of The Football Association. London: Heinemann.

Welsh, A., 1999, In *The Soccer Goalkeeping Handbook: An Authoritative Guide for Players and Coaches*. Chicago: Masters Press.

# CHAPTER TWELVE

# Characteristics of the kicking motion in female soccer players

K. Sakamoto[1], S. Hong[1] and T. Asai[2]

[1]Doctoral Program, University of Tsukuba, Japan, [2] University of Tsukuba, Japan

## 1. INTRODUCTION

Many studies have examined soccer kicking techniques in regard to swing action and joint torque. Shinkai *et al.* (2009) estimated the force of impact that occurs during instep kicks, and Ishii and Maruyama (2009) analyzed external rotation angle of the foot during inside kicks. However, to date, most of the participants in studies on soccer kicking techniques have been male soccer players, and the number of studies that have examined the kicking action of female soccer players is limited (Barfield *et al.*, 2002; Clagg *et al.*, 2009).

In recent years, the number of female soccer players has been increasing worldwide (The International Federation of Association Football, 2007). Consequently, elucidating the characteristics of female player techniques is an interesting research topic. Accordingly, in this study, we used three high-speed video cameras set at 1000 fps to compare the ball velocity, foot velocity, repulsion ratio (Nunome *et al.*, 2006), and angular displacement at ball impact of the instep kick and inside kick of female and male soccer players. Through these measurements, we attempted to identify the mechanical and technical characteristics of female players at ball impact.

## 2. METHODS

The participants in this study comprised 17 male soccer players who had at least 10 years of soccer experience (height: $172.0 \pm 4.4$ cm, weight: $65.7 \pm 4.8$ kg) and 17 female soccer players who had at least 5 years of soccer experience (height: $161.4 \pm 4.5$ cm, weight: $56.0 \pm 3.4$ kg). Permission for the soccer players to participate was obtained from the participants and from the Ethics Committee for the Institute of Health and Sport Sciences, the University of Tsukuba, Japan. Informed written consent was obtained from each participant. All participants preferred to kick the ball using their right leg.

The participants were instructed to kick a stationary soccer ball (FIFA-approved size 5 ball, weight: 430 g, pressure: 900 hp; Adidas, Herzogenaurach, Germany) with their dominant foot at full strength towards the goal, which was located at a distance of 11m in front of them (height: 2.44 m, width: 7.32 m). The kicking techniques that they used were the instep kick and the inside kick (Figure 1). Test kicks were recorded with three high-speed video cameras (FASTCAM 1024 PCI model 100KC, speed: 1000 fps, exposure time: 1/5000 s, resolution: 1024 × 1024 pixels; Photron, Tokyo, Japan). A camera was installed on the right side of each participant's leg (their kicking leg). Another camera was installed on the right rear side of each person's leg with respect to the kicking direction, and this was used to record data synchronously (Figure 2). A third camera was set up normal to the swing plane of the kicking foot and was used to measure the horizontal velocity of the person's foot.

Three-dimensional motions of the foot and ball were measured using the direct linear transformation (DLT) method. The calibrated range covered an area of 0.75 m ($x$-axis) × 1.25 m ($y$-axis) × 0.7 m ($z$-axis). A coordinate system was established with the horizontal kicking direction as the $y$-axis, the vertical direction as the $z$-axis, and the direction perpendicular to the $y$-axis and the $z$-axis as the $x$-axis. To investigate the relationships among the ball velocity, foot velocity, ball-to-foot speed ratio, distance between the impact point and the centre of gravity of the foot, and angular displacement, quadratic regression analysis was performed on each data set. Moreover, to investigate the relationship between the parameters for male and female participants, Welch's method was used, and the level of significance was set at five percent.

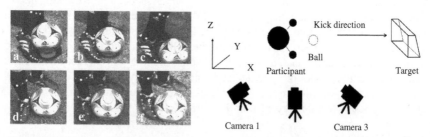

**Figure 1** Kick impact points, where a, b, and c denote the instep kick, and d, e, and f denote the inside kick.

**Figure 2** Experimental setup.

## 3. RESULTS AND DISCUSSION

### 3.1. Comparison of male and female players

The average ball velocity for the instep kick of the female players was 22.0 ± 2.6 m/s and that of the inside kick it was 19.0 ± 2.1 m/s. Those values for male players were 26.6 ± 2.6 m/s and 21.9 ± 2.0 m/s, respectively (Figure 3a). Thus, the average ball velocity of the female players was 17% lower than that of the male players for the instep kick and 13% lower than that of the male players for the inside kick, both of which were significantly different ($p < 0.05$) between the male and female players. The average ball velocity of the instep kick of the male players was 24.7 ± 2.5 m/s; this was slightly higher (1.9 m/s) than that reported for male players by Dörge *et al.* (2002). Further, the average ball velocity of the inside kick of the male players was 23.4 ± 1.7 m/s; this was slightly lower (1.5 m/s) than that reported for male players by Nunome *et al.* (2002).

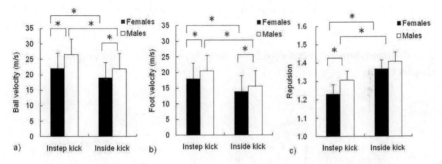

**Figure 3** Comparisons of kicking parameters for female and male players [a = ball velocity; b = foot velocity; c = coefficient of restitution; d = reduced mass]. The bars and asterisks represent significant differences between males and females, instep and inside kick (*$p < 0.05$ ); significant differences between kicks are not shown on the graphs.

For female players, the average foot velocity immediately prior to impact was 18.0 ± 1.8 m/s for the instep kick and 14.0 ± 1.3 m/s for the inside kick (Figure 3b). One possible reason for this difference might be that it is easier for players to achieve faster leg swing speed during the instep kick compared to the inside kick because the inside kicking requires a more complex series of joint rotations (Nunome *et al*, 2002). In this study, the average foot velocity of the instep kick for the female players (16.2 ± 2.3 m/s) was slightly higher (1.8 m/s) than that for female players reported by Barfield *et al.* (2002). The foot velocities of the female players in our study immediately prior to impact were roughly 12% and 10% lower than those for male players for the instep kick and the inside kick, respectively and both the values were significantly different ($p < 0.05$) (between males and females) (between instep and inside kick). It can be assumed that these results reflect the gender differences with respect to physical characteristics such as leg extension power as well as differences in swing technique.

The average repulsion ratio of the instep kick was 1.23 ± 0.16 for the female players and 1.31 ± 0.18 for the male player. The value of the female was significantly lower (6%) than that of the male players ($p < 0.05$; Figure 3c). The average repulsion ratio reported for the male players in Kellis *et al.* (2006) was slightly higher (1.40 ± 0.12) than the value of the present study. The significant difference in the repulsion ratios of the instep kick between males and females in our study may attribute to reduced stiffness of the ankle joint of the female players on impact compared to the male players. Thus, we should discuss these parameters in more details. The average repulsion ratio of the inside kick was slightly lower for the female players than that of the male players at $1.37 \pm 0.14$ versus $1.41 \pm 0.16$, respectively, although the difference was not significant. On comparing this average value with that of the instep kick, it was seen that the repulsion ratios of the inside kick tended to be larger. The differences in the ball impact location are expected to have a large effect on the repulsion ratio. Consequently, investigating the relationship between the repulsion ratio and ball impact location would be valuable.

## 3.2. Relationships between repulsion ratio, impact point, and angular displacement

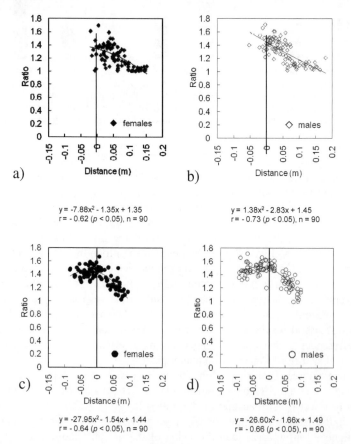

$$y = -7.88x^2 - 1.35x + 1.35$$
$$r = -0.62 \ (p < 0.05), n = 90$$

$$y = 1.38x^2 - 2.83x + 1.45$$
$$r = -0.73 \ (p < 0.05), n = 90$$

$$y = -27.95x^2 - 1.54x + 1.44$$
$$r = -0.64 \ (p < 0.05), n = 90$$

$$y = -26.60x^2 - 1.66x + 1.49$$
$$r = -0.66 \ (p < 0.05), n = 90$$

**Figure 4** The relationships between the impact distance and repulsion [a = the instep kick of female; b = the instep kick of the males; c = the inside kick of the females; d = the inside kick of the males].

The repulsion ratio for the instep kick when the foot hit the ball with near the centre of gravity was ~1.35 for the female players (the $y$-intercept of the quadratic regression curve), which was slightly lower than that of the male players (~1.45) (Figure 4a, b). The angular displacement (dorsi-plantar flexion) in the ankle joints of female players tended to be greater than that in male players when the impact point was farther from the foot's centre of gravity (Figure 5a, b). In terms of the mechanical characteristics at impact, these results suggest that the female players have lower foot mass and lower dynamic stiffness than those of the male players. It can be assumed that the quality of ball impact of female players is more susceptible for the offset distance from the centre of gravity of the foot because they have lower dynamic stiffness of the ankle joint.

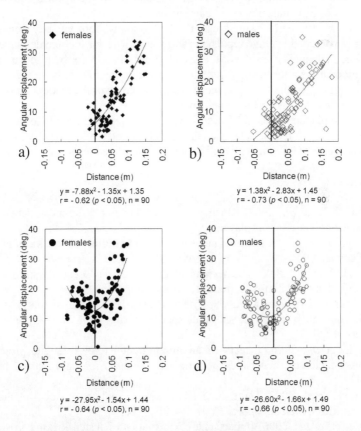

**Figure 5** The relationships between the impact distance and angular displacement [a = the instep kick of female; b = the instep kick of male; c = the inside kick of female; d = the inside kick of male].

For all of the test kicks, a trend was seen whereby the repulsion ratio was higher when the foot hit the ball with near the centre of gravity regardless of the kicking techniques: the instep and inside kicks. Consequently, it is conceivable then that for both male and female players and for both the instep and inside kicks that impacting the ball at the centre of gravity of the foot is an important technical point, as it increases the repulsion ratio.

## 4. CONCLUSIONS

In this study, we used three high-speed video cameras set at 1000 fps to compare the ball velocity, foot velocity, repulsion ratio, and angular displacement at ball impact of the instep kick and inside kick of female and male soccer players. From the data that we collected, we attempted to elucidate the mechanical and technical characteristics of female players at ball impact.

For the instep and inside kicks, the ball velocity, foot velocity immediately prior to impact, and average repulsion ratio were lower for the female players than that of the male players ($p < 0.05$). For both types of kicks for both sets of players, there tended to be a lower repulsion ratio the further the impact point was from the centre of gravity of the foot. The mechanical properties of the ankle joint of female players during the instep kick may involve slightly lower dynamic stiffness than that of male players. Thus, the lower dynamic stiffness of the ankle joint of female players was suggested to have a comparatively greater effect on the instep kick. The importance of ball impact position may be reinforced for female players.

## References

Barfield, W.R. *et al.*, 2002, Kinematics instep kicking differences between elite female and male soccer players. *J Sports Sci Med*, **1**, 72–79.

Clagg, S.E. *et al.*, 2009, Kinetic analyses of maximal effort soccer kicks in female collegiate athletes. *Sports Biomechanics*, **8**, 141–153.

Dörge, H.C. *et al.*, 2002, Biomechanical differences in soccer kicking with the preferred and the non-preferred leg. *J Sports Sci*, **20**, 293–299.

Ishii, H. and Maruyama K., 2008, Effect of abduction angle of foot and impact point on ball behavior in side-foot soccer kicking. *Jpn Biomechanics Sports Exerc*, **12**, 9–21.

Kellis, E. *et al.*, 2006, Effects of an intermittent exercise fatigue protocol on biomechanics of soccer kick performance. *Scand J Med Sci Sports*, **16**, 334–344.

Nunome, H. *et al.*, 2002, Three-dimensional kinetic analysis of side-foot and instep soccer kicks. *Med Sci Sports Exerc*, **34**, 2028–2036.

Nunome, H. *et al.*, 2006, Impact phase kinematics of instep kicking in soccer. *J Sports Sci*, **24**, 11–22.

Shinkai, H. *et al.*, 2009, Ball impact dynamics of instep soccer kicking. *Med Sci Sports Exerc*, **41**, 889–897.

# Part II
# Exercise physiology

# CHAPTER THIRTEEN

# The physiological effects of soccer training in elite youth soccer players

M. Green[1], W. Gregson[2] and B. Drust[2]

[1]West Bromwich Football Club, UK, [2]Research Institute for Sport and Exercise Sciences, Liverpool John Moores University, UK

## 1. INTRODUCTION

The purpose of soccer training is to improve the technical, tactical, psychological and physical qualities of the player (Dupont *et al.,* 2004). Coaches must attempt to achieve these outcomes using a variety of different training sessions. The extent that in-season soccer training may impact components of physical fitness is relatively unknown. Little specific research examining the structure and effects of the training process upon the physical qualities of elite players is therefore available. The present study aims to examine the structure and effects of in-season training in elite youth soccer players by (a) quantifying the loads associated with the soccer training and (b) determining the effect of this activity on jump performance, speed, agility, repeated sprint ability and aerobic performance.

## 2. METHODS

Seventeen elite youth team soccer players (age $16 \pm 1$, body mass $70.8 \pm 10.7$ kg, height $1.77 \pm 0.07$ m) participated in the study. All participants were training full time with the same Premier League soccer team. Goalkeepers were excluded from the study. Each participant provided written consent following a verbal and written explanation. Liverpool John Moores Ethics Committee approved the study.

The participants completed 7-weeks of in-season soccer training. The daily training activities completed were classified as follows. Tactical training aimed to improve match understanding and decision making. Technical work was associated with the teaching and refinement of a skill. Physical training prioritised the improvement of physical fitness. Training games was training time involved in match play, whereas competitive match play was identified as competitive 11 a-side league fixtures. The classification of training sessions was based upon discussions with the coach. No other additional training was completed by the participants.

All participants wore a Polar Team System heart rate belt (Polar Electro, Kempele, Finland) throughout all training sessions. Heart rate was recorded every 5-sec during training. This data was used to calculate an average percentage of maximum heart rate (%HRmax) and the relevant training impulse (TRIMP) for each training session (Edwards, 1993). TRIMP was calculated from assigning an intensity of 1–10 to the time spent in each of the ten 5% zone from 50–55% – 95–100% of maximum heart rate. The duration spent in each zone was multiplied by the intensity value and then each added together, producing the overall TRIMP for the session. Subjective ratings of perceived exertion (RPE) were gathered from each participant using Borg's CR10 RPE scale (Foster, 1998) 30-min after each training session. The duration of the session was noted, which enabled a session RPE to be calculated. All participants were previously familiarised with the use of all monitoring methods for the 12-month period before the study commenced.

Field based fitness assessments were conducted before and one week after the training phase. The assessments were scheduled following a 24-hour rest period. All tests were completed in one day and took place in a controlled indoor environment on a third generation astroturf surface. The environmental conditions were consistent for each testing day. Participants were instructed to keep their nutritional preparation 24-hours prior to the testing similar on each occasion. All players had been familiarised to the testing protocols in a previous pilot testing session. Prior to the assessments a standardised 10-min warm up was completed.

Firstly, each participant's lower limb muscular power was evaluated using a countermovement jump without the use of arms. The participant fixed their hands upon their hips and completed a maximal jump on a jump mat (Probotics, USA). The jump was repeated three times with 5-min rest between each trial. The best score of the three trials was recorded as the criterion measure of jump performance.

Following a 5-min break sprint tests were completed to evaluate both acceleration (10 m) and speed (15 m & 30 m) (Strudwick *et al.,* 2002). Participants were required to sprint maximally for 30 m in a straight line, along a prepared course. A time for 10 m, 15 m and 30 m was recorded. A t-test to assess agility was completed following a 5-min break. The t-test required participants to sprint around a predetermined course shaped like a 'T'. The participant began by sprinting forwards for 10 m, they then turn left and sprint for 5 m, turn 180° and sprint 10 m to the opposite side before once again turning back 180° to sprint 5 m and finally backpedalling to the left 10 m to where the test started. Electronic timing gates were utilised to assess both of the sprint tests to the nearest 0.01 sec (Brower, USA). The speed and agility tests used a 1 m lead in prior to the actual assessment distance. The speed and agility tests were each repeated three times with a 5-min rest period between trials. The fastest of the three trails was recorded.

The participants then completed a 6 x 30 m repeated sprint test (Pyne *et al.,* 2008). The test required participants to sprint 30 m, before turning around during a 20-sec recovery period and sprinting back to the where the test started. This process was repeated two more times. The time of each of the six sprints was recorded using electronic timing gates and a hand held transmitter (Brower, USA) to the nearest 0.01 sec. A mean 30 m sprint time for the 6 attempts was calculated.

An indirect estimation of maximal aerobic power was determined using the multistage fitness test (MSFT) (Ramsbottom *et al.,* 1988). The MSFT was started following a 15-min rest period. Participants were required to run back and forth along a 20 m track in time with audio signals played from a CD (Sports Coach, UK). Each participant continued running until they could no longer maintain the required running speed or until voluntary exhaustion occurred.

The mean value and standard deviation (mean ± SD) was produced for each set of data using descriptive statistics. A normality test using Shapiro-Wilk methods was conducted and the data sets were found to be normally distributed. As a result a paired sample t-test was used along with Cohen's effect sizes to compare the pre and post training fitness testing results. Only the data from participants who performed both the pre and post phase tests and adhered to the training programme were computed. Significance level was set at $p \leq 0.05$.

## 3. RESULTS

### 3.1. Overview of the soccer training completed

The daily training sessions were 75.5 ± 21.4 min (mean ± SD) in duration, with an average 444.3 ± 77.9 min of soccer training and matches each week. The largest proportion of organised coaching time was spent in variations of training games (32%). Competitive match play was the second most common soccer activity (30%). The other three areas of training had smaller amounts of time dedicated to them (tactical: 17%; technical: 10%; physical: 11%) (see Figure 1). The highest mean %HR max, observed over the 7-week training study was observed for competitive match play (84 ± 1%). The values associated with training games (76 ± 3%), technical training (67 ± 4%) and tactical training (65 ± 4%) were lower (see Figure 2). The heart rates associated with each training type were all significantly different from each other ($p < 0.05$), except between technical and tactical training methods ($p > 0.05$).

### 3.2. Daily variations of training loads

Wednesdays (267.6 ± 119.2 au) and Fridays (284.6 ± 59.7 au) were associated with the lowest training loads when the TRIMPs were compared to the other training days (Monday (431.6 ± 168.0 au) ($p > 0.05$), Tuesday (443.9 ± 148.0 au) ($p < 0.05$), Thursday (429.3 ± 106.6 au) ($p < 0.05$) and Saturday (450.7 ± 158.4 au) ($p > 0.05$)) (see Figure 3). When assessing the daily session RPEs, Friday (288.6 ± 116.1 au) was rated significantly lower than Monday (413.1 ± 154.9 au) and Thursday (479.7 ± 105.4 au) ($p < 0.05$). RPE for Wednesday's session (312.0 ± 119.6 au) was also significantly lower than the load associated with a Thursday ($p < 0.05$).

### 3.3. Performance test results

Pre and post fitness testing data indicated that aerobic performance significantly increased ($p < 0.05$) over the training period (see Table 1). The 10 m, 15 m and 30 m sprint times and t-test agility performance did not change following the soccer training period ($p > 0.05$). A significant increase ($p < 0.05$) in the mean sprint time was observed during the repeated sprint ability testing. The height of the countermovement jump without the use of arms also decreased significantly ($p < 0.05$) by around 5.2%.

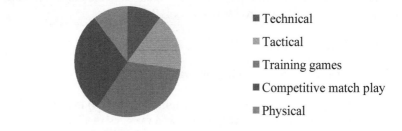

Figure 1 Proportion of time spent on each type of training or match play.

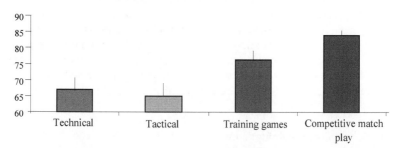

**Figure 2** Mean ± SD % heart rate max of values associated with technical training, tactical training, training games and competitive match play.

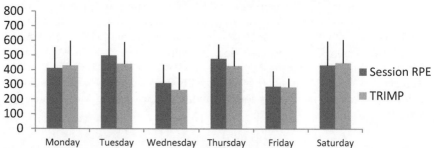

**Figure 3** Mean ± SD session RPE and TRIMP associated with each training day.

**Table 1** Fitness assessment data before and after the training phase (mean (SD)).

|  | N | Pre training mean *(SD)* | Post training mean *(SD)* | Effect size (d) |
|---|---|---|---|---|
| Multistage fitness test level | 10 | 14/3 (1/0) | 14/12 (0/10) | -0.69 |
| 10m sprint (sec) | 12 | 1.70 (0.08) | 1.70 (0.05) | 0.00 |
| 15m sprint (sec) | 12 | 2.34 (0.10) | 2.35 (0.06) | -0.10 |
| 30m sprint (sec) | 12 | 4.13 (0.18) | 4.18 (0.12) | -0.28 |
| T-test (sec) | 13 | 8.99 (0.33) | 9.01 (0.31) | -0.06 |
| Repeated sprint test – mean (sec) | 12 | 4.37 (0.17) | 4.52 (0.23) | -0.88 |
| Counter movement jump (cm) | 16 | 58.6 (5.9) | 55.5 (6.1) | 0.53 |

## 4. DISCUSSION AND CONCLUSION

The results imply that the majority of the young soccer players' time was spent in match play or replicated match related games during training. The time spent in an isolated technical or tactical setting was minimal by comparison. The match related types of activities were associated with the greatest physiological stress. The mean %HR max measured during competitive match play and training games demonstrate the increased cardiovascular load that is present during these modes of soccer. When the related heart rate responses were analysed, the less common technical and tactical training methods displayed a smaller physiological demand.

The fitness assessments completed pre and post the 7-week training period suggests that the training structure studied may be beneficial for the development of aerobic performance. However, other fitness test results suggest that the training programme may be detrimental to repeated sprint and jumping ability. There was no change in the participant's sprint performances.

There is very little other published literature that has examined the adaptations to full time soccer training as prescribed by coaches in the 'real world' without the addition of any additional training manipulations. Comparisons to data within the literature are therefore difficult to draw. One study that has published data on the effects of soccer training in young professional soccer players was Helgerud *et al.* (2001). This study found that such training periods did not significantly affect the group's fitness. These findings do not support the current research that showed an increase in aerobic performance as a result of 7-weeks of soccer training. The previous study did not, however, detail the type and intensity of the soccer training included in the investigation. This makes it difficult to draw true comparisons between the outcomes of the investigations.

The improvements in the multistage fitness test following the training period of the current study may be a reflection of the high aerobic demand of the training methods undertaken. If lower intensity training methods such as technical and tactical training were more commonly present, these beneficial adaptations may not be expected. The high physiological loads of the training activities undertaken, however, do not promote physiological adaptations in other areas of fitness. Soccer training alone was an insufficient load to maintain the jumping ability of participants. The reduction of lower limb power, therefore, may be explained by the absence of any specific strength or power training in the programme. This detriment, however, was not reflected in sprint performances. The large amount of maximal sprinting required during the training games and match play may have ensured speed maintenance. This was not echoed in the 30 m repeated sprint testing, however, which deteriorated. This may be explained by the nature of the most common training activity, training games, which are often completed within small sided areas. These activities, therefore, limited the participant's exposure to repeated sprints over this extensive distance. This study's findings imply that if adaptations in areas of fitness other than aerobic ability are desired, supplementary training should be prescribed. Such supplementary training should include elements of strength, power and speed.

### References

Dupont, G. *et al.*, 2004, The effect of in-season, high-intensity interval training in soccer players. *J Strength Cond Res*, **18**, 584–589.

Edwards, S., 1993, High performance training and racing. In *The Heart Rate Monitor Book*, Sacremento CA: Feet Fleet Press, pp. 113–123.

Foster, C., 1998, Monitoring training in athletes with reference to overtraining syndrome. *Med Sci Sports Exerc*, **30**, 1164–1168.

Helgerud, J. *et al.*, 2001, Aerobic endurance training improves soccer performance. *Med Sci Sports Exerc*, **33**, 1925–1931.

Pyne, D.B. *et al.*, 2008, Relationships between repeated sprint testing, speed and endurance. *J Strength Cond Res*, **22**, 1633–1637.

Ramsbottom, R. *et al.*, 1988, A progressive shuttle run test to estimate maximal oxygen uptake. *Brit J Sport Med*, **22**, 141–144.

Strudwick, A. *et al.*, 2002, Anthropometric and fitness profiles of elite players in two football codes. *J Sport Med Phys Fit*, **42**, 239–242.

# CHAPTER FOURTEEN

# The physiological responses to a laboratory-based soccer-specific training simulation (LSSTS) on a motorized treadmill

T. S. Jeong[1,2], T. Reilly[1], J. P. Morton[1] and B. Drust[1]

[1]Research Institute for Sport and Exercise Sciences, Liverpool John Moores University, Liverpool, UK, [2]Dept. of Physical Medicine & Rehabilitation, College of Medicine, SCH University and Hospital, Gumi, Korea

## 1. INTRODUCTION

Soccer is separated from other sports by its intermittent activity profile. This results in the physiological demands being more complex than continuous exercise (Drust *et al.*, 2000). The demands of soccer-specific intermittent exercise have been obtained by measuring physiological and metabolic responses during competitive and practice games (Rhode and Espersen, 1988; Bangsbo, 1994; Impellizzeri *et al.*, 2005). Such direct monitoring of actual physiological responses to match-play would seem to be the most effective way of determining the physiological cost of soccer-specific intermittent activity (Drust *et al*, 2007). In reality these procedures are limited by a number of theoretical and practical methodological issues. This may therefore limit the usefulness of the data in terms of its ability to accurately describe the physiological requirements of the sport. An alternative model to this approach is to attempt to recreate the demands of the sport using laboratory-based simulations. This approach provides the controlled conditions required in experimental investigations and/or the depth of understanding associated with laboratory-based analytical procedures (Drust *et al.*, 2000). A small number of researchers have attempted to devise soccer-specific laboratory-based protocols that replicate the exercise patterns observed during match-play using both motorized (Drust *et al.*, 2000) and non-motorized treadmills (Clarke *et al.*, 2005). Such protocols elicit broadly similar physiological responses to those observed in games thereby supporting their efficacy as suitable experimental models to apply to the sport.

The physiological demands associated with matches and training sessions are different (Rhode and Espersen, 1988; Impellizzeri *et al.*, 2005). Recent observations of training in Korean professional players (Jeong et *al.*, 2011)

supports this view by indicating lower physiological strain compared to previously published data on match-play (Bangsbo, 1994; Rienzi *et al.*, 2000). These variations may ultimately lead to differences in the internal training loads placed on individual players (Impellizzeri *et al.*, 2005). This information would suggest that soccer-specific treadmill simulations that are currently published in the literature may not be appropriate to simulate the physiological loads associated with soccer training.

This study aimed to evaluate the validity of a laboratory-based soccer-specific training simulation (LSSTS) on a motorized treadmill and to examine metabolic responses to the LSSTS.

## 2. MATERIALS AND METHOD

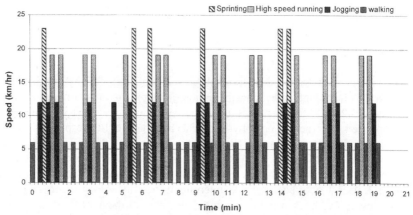

**Figure 1** The graphical representation of the activity patterns undertaken during one bout (20 min 36 s) of a soccer-training specific intermittent exercise protocol. A block of exercise incorporated 93 discrete activities; these included 26 static pauses, 28 walks, 17 jogs, 16 high speed runs and 6 sprints. This block was then repeated a total of 3 times in order to complete the LSSTS.

Ten professional players (mean±SD age: 24±3 years, body mass: 73±4 kg, height: 1.78±0.06 m) were monitored during a physical training session by measuring heart rate using a short-range telemetry system (Polar Team System®, Kempele, Finland). The rating of perceived exertion (RPE)-based training load was also evaluated after the completion of training using a modified 10-point rating Borg scale (Borg *et al.*, 1987; Jeong *et al.*, 2011). Six players (2 defenders, 2 mid-fielders, 2 forwards) were filmed using one video camera per player for the entire duration of training and their activity profiles were analysed using video-based notation system. The activities completed during training were classified into specific movement categories based on the intensity of action including sprinting (maximal running) (Sp), high speed running (HSR), jogging (J), walking (W) and static pause (St) (Bangsbo, 1994; Rienzi *et al.*, 2000). The categorization of movement was based around the stride counts observed per second in each activity. The stride counts associated with sprinting, high speed running, and jogging were above 4 strides·s⁻¹, between 3 strides·s⁻¹ and 4 strides·s⁻¹ and below 3 strides·s⁻¹, respectively (Rienzi *et al.*, 2000). Movement categories were determined on a second by second basis using the computerized coding system developed (Sportscode Gamebreaker® software, Sportec Ltd, Australia). The total time associated with each movement category was summated thereby permitting the calculation of the activity profile for an entire training session to be determined. Overall activity profiles and patterns of discrete actions obtained in training were then re-created on a treadmill (Jeong *et al.*, 2009). The speeds of each movement on the treadmill were based on previous observations obtained during match play (Mohr *et al.*, 2003). The relevant speeds utilized for W, J, HSR and Sp were 6 km·h⁻¹, 12 km·h⁻¹, 19 km·h⁻¹ and 23 km·h⁻¹, respectively (Figure 1).

The validity of LSSTS was subsequently evaluated by comparing the physiological loads of the professional players with those of 16 healthy subjects (mean±SD age: 25±5 years, body mass: 74±6 kg, height: 1.77±0.06 m). Heart rate and RPE-based training load were monitored to evaluate the physiological stress associated with the LSSTS in the laboratory. The time spent within specific HR zones was also calculated. Blood samples were collected from 10 of the 16 subjects who participated. Blood metabolites such as glucose, lactate, non-esterified fatty acid (NEFA) and glycerol were measured pre-, during and post-LSSTS to provide further evidence of the metabolic response to the simulation.

Independent t-tests were used to analyse the validity of the LSSTS compared to the actual physiological responses to the training. The responses of blood metabolites to the LSSTS were evaluated using one-way analysis of variance (ANOVA) for repeated measures and *p*-values <0.05 were considered significant.

## 3. RESULTS

### 3.1 Physiological responses to the LSSTS and its validity

The mean HR during the simulation (137±10 b·min⁻¹, 71±5 % of $HR_{max}$) was similar to that obtained in actual training (137±8 b·min⁻¹, 72+3 % of $HR_{max}$) (*p>0.05*). One±1% and 23±13% of the total time during the LSSTS was spent in the HR zones between 90~100 and 80~90% of $HR_{max}$, respectively. Around 60% of the time was spent in HR zones between 60~80% of $HR_{max}$. Seventeen percent of the time was in the relatively low-intensity HR zones (below 60% of $HR_{max}$). There was, however, no significant difference in time spent in all HR zones between either groups (*p>0.05*). The mean RPE-based training load in the protocol was also similar to those observed in the actual training session (simulation, 341±68 AU vs. training, 365±63 AU) (*p>0.05*) (Table 1).

**Table 1** The physiological responses during the laboratory-based soccer-specific training simulation and the actual training session observed.

| | Mean HR (b·min⁻¹) | Mean % of HR$_{max}$ | % of time spent in the HR zone (% of HR$_{max}$) | | | | | | RPE-TL (AU) |
|---|---|---|---|---|---|---|---|---|---|
| | | | 100~90 | 90~80 | 80~70 | 70~60 | 60~50 | <50 | |
| Training (n=10) | 137±8 | 72±3 | 0.4±1 | 22±12 | 41±8 | 19±3 | 15±7 | 2±2 | 365±63 |
| Simulation (n=16) | 137±10 | 71±5 | 0.8±1 | 23±13 | 35±7 | 25±7 | 13±8 | 4±6 | 341±68 |

Values are ± standard deviation (SD), Training; training group, Simulation; simulation group, HR; heart rate, HR$_{max}$; maximal heart rate, RPE-TL; RPE based-training load.

## 3. 2 Metabolic responses to LSSTS

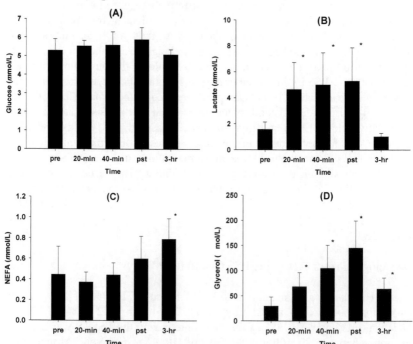

**Figure 2** The responses of blood metabolites to the laboratory-based soccer-specific training simulation; (A) glucose, (B) lactate, (C) NEFA and (D) glycerol.
* $p<0.05$, significant difference compared to pre-exercise.

The blood lactate concentration was significantly increased during (20-min, 4.6±2.1 mmol·l⁻¹) and immediately after exercise (5.3 ±2.6 mmol·l⁻¹), compared with rest (1.6±0.6 mmol·l⁻¹) ($p<0.05$). There were also significant changes in NEFA and glycerol following exercise. The concentration of NEFA was significantly higher at 40-min (0.5±0.1 mmol·l⁻¹), immediately after exercise (0.6±0.2 mmol·l⁻¹) and 3-hr after completion of exercise (0.8±0.2 mmol·l⁻¹)

compared with the pre-exercise value $(0.4\pm0.3$ mmol·l$^{-1}$) $(p<0.05)$. The concentration of glycerol during $(20\text{-min}, 69\pm28$ μmol·l$^{-1}$; $40\text{-min}, 105\pm46$ μmol·l$^{-1}$), immediately after $(145\pm54$ μmol·l$^{-1}$) and 3-hr after completion of exercise $(64\pm22$ μmol·l$^{-1}$) was also significantly higher than that observed pre-exercise levels $(29\pm19$ μmol·l$^{-1}$) $(p<0.05)$. Blood glucose concentration, however, did not change either during or following the LSSTS (Figure 2).

## 4. DISCUSSION

This study aimed to evaluate physiological stress and metabolic response to a laboratory-based soccer-specific training simulation. The LSSTS initiated similar heart rate responses and training loads to those observed in professional soccer training. The metabolic profiles obtained in the stimulation were also similar to those associated with match-play. These findings indicate that the simulation is a valid model for lab-based investigations on soccer-specific training.

The physiological responses to the LSSTS were similar to those recorded in the physical training session of the elite professional players. The actual training session included mainly physical training activities such as small-a-side games and short speed and speed endurance work. No significant differences between the mean values for HR and RPE-based TL were observed between the two conditions. The time spent in high intensity HR zones $(80\sim100\%$ of HR$_{max}$) was also equivalent between both groups (training group, 22.4% vs. simulation group, 23.8%). Such similarities in the physiological responses between the actual training session and the simulation would seem to be indicative of the suitability of the protocol to act as a recreation of a real world training session. The physiological indicators used in this investigation were, however, limited in their ability to determine the 'true' physiological cost of the exercise as the measurement strategies employed are not always fully representative of the load. That is, the simulation did not include utility movements (backwards and sideways) and soccer-specific technical elements (e.g. ball touches, jumping, dribbling, kicking, heading etc).

These omissions may cause a reduction in the physiological cost of exercise compared to that associated with actual field based training. The independent groups' experimental design that was employed is also a limitation as the two populations included in the investigation are likely to vary in a number of parameters (e.g. fitness, training history) that may influence the physiological responses to the exercise. Such issues are very difficult to address in studies of this nature as a consequence of the unavailability of players to attend laboratory trials. Therefore, the available data may well represent the most realistic and therefore effective evaluation of the simulation that could be performed. These findings suggest that the LSSTS was valid enough to re-create the relevant physiological strains during the actual training session of professional players.

No previous attempt has been made to evaluate the metabolic responses to a laboratory-based soccer-specific training simulation. The metabolic responses to the LSSTS showed similar patterns observed in both match-specific simulations (Clarke *et al.*, 2005) and model matches (Bangsbo, 1994). This data would therefore suggest that soccer-specific training sessions offer similar patterns of metabolic stress associated with match-play. This would seem to indicate that the pattern of exercise and the physiological load associated with soccer training sessions provides a basis for metabolic adaptations that are suitable for supporting performance in the game. This pattern of response would also indicate that the protocol provides a suitable model of 'real world' soccer-specific training.

In conclusion, the laboratory-based soccer-specific training simulation may present a valid model representing soccer-specific training sessions and could be used as a model for laboratory-based investigations.

## References

Bangsbo, J., 1994, The physiology of soccer, with special reference to intense intermittent exercise. *Acta Physiol Scand*, **151**, 1–155.

Borg, G. *et al.*, 1987, Perceived exertion related to heart rate and blood lactate during arm and leg exercise. *Eur J Appl Physiol Occup Physiol*, **56**, 679–685.

Clarke, N.D. *et al.*, 2005, Strategies for hydration and energy provision during soccer-specific exercise. *Int J Sport Nutr Exerc Metab*, **15**, 625–640.

Drust, B. *et al.*, 2000, Physiological responses to laboratory-based soccer-specific intermittent and continuous exercise. *J Sports Sci*, **18**, 885–892.

Drust, B. *et al.*, 2007, Future perspectives in the evaluation of the physiological demands of soccer. *Sports Med*, **37**, 783–805.

Impellizzeri, F.M. *et al.*, 2005, Physiological assessment of aerobic training in soccer. *J Sports Sci*, **23**, 583–592.

Jeong, T.S. *et al.*, 2009, The development of a laboratory-based soccer-specific training simulation. *Brit J Sports Med*, **43**, e2.

Jeong, T.S. *et al.*, 2011, Quantification of the physiological loading of one week of 'pre-season' and one week of 'in-season' training in professional soccer players. *J Sports Sci*, **29**, 1161–1166.

Mohr, M. *et al.*, 2003, Match performance of high-standard soccer players with special reference to development of fatigue. *J Sports Sci*, **21**, 519–528.

Rhode, H.C. and Espersen, T., 1988, Work intensity during soccer training and match-play. In *Science and Football*, London: E. & F.N. Spon, pp. 68–75.

Rienzi, E. *et al.*, 2000, Investigation of anthropometric and work-rate profiles of elite South American international soccer players. *J Sports Med Phys Fit*, **40**, 162–169.

# CHAPTER FIFTEEN

# Elite-youth and university-level versions of SAFT[90] simulate the internal and external loads of competitive soccer match-play

S. Barrett[1,2], A. Guard[1,3] and R. Lovell[1,4]

[1]Department of Sport, Health and Exercise Science, The University of Hull, UK
[2]Perform Better, Warwickshire, UK, [3]Celtic Football Club, Scotland, UK
[4]School of Science and Health, University of Western Sydney, Australia

## 1. INTRODUCTION

The motion demands of competitive soccer match-play have been published extensively. The recent development of semi-automated systems has enabled researchers and practitioners to collect and manage large volumes of data, which has furthered our understanding of the physical requirements. It is increasingly acknowledged that players perform within their physical capabilities (Drust et al., 2007) and that extrinsic factors such as tactical approach, quality of opposition, match status and crowd support create a large degree of inter-match variability in the physical data (Gregson et al., 2010). The myriad of factors that affect physical match performances makes it difficult for researchers to adopt these outcome measures to determine the efficacy of a given physical training intervention or ergogenic aid.

Consequently, researchers have developed laboratory and field-based match-play simulations to enable them to examine the efficacy of nutritional, training, and thermoregulatory interventions. Motorised treadmill (Drust et al., 2000), shuttle running (Nicholas et al., 2000), and field-based (Williams et al., 2010) simulations have generally required the participants to cover more total and high speed running distances than those typically observed in match-play (Drust et al., 2000; Williams et al., 2010). This can be attributed to their linear nature, which precludes non-uniform locomotor patterns, changes in direction and utility movements, all of which significantly increase the energetic cost (Drust et al., 2007). In addition, motorised treadmill protocols (Drust et al., 2000) have not always mimicked the high frequency of activity changes in match-play (~1400), hence changes in velocity from acceleration and deceleration movements are not inherent features of many simulations. This is a particularly important omission since players engage in these movements frequently and they are also more energetically demanding than constant velocity running (Osgnach *et al.*, 2010). Non-motorised treadmill simulations (Thatcher and Batterham, 2004) have been more successful as players are required to perform acceleration and deceleration actions. However, the resistance of the treadmill belt allows only 80% of the player's peak velocity to be achieved during sprint efforts, and the utility movements are absent in non-motorised treadmill simulation, hence the mechanical demands are not indicative of match-play.

Accordingly a 90-min soccer-specific aerobic field test (SAFT[90]) was developed to address these limitations, based on match-analysis data taken (Prozone®) from English Championship matches. SAFT[90] is a fixed-intensity shuttle running simulation around an agility course, with the intermittent exercise demands prescribed by an audio CD. During the 90-min simulation, the players cover 10.78 km, with frequent changes in intensity (1269 changes, every 4.3 seconds) and multi-directional activities (1350 changes in direction), eliciting internal loads similar to those reported from competitive match play (Lovell *et al.*, 2008). Comparing the physiological and/or mechanical responses to a soccer-specific protocol with actual match-play data is a common experimental approach to validate simulations, however, there are limitations with this approach: 1) internal and external demands of soccer match-play are often obtained from single match observations of 'non-competitive' fixtures, which does not account for the high-degree of match-to-match variability in physical performances (Gregson *et al.*, 2010); and 2) most attempts to validate a soccer-specific simulation (with the exception of Thatcher and Batterham, 2004) have used a different population to that from which the activity profile data was ascertained (e.g. Drust *et al.*, 2000; Lovell *et al.*, 2008).

Hence, this study had three aims: 1) to determine the internal (physiological) and external (motion analysis) loads of elite-youth (English Championship Team) and university players during competitive soccer match-play; 2) to create squad-specific soccer simulations using the SAFT[90] model (Lovell *et al.*, 2008); and 3) to validate the simulations from the players' internal (HR) and external (tri-axial accelerometer) loads using their respective match-play data.

## 2. METHODS

Nine elite-youth (Age: 17 ± 1 years; $\dot{V}O_{2max}$: 60.5 ± 4.1 ml.kg$^{-1}$.min$^{-1}$), and six University male soccer players (21 ± 1 years; $\dot{V}O_{2max}$: 56.7 ± 4.6 ml.kg$^{-1}$.min$^{-1}$) wore heart rate monitors (HR; Team System, Polar, Kempele, Finland) and 5 Hz GPS (MinimaxX, Catapult, Australia) units during 14 and 8 competitive league fixtures, respectively. Data were included if the player completed the 90-min match in the same tactical position, and only data from players completing three full 90-minute matches were included in the creation and subsequent validation of the squad-specific soccer simulations. Locomotor activities were categorised as standing (0.0–0.7 km·h⁻¹), walking (0.7–6.0 km·h⁻¹), jogging (6.0–15.0 km·h⁻¹), running (15.0–25.0 km·h⁻¹) and sprinting (> 25.0 km·h⁻¹). A 100 Hz tri-axial accelerometer that resides inside the GPS system was used to determine the external load of the player (PL), because of its capacity to detect instantaneous accelerations that are energetically taxing, which are not typically detected using velocity bands *per se* (Osgnach *et al.*, 2010). The accelerometer data was reported as a vector magnitude, which sums the frequency and magnitude of accelerations in all three axial planes.

The squad mean distance and time spent in each velocity category were aligned to a previous intermittent and multi-directional model (SAFT⁹⁰; Lovell *et al.*, 2008) which incorporates acceleration, deceleration, cutting, side-stepping, backwards and forwards running, to create an elite youth- (Y-SAFT⁹⁰) and University- (U-SAFT⁹⁰) squad-specific match-play simulation. After *a priori* familiarisation, players were fitted with a HR and GPS device and performed their respective squad-specific version of SAFT⁹⁰. The players performed their typical pre-match routines in terms of rest, nutrition, hydration and physical preparation, before performing the 90-min simulation, which was interceded by a 15-min passive half-time interval. The simulation was performed on an indoor 3G surface whilst wearing typical playing attire. The pace and nature of the utility movements required were directed by verbal signals from an audio CD.

Paired t-test was used to compare the players' mean PL and HR elicited by competitive match-play and the squad-specific SAFT⁹⁰ simulation. Their relationship was subsequently assessed via Pearsons correlation ($r$). Data are presented as the mean (SD).

## 3. RESULTS

The time motion data collected, together with the intensity distribution of the Y-SAFT⁹⁰ and U-SAFT⁹⁰ simulations are shown in Table 1. Due to the incorporation of utility movement and frequent accelerations and decelerations, the velocity of each movement category shown in Table 1 for the respective SAFT⁹⁰ simulation refers to the average velocity required to maintain the desired intensity.

There were no significant differences between the internal (HR) and external (PL) load measures recorded during match play and the squad-specific SAFT⁹⁰ simulation ($p > 0.05$; Table 2). A weak association was denoted for the players' average HR response to match-play and their respective SAFT⁹⁰ protocol (Elite youth players: $r = 0.222$; University 1ˢᵗ XI players $r = 0.109$). The players' mean PL denoted from match-play showed a moderate relationship ($r = 0.418$) to that elicited by Y-SAFT⁹⁰, whereas a weak association was detected for U-SAFT⁹⁰ ($r = 0.204$).

**Table 1** A comparison of the average match demands of elite youth (Y-SAFT$^{90}$) and University (U-SAFT$^{90}$) players. The squad-specific SAFT$^{90}$ distance and velocity for each locomotor category is also presented.

| | | Movement Category | | | | | |
|---|---|---|---|---|---|---|---|
| | | Stand | Walk | Jog | Run | Sprint | Total |
| | | | | Y-SAFT$^{90}$ | | | |
| Distance | Match-play | 467 | 2281 | 5035 | 1687 | 170 | 9640 |
| (m) | Y-SAFT$^{90}$ | 0 | 2760 | 5100 | 1650 | 240 | 9750 |
| Velocity (km·h$^{-1}$) | | 0 | 4.48 | 10.94 | 16.32 | 20.75 | - |
| | | | | U-SAFT$^{90}$ | | | |
| Distance | Match-play | 466 | 2318 | 5048 | 1456 | 137 | 9425 |
| (m) | U-SAFT$^{90}$ | 0 | 2760 | 4920 | 1500 | 240 | 9420 |
| Velocity (km·h$^{-1}$) | | 0 | 5.76 | 7.76 | 14.16 | 19.83 | - |

**Table 2** Player mean internal and external load responses from squad-specific match play and respective SAFT$^{90}$ simulation.

| | Elite Youth Players | | University Players | |
|---|---|---|---|---|
| | Match-play | Y-SAFT$^{90}$ | Match-play | U-SAFT$^{90}$ |
| Mean HR (bpm$^{-1}$) | 165 (4) | 165 (9) | 164 (8) | 162 (6) |
| %HR maximum | 82.2 (2.4) | 82.2 (5.4) | 87.8 (4.8) | 85.9 (3.7) |
| PL (au) | 1245 (223) | 1281 (304) | 1142 (382) | 1156 (200) |

## 4. DISCUSSION

Using the SAFT$^{90}$ model, both the internal and external loads from soccer match-play can be mimicked in a laboratory or field environment. In this study, two different versions of the simulation were created, based on time-motion data collected from serial competitive match-play fixtures.

The Y-SAFT$^{90}$ and U-SAFT$^{90}$ elicited both the internal (heart rate) and external (tri-axial accelerometer data) loads that were observed in their respective matches, which suggests that they are a valid representation of the physical performances required in soccer. The experimental approach adopted here to validate the Y-SAFT$^{90}$ and U-SAFT$^{90}$ is similar to that undertaken by other researchers (Drust *et al.*, 2000; Thatcher and Batterham, 2004), however, the strengths of the current study are that the time motion data was collected using repeated match observations, and that the same players were used to validate the protocols. The repeated match-play observations collected in this study accounts (to some extent) for the high degree of variability in player physical match performances (Gregson *et al.*, 2010), likely caused by situational factors such as match-status, standard of opposition, environmental conditions, and tactical considerations. The individual players whose data was used to create the squad-specific protocols, subsequently performed them during the in-season approximately three weeks after the final match-play data was collected, therefore the training status of these individuals was not altered. Surprisingly, only one other study to date has used the same sample of players to validate a simulation that was based on their own time-motion characteristics (Thatcher and Batterham, 2004), which may be a compromising feature of many of the other available simulations.

The SAFT$^{90}$ model emulates the intermittent and multi-directional nature of soccer match-play, with frequent changes in direction and activity. Though previous protocols have successfully demonstrated external validity by eliciting the physiological costs observed from match-play scenarios, they have not well represented the mechanical nature of the game, which has ~1400 changes in activity and over 500 turns. These movements, along with unorthodox running and rapid changes in velocity (Osgnach *et al.*, 2010) have a high energetic cost. Therefore to simulate the physiological demands of match-play, simulations have often exceeded either the total distance covered, or the distance covered at high-speeds, which compromises their ecological validity. The mean cardiovascular response to Y-SAFT$^{90}$ and U-SAFT$^{90}$ was almost identical to that recorded in the corresponding fixtures. This was achieved without compromising the mechanical demands of match-play, evidenced by the similar PL's reported.

To our knowledge, this is the first study to report the external loads of soccer match-play using a tri-axial accelerometer. This technique may provide a more rigorous assessment of the mechanical demand than traditional methods of time-motion data using arbitrary velocity categories, which neglect many high-intensity activities that may occur at low velocity (Osgnach *et al.*, 2010). The similar mean PL's observed in this study provides further support for both the external and ecological validity of the Y-SAFT$^{90}$ and U-SAFT$^{90}$ protocols.

Whilst the mean responses to Y-SAFT$^{90}$ and U-SAFT$^{90}$ were very similar to competitive matches, there was a weak correlation for both heart rate and player load. This was a result of using squad-mean GPS data to create the simulations, an approach which neglects the positional variation inherent to the game. Therefore, when performing their respective SAFT$^{90}$ some players will be performing more physical work than they would normally undertake in matches, and vice versa. In the current study, these differences were broadly position specific; for example, central defenders demonstrated a lower internal and external load in match-play than in SAFT$^{90}$, with the opposite trend denoted in midfield players. Therefore the SAFT$^{90}$ versions examined in this study are representative of the mean match demands, and given the considerable positional variation this is a limitation of the current approach. Researchers might consider developing position-specific simulations, or alternatively refine the free-paced protocols available in the literature (Nicholas *et al.*, 2000; Williams *et al.*, 2010). Whilst the fixed-paced nature of the SAFT$^{90}$ protocols precludes an intrinsic measure of performance, sprint performance can be determined with photocells and other measures can be achieved simply by pausing the simulation. Fixed-intensity simulations are also inherently reproducible and enable researchers to detect changes in response to an intervention with scientific rigour. For this reason, the SAFT[90] protocols do not include ball involvements, contact with other players and certain purposeful movements such as jumping and lunging, as the performance of these aspects might vary within and between experimental trials. However, researchers and practitioners can add these features into the protocol as desired.

In summary, this study has demonstrated both the external and ecological validity of Y-SAFT[90] and U-SAFT[90]. For scientists and practitioners, the current model can be applied to rigorously assess intervention strategies, especially since the sample populations used here are often recruited for research studies. Furthermore, it provides a non-contact exercise for late-stage rehabilitating players, specific to their match-play demands without the risk of contact injury. Future research may be warranted in developing position-specific match-play simulations, or to improve the ecological validity of free-paced protocols to better simulate the mechanical demands of soccer match-play.

## References

Drust, B. *et al.*, 2000, Physiological responses to laboratory-based soccer-specific intermittent and continuous exercise. *J Sports Sci*, **18**, 885–892.

Drust, B. *et al.*, 2007, Future perspectives in the evaluation of the physiological demands of soccer. *Sports Med*, **37**, 783–805.

Gregson, W. *et al.*, 2010, Match-to-match variability of high-speed activities in premier league soccer. *Int J Sports Med*, **31**, 237–242.

Lovell, R. *et al.*, 2008, Physiological responses to SAFT[90]: a new soccer-specific match simulation. *Coaching Sports Sci*, **3**, 46–67.

Nicholas, C.W. *et al.*, 2000, The Loughborough intermittent shuttle test: a field test that simulates the activity pattern of soccer. *J Sports Sci*, **18**, 97–104.

Osgnach, C. *et al.*, 2010, Energy cost and metabolic power in elite soccer: a new match analysis approach. *Med Sci Sports Exerc*, **42**, 170–178.

Thatcher, R. and Batterham, A.M., 2004, Development and validation of a sport-specific exercise protocol for elite youth soccer players. *J Sports Med Phys Fit*, **44**, 15–22.

Williams, J.D. *et al.*, 2010, Ball-Sport Endurance and Sprint Test (BEAST90): Validity and reliability of a 90-minute soccer performance test. *J Strength Cond Res*, **24**, 3209–3218.

# CHAPTER SIXTEEN

# Yo-Yo intermittent recovery level 2 test in young soccer players from U-13 to U-18

K. Chuman[1,2], T. Ikoma[1], Y. Hoshikawa[3],
T. Iida[3] and T. Nishijima[4]

[1]Yamaha Football Club Co. Ltd., Japan
[2]Doctoral Program Health and Sport Science, University of Tsukuba, Japan
[3]Sports Photonics Laboratory, Hamamatsu Photonics K.K., Japan
[4]Institute of Health and Sport Science, University of Tsukuba, Japan

## 1. INTRODUCTION

The Yo-Yo intermittent recovery level 2 test (Yo-Yo IR2) is widely utilized to evaluate high-intensity intermittent endurance in high-level soccer players (Randers *et al.*, 2009). Yo-Yo IR2 results improve with age during adolescence. According to Bangsbo *et al.* (2008), the Yo-Yo IR2 applies a heavy load to both the aerobic and anaerobic energy systems of players. Adolescent development in aerobic and anaerobic fitness occurs at different timings and tempos (Chuman *et al.*, 2009; Malina and Bouchard, 1991). In general, anaerobic fitness improves gradually with age during adolescence (Malina and Bouchard, 1991) and young soccer players aged 12–13 years have already achieved aerobic fitness equivalent to that of professional players (Chuman *et al.*, 2009). Both Yo-Yo IR2 and anaerobic fitness are closely correlated to age (Chuman *et al.*, 2009), but aerobic fitness may not be. Therefore, improvement in Yo-Yo IR2 results in young soccer players seems due mainly to the development of anaerobic fitness. However, whether anaerobic fitness is more important than aerobic fitness for Yo-Yo IR2 performance after taking the age factor into account is unknown. We hypothesized that Yo-Yo IR2 performance in youth soccer players (U-13 to U-18) was affected by anaerobic fitness rather than aerobic fitness, and was affected by aerobic fitness even after taking the player age into account (Figure 1). The purpose of this study was to confirm the hypothetical models.

## 2. METHODS

The participants were 86 members (age; 12 to 18 years) of an academy team managed by a club belonging to the Japan Professional Football League Division 1 (J1-League). The participants were divided into six age groups: U-13 (N=16), U-14 (N=15), U-15 (N=15), U-16 (N=14), U-17 (N=16) and U-18 (N=10), and performed Yo-Yo IR2 on artificial turf with the players wearing soccer shoes in each group. The test was supervised by soccer coaches, and controlled by the physical coach. The air temperature was 15–20°C.

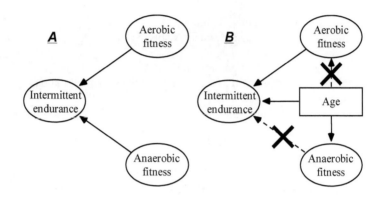

**Figure 1** Hypothetical models in young soccer players from U-13 to U-18.

*A,* Intermittent endurance is affected by anaerobic fitness to a greater extent than aerobic fitness in young soccer players from U-13 to U-18.

*B,* Aerobic fitness affected intermittent endurance even after taking the player age into account.

Within 1 week after the Yo-Yo IR2, aerobic and anaerobic fitness were measured by $\dot{V}O_{2max}$ (mL·min$^{-1}$·kg$^{-1}$) and Wingate tests (W·kg$^{-1}$), respectively. $\dot{V}O_{2max}$ was determined by an incremental exercise test to exhaustion on a treadmill. Oxygen uptake was measured continuously by a Meta Max system (Cortex Biophysic GmbH, Germany). The running velocity for determining $\dot{V}O_{2max}$ was set to 280 m· min$^{-1}$ for U-13 to U-18 groups. The treadmill inclination was increased by 1% per minute after 3 min of running until volitional exhaustion. The Wingate test was performed for 30 seconds at a load of 7.5% body mass (Bar-Or, 1987) using an electrically braked cycle ergometer (Powermax VII, Combi Wellness Co. Ltd., Japan). The pedal rotation was recorded at 10 Hz and the exerted power was calculated by multiplying the load by the rotation. One-way ANOVA was performed to examine differences among the six age groups. Structural equation modelling (SEM) was implemented to confirm our hypothetical models (Figure 1). The $x^2$, GFI, AGFI, CFI, NFI, RFI and RMSEA that show coefficient of determination for data variance and covariance were used for the model fitting indication (Kano, 1997; Yamamoto, 1999). SPSS 12.0J and Amos 5.0 were used for all statistical analyses. Significance level was set at $p<0.05$.

## 3. RESULTS

Table 1 shows descriptive statistics. The results of Wingate test for the U-13 to U-18 were 7.8(0.5), 7.9(0.7), 8.7(0.6), 9.0(0.5), 9.5(0.4) and 9.5(0.5) W · kg$^{-1}$, respectively. The $\dot{V}O_{2max}$ were 65.4(3.9), 66.0(6.9), 69.9(6.7), 68.3(3.6), 67.4(3.8) and 66.7(5.2) mL · min$^{-1}$ · kg$^{-1}$. The Yo-Yo IR2 results were 420(86), 683(120), 733(168), 814(184), 953(230) and 1172(171) m (Figure 2). When one-way ANOVA was performed to examine differences among the six age groups (U-13 to U-18), main effects were found in height, body mass, Yo-Yo IR2 and Wingate test, but not in $\dot{V}O_{2max}$.

**Table 1** Descriptive statistics.

| Item | Young soccer players | | | | | | F value |
|---|---|---|---|---|---|---|---|
| | U-13 | U-14 | U-15 | U-16 | U-17 | U-18 | |
| Height (m) | 1.59 (0.09) | 1.65 (0.07) | 1.69 (0.06) | 1.72 (0.04) | 1.72 (0.03) | 1.72 (0.04) | 11.6 * |
| Body mass (kg) | 47.1 (8.6) | 52.9 (9.1) | 59.0 (8.2) | 64.4 (7.3) | 65.4 (5.4) | 65.2 (4.7) | 15.1 * |
| Wingate test (W·kg$^{-1}$) | 7.8 (0.5) | 7.9 (0.7) | 8.7 (0.6) | 9.0 (0.5) | 9.5 (0.4) | 9.5 (0.5) | 25.8 * |
| $\dot{V}O_2$max (mL·min$^{-1}$·kg$^{-1}$) | 65.4 (3.9) | 66.0 (6.9) | 69.9 (6.7) | 68.3 (3.6) | 67.4 (3.8) | 66.7 (5.2) | 1.2 |

Mean(S.D.), *; significant differences ($p<0.05$)

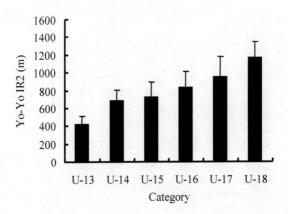

**Figure 2** Yo-Yo IR2 results in young soccer players from U-13 to U-18 ($F$=32.1, $p<0.05$).

Figure 3 shows the effects of aerobic and anaerobic fitness on intermittent endurance in young soccer players from U-13 to U-18. Here, the $x^2$ which is a model fitting indicator, was 1.906 (*P* value=0.167), GFI was 0.985, AGFI was 0.913, CFI was 0.980, NFI was 0.961, RFI was 0.882, and RMSEA was 0.103. The path coefficients from $\dot{V}O_{2max}$ and Wingate test to Yo-Yo IR2 were 0.35 and 0.52, respectively. Both path coefficients were significant.

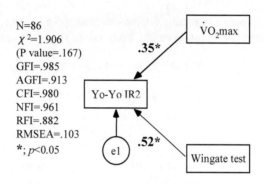

**Figure 3** Effects of aerobic and anaerobic fitness on intermittent endurance in young soccer players from U-13 to U-18.

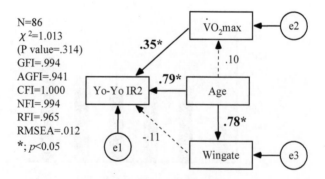

**Figure 4** Effects of aerobic and anaerobic fitness on intermittent endurance taking age into account among young soccer players from U-13 to U-18.

Figure 4 shows effects of aerobic and anaerobic fitness on intermittent endurance when the age of young soccer players from U-13 to U-18 is taken into account. Here, the $x^2$ was 1.013 (*P* value=0.314), GFI was 0.994, AGFI was 0.941, CFI was 1.000, NFI was 0.994, RFI was 0.965, and RMSEA was 0.012. Path coefficients from age to Yo-Yo IR2, $\dot{V}O_{2max}$ and Wingate test were 0.79, 0.10 and 0.78, respectively. The path coefficients from age to Yo-Yo IR2 and Wingate test were significant. Path coefficients from $\dot{V}O_{2max}$ and Wingate test to Yo-Yo IR2 were 0.35 and 0.52, respectively. The path coefficient from $\dot{V}O_{2max}$ to Yo-Yo IR2 was significant.

## 4. DISCUSSION

The model fitting indicators for the hypothetical models (Figure 1) showed significant values and these causal structural models were confirmed (Figure 3 and 4). Significant path coefficients from $\dot{V}O_{2max}$ and Wingate test result to Yo-Yo IR2 result were confirmed in one model (Figure 3). The Yo-Yo IR2 test does apply a heavy load to both the aerobic and anaerobic energy systems (Bangsbo *et al.*, 2008). Both Yo-Yo IR2 and anaerobic fitness are closely correlated with age (Table 1), but young soccer players aged 12-13 years have already achieved a high-level of $\dot{V}O_{2max}$ equivalent to professional soccer players (Chuman *et al.*, 2009). These results suggest that intermittent endurance (Yo-Yo IR2 performance) is affected by anaerobic fitness (Wingate test performance) to a higher degree than aerobic fitness ($\dot{V}O_{2max}$).

In the other model, significant path coefficients from age to Yo-Yo IR2 and Wingate test results and from $\dot{V}O_{2max}$ to Yo-Yo IR2 results were confirmed, however, those from age to $\dot{V}O_{2max}$ and Wingate test result to Yo-Yo IR2 result were not confirmed (Figure 4). The above results all suggest that intermittent endurance (Yo-Yo IR2 result) is affected by anaerobic fitness to a greater degree than aerobic fitness in young soccer players from U-13 to U-18, while only aerobic fitness affects intermittent endurance (Yo-Yo IR2 result) even after taking the player age into account. Generally, young soccer players are categorized by age, performing soccer training and games. Therefore, it was thought that the higher the aerobic fitness, the greater intermittent endurance was in each age category. We therefore also suggest that achievement of high-level aerobic fitness is very important in young soccer players.

## 5. CONCLUSIONS

- Intermittent endurance is affected by anaerobic fitness to a greater extent than aerobic fitness in young soccer players from U-13 to U-18.
- Aerobic fitness affected intermittent endurance even after taking the player's age into account.

## References

Bangsbo, J. *et al.*, 2008, The Yo-Yo intermittent recovery test: A useful tool for evaluation of physical performance in intermittent sports. *Sports Med*, **38**, 37–51.

Bar-Or, O., 1987, The Wingate anaerobic test: An update on methodology, reliability and validity. *Sports Med*, **4**, 381–394.

Chuman, K. *et al.*, 2009, Yo-Yo intermittent recovery level 2 test in pubescent soccer players with relation to maturity category. *Football Science*, **6**, 1–6.

Kano, Y., 1997, *Graphical Multi Validate Analysis*, Kyoto: Gendaisugakusya (in Japanese), pp. 186–224.

Malina, R.M. and Bouchard, C., 1991, *Growth, Maturation and Physical Activity*. Champaign, IL: Human Kinetics.

Randers, M.B. *et al.*, 2009, Match performance and Yo-Yo IR2 test performance of players from successful and unsuccessful professional soccer teams. In *Science and Football VI*, New York: Routledge pp, 345–349.

Yamamoto, K., 1999, *Covariance Structure Analysis and Cases using Amos*, Tokyo: Nakanishiya-syuppan (in Japanese), pp. 83–96.

# CHAPTER SEVENTEEN

# The assessment of repeated sprint ability using a combined sub-maximal and exhaustive treadmill protocol

B. Drust[1], C. Cullen[1] and R. Di Michele[2]

[1]Research Institute for Sports and Exercise Sciences,
Liverpool John Moores University, UK
[2]Department of Histology, Embryology and Applied Biology,
University of Bologna, Italy

## 1. INTRODUCTION

Repeated sprint ability (RSA) is a key capacity for a football player (Spencer et al., 2005). Repeated sprint performance is therefore an important component of any physiological test battery used within the sport of soccer.

Common RSA tests have focused primarily on performance assessment, with outcomes usually consisting of indicators of mean speed and/or the speed decrease in a series of brief maximal sprints interspersed by short recovery periods (Wragg et al., 2000; Aziz et al., 2007; Brown et al., 2007; Impellizzeri et al., 2008). In addition to maximum sprinting performance, it seems useful for a more in-depth evaluation of RSA to consider the physiological responses to high-intensity intermittent running. Such information may provide useful information on the important physiological characteristics that may relate to RSA (Rampinini et al., 2009).

Despite the need to frequently evaluate RSA in the laboratory, the majority of assessments for RSA have been designed for field based testing (e.g. Wragg et al., 2000; Impellizzeri et al., 2008). Only a few studies have evaluated RSA with treadmill tests (Aziz et al., 2007; Brown et al., 2007). These tests were performed on a non-motorised treadmill which is not frequently available in the majority of laboratories. This makes it difficult for a large number of scientists and practitioners to replicate the protocols.

Therefore, the purpose of this study was to analyze the reliability and validity of a new RSA test (RST) for a motorised treadmill. This test included both a sub-maximal phase followed by an exhaustive effort. The effect of acute hypoxia exposure on RSA outcomes was also assessed to provide some information on the sensitivity of the test to an environmental manipulation.

## 2. METHODS

### 2.1. Subjects

Nine amateur football players were recruited. Their mean ± standard deviation age, body mass, and body height were, respectively, 25 ± 3 yrs, 72.6 ± 5.1 kg, and 1.74 ± 0.05 m. The subjects were required to refrain from any intense exercise for at least two days before each session, and to avoid caffeine and alcoholic beverages in the testing days. Before the study, participants were informed about the procedures and signed their written consent to participate. The study was approved by the institutional ethical committee.

### 2.2. Procedures

All participants completed a $\dot{V}O_{2max}$ assessment and a Yo-Yo IR2 test. Participants then completed the RST twice in normoxia and once in hypoxic conditions in a normobaric hypoxic chamber (at a height corresponding to a 3600-m altitude). The five tests were performed in different sessions. The subjects were familiarised to all testing procedures prior to the completion of the experimental trials.

#### 2.2.1. $\dot{V}O_2max$ test and Yo-Yo IR2 test

An incremental exhaustive running test was performed on a treadmill (Cosmos, Nussdorf-Tarunstein, Germany). After a 5 minute warm-up at 8 km·h$^{-1}$, the subjects ran at 8 km·h$^{-1}$ for 2 min at level grade. The speed was then increased by 2 km·h$^{-1}$ every 2 min, with the grade remaining at 0%. The test continued upon voluntary exhaustion. $\dot{V}O_2$ was monitored with a Metamax gas analyser (Metamax, Cortex, Biophysik, Leipzig, Germany), properly calibrated before each test. In the test, all the subjects reached a $\dot{V}O_2$ plateau, and $\dot{V}O_2$ was recorded as the highest of 30-s averaged $\dot{V}O_2$ values. All subjects carried out a Yo-Yo IR2 test on an indoor track (Krustrup *et al.*, 2006).

#### 2.2.2. RST

The RST was performed on a Cosmos motorised treadmill (Cosmos, Nussdorf-Tarunstein, Germany), at 0% gradient after a 2 min warm-up. The first, sub-maximal phase of the RST protocol consisted of ten 15-s sprints at 23 km·h$^{-1}$, interspersed by a 15-s static pause. Thereafter, the duration of each sprint and recovery period was increased and decreased by 5 s respectively every 5 sprints. The test was terminated upon volitional exhaustion.

Throughout the test, the heart rate was continuously measured with a Polar S610 heart rate monitor (Polar Electro Oy, Tampere, Finland). The maximum achieved heart rate ($HR_{MAX}$) during the test, and the end heart rate after the 10$^{th}$

sprint ($HR_{10}$) were collected. Ratings of perceived exertion ($RPE_{10}$) were recorded using a 15 points (from 6 to 20) Borg scale. Upon the termination of exercise, the number of completed sprints ($N_{SP}$) was recorded, and blood lactate concentration (LA) was measured with a Lactate Pro analyser (Arkray, Tokyo, Japan).

## 2.3. Statistical analysis

All the data are reported as mean ± standard deviation. In order to assess the reliability of the RST, 95% limits of agreement were computed between the values of each dependent variable measured in the first RST trial and the second trial. Spearman's rho correlation coefficients were used to analyse the relationships between the RST variables and the outcomes of the other tests, i.e. the Yo-Yo IR2 and the $\dot{V}O_{2max}$ test. This permitted an evaluation of the validity of the RST. Finally, the sensitivity to hypoxia exposure was assessed by comparing the results of the hypoxia RST with those of the first normoxia RST trial, using paired Student's t-tests and effect sizes. For all the tests, the significance was set at α=0.05.

## 3. RESULTS

### 3.1. Reliability

The 95% limits of agreement for the first and the second RST trial were 0 ± 3 sprints ($N_{SP}$), 0 ± 4 ($RPE_{10}$), 0.3 ± 2.6 bpm ($HR_{MAX}$), and 1.2 ± 7.3 bpm ($HR_{10}$). For all these variables, the bias was not significantly different from the zero value (p>0.05).

### 3.2. Validity

The $\dot{V}O_{2max}$ of the subjects was 56.9 ± 6.3 ml·min$^{-1}$·kg$^{-1}$. The distance covered in the Yo-Yo IR2 test was 471 ± 144 m. The number of completed sprints was highly correlated to both $\dot{V}O_{2max}$ ($r_s$=0.79, p<0.01) and Yo-Yo IR2 performance ($r_s$=0.88, p<0.001).

### 3.3. Sensitivity

Six subjects did not manage to complete ten or more sprints due to fatigue in the hypoxic condition. $HR_{10}$ and $RPE_{10}$ were therefore only measured in three subjects. As a result this data was not considered in the formal sensitivity analysis. $HR_{MAX}$, LA, and $N_{SP}$ were analysed. Table 1 displays both the mean values and the effect sizes of these variables.

**Table 1** Mean values in the normoxia and hypoxia trial of the RST variables, and effect sizes.
*significantly different from normoxia (p<0.05).

|  | Normoxia | Hypoxia | Effect size |
|---|---|---|---|
| $N_{SP}$ (sprints) | 14 ± 3 | 9 ± 3* | 0.78 |
| $HR_{MAX}$ (bpm) | 189.4 ± 5.2 | 176.5 ± 6.3* | 2.39 |
| LA (mmol·l$^{-1}$) | 13.6 ± 2.2 | 11.6 ± 1.5* | 1.11 |

Significantly lower values of $N_{SP}$, $HR_{MAX}$, and LA were observed in hypoxia. There was a medium effect size for $N_{SP}$, whereas the effect size was large for LA and especially for $HR_{MAX}$.

## 4. DISCUSSION AND CONCLUSION

This study aimed to analyze the reliability, validity and sensitivity of a new RSA test for a motorised treadmill. Taken together, the results would seem to indicate acceptable levels of reliability for all the key outcome variables, a good concurrent validity for the test against frequently used assessments of aerobic and anaerobic performance and sensitivity of the test to acute hypoxia exposure. To our knowledge, despite the need to frequently evaluate RSA in the laboratory, the RST is the first RSA test designed for a motorised treadmill. A further novelty of the RST is the ability to assess the physiological responses to a set bout of high-intensity repeated sprints along with a maximal performance outcome, i.e. the number of sprint carried out before exhaustion.

The validity of the RST have been evaluated by comparing performance with $\dot{V}O_{2max}$, an indicator of aerobic power, and to distance covered in the Yo-Yo IR2 test. These parameters were selected for the validity assessment as both the aerobic and anaerobic energy systems can limit the repeated sprint performance in soccer players (Brown *et al.*, 2007; Meckel *et al.*, 2009). The high correlation observed between $N_{SP}$ and each of the two aforementioned parameters supports the validity of this index as a measure of the different physiological aspects related to RSA.

All the examined indices showed good levels of repeatability, with insignificant bias between the first and second assessments. The 95% agreement intervals can be considered sufficiently narrow for all the parameters except $HR_{10}$. In fact, the observed 95% random error component of 7.3 bpm is higher than the 2-4 bpm change considered to be the normal intra-individual day-to-day variability in HR under controlled conditions (Acthen and Jeukendrup, 2003). This value may reflect the influence of a single subject on the data as only one individual showed a difference in HR between the two trials higher than 5 bpm. Further studies with a larger sample size could therefore demonstrate acceptable reliability for $HR_{10}$.

Acute hypoxia exposure has been shown to impair the performance in RSA (Smith and Billaut, 2010). It was therefore expected that the outcomes of the RST would be sensitive to a simulated 3600-m altitude. This was confirmed by our results with lower values of $N_{SP}$, $HR_{MAX}$, and LA in the hypoxia trial.

In conclusion, the RST seems to provide an effective tool for an RSA assessment in a laboratory setting using a motorised treadmill. This may make the test useful as both a tool in experimental investigations and also for the assessment of RSA performance in different playing populations.

## References

Achten J. and Jeukendrup A.E., 2003, Heart rate monitoring: Applications and limitations. *Sports Med*, **33**, 517–538

Aziz, A.R. *et al.*, 2007, Relationship between measured maximal oxygen uptake and aerobic endurance performance with running repeated sprint ability in young elite soccer players. *J Sports Med Phys Fit*, **47**, 401–407.

Brown, P.I. *et al.*, 2007, Relationship between $VO_2$max and repeated sprint ability using non-motorised treadmill ergometry. *J Sports Med Phys Fit*, **47**, 186–190.

Impellizzeri, F.M. *et al.*, 2008, Validity of a repeated-sprint test for football. *Int J Sports Med*, **29**, 899–905.

Krustrup, P. *et al.*, 2006, The Yo-Yo IR2 test: Physiological response, reliability, and application to elite soccer. *Med Sci Sports Exerc*, **38**, 1666–1673.

Meckel, Y. *et al.*, 2009, Relationship among repeated sprint tests, aerobic fitness, and anaerobic fitness in adolescent soccer players. *J Strength Cond Res*, **23**, 163–169.

Rampinini, E. *et al.*, 2009, Repeated-sprint ability in professional and amateur soccer players. *Appl Physiol, Nutr Metab*, **34**, 1048–1054.

Smith, K.J. and Billaut, F., 2010, Influence of cerebral and muscle oxygenation on repeated-sprint ability. *Eur J Appl Physiol*, **109**, 989–999.

Spencer, M. *et al.*, 2005, Physiological and metabolic responses of repeated-sprint activities: specific to field-based team sports. *Sports Med*, **35**, 1025–1044.

Wragg, C.B. *et al.*, 2000, Evaluation of the reliability and validity of a soccer-specific field test of repeated sprint ability. *European J Appl Physiol*, **83**, 77–83.

# CHAPTER EIGHTEEN

# Effect of a 2-week preseason conditioning program on repeat sprint ability on male collegiate soccer athletes

T. Favero, G. Rouse and A. Kraus

Department of Biology, University of Portland, Portland Oregon, USA

## 1. INTRODUCTION

Soccer training is divided into seasonal component parts, the preseason, competitive season, and off-season. Preseason is the period immediately prior to the competitive season. During this time, technical and tactical training are emphasized along with the development of agility, speed and soccer specific endurance capacities. While professional teams typically take 6 weeks to prepare for an upcoming season, collegiate athletes in the US only get 16 days of preseason before their first competition. Historically, preseason in the United States for collegiate athletes includes two workouts per day as coaches try to maximize the time available for training. Teams typically train with the ball in the morning session and condition with or without the ball in the afternoon session. Every three or four days athletes commonly complete a comprehensive strength training session.

However, while necessary for preseason training, concentrated, repetitive, and demanding training activities can reduce the strength and power of the lower extremities, which are critical to soccer performance (Woods et al., 2002). Little time for daily recovery can lead to fatigue. Moreover, recovery interventions planned between sessions have little effect on anaerobic performance (Tessitore et al., 2007). Such intensive training during preseason potentially puts athletes in an overreached state leading to performance declines (Coutts et al., 2007). A demanding preseason without adequate recovery could reduce lower extremity power and affect performance in the first game. The aim of this study was to track the changes on repeated sprint ability (RSA) and lower extremity power production during an intense preseason program in a male collegiate soccer team.

## 2. METHODS

### Subjects and test administration

Sixteen Division I men's collegiate soccer athletes were recruited for the study (age 20.2 ± 1.4 years; range 18–22). Before performing any testing, all players were required to complete a medical screening questionnaire to ensure they were in good health. Additionally, after receiving verbal and written explanation of the study procedures and potential risks, participants signed a written consent form. This study was approved by the University of Portland Institutional Review Board.

Following test familiarization, the athletes performed a standing long jump (SLJ) and a countermovement jump (CMJ) as described by Mujika *et al.* (2009)(Vertec, USA). Each athlete was given three attempts separated by 1 minute and the best jump was recorded. A repeated sprint ability (RSA) test was conducted as described by Mujika *et al.* (2009). Athletes ran 6 x 30 m sprints followed by a 20 meter deceleration zone. Each successive sprint was started every 30 seconds. Post RSA lactate (Lactate Plus, Nova Biomedical, Waltham Mass) measurements were taken three minutes following the last sprint.

Total daily workload was calculated by multiplying a session RPE by duration of training session in minutes (Foster, *et al.*, 2001; Day *et al.,* 2004). Athletes were individually queried at the end of each training session coming off the field or at the end of the day and asked to note the difficulty of the session using the Borg (1998) RPE scale (6–20). Athlete RPE values were averaged and multiplied by the session duration. Morning and afternoon workload values were summed to produce a daily workload value. This rating has been shown to be an effective indicator of the demands of the training session (Impellizzeri *et al.*, 2004). Data for workload appears as Arbitrary Units (AU).

### Test protocols

Tests were conducted 2 days prior to the beginning of preseason training when the athletes were rested for at least 24 hours. This test is referred to as pre-preseason. The post-preseason test occurred 15 days later, 2 days prior to the first game. All tests were performed on a synthetic soccer field at approximately the same time in the morning on both days. Environmental conditions were similar on the two testing days. Players were instructed not to eat or drink within 2 hours of the testing.

### Statistical analysis

Descriptive statistics are presented as mean ± SD unless otherwise indicated. Student's t-test were used to determine differences. Significance was initially set at

$p < 0.05$. Excel 2010 (Microsoft Corporation, Redmond, USA) was used for data preparation and statistical analysis.

## 3. RESULTS

The athletes lost, on average, 0.5kg (0.65%) body weight from pre-preseason to post-preseason but the result was not significant ($p = 0.07$) (Table 1). Table 1 shows test results from RSA testing. We found there was no change in best sprint time between the pre-preseason and post-preseason tests ($p = 0.37$). Additionally, there was no change noted in mean sprint time between the pre-preseason and post-preseason ($p = 0.48$). The participants showed a slightly higher percentage decline over the course of six sprints in the post-preseason test, a 0.08% decline in total, however, these results were not significant ($p = 0.43$). A small, 0.2mM (1.57%), but insignificant, decline in lactate levels was observed following the RSA tests in the post-preseason versus the pre-preseason ($p = 0.40$).

**Table 1** Repeat sprint ability and lactate.

| Test | Pre-Preseason | Post-Preseason |
|---|---|---|
| Weight (kg) | 77.2 ± 7.3 | 76.7 ± 7.1 |
| Best Sprint Time (sec) | 4.36 ± 0.13 | 4.36 ± 0.14 |
| Mean Sprint Time (sec) | 4.46 ± 0.14 | 4.46 ± 0.15 |
| % Decline in RSA | 4.07 ± 1.90 | 4.15 ± 2.19 |
| Lactate (mM) | 12.9 ± 2.9 | 12.7 ± 2.1 |
| Countermovement Jump (cm) | 63.5 ± 6.3 | 61.4 ± 7.9 |
| Standing Long Jump (cm) | 245.5 ± 15.3 | 248.4 ± 15.1 |

Results presented as mean ± SD. n = 16.

Lower extremity power production variables are listed in Table 1. Although we observed a 2.04 cm (3.42%) reduction in countermovement jump performance, this result was not significant ($p = 0.18$). Post-preseason standing long jump performance improved by 2.9 cm (1.20 %) versus the pre-preseason, but this result was not significant ($p = 0.20$).

Daily workload calculations are shown in Figure 1. Morning and afternoon session data were calculated independently and added to produce a total daily workload. While not reported, morning sessions were typically 90 minutes in length and afternoon sessions lasted between 60–75 minutes. With few exceptions the RPE values for the morning sessions were typically higher than those reported for the afternoon sessions. Training blocks typically lasted 3 or 4 days without a significant break or recovery day. Testing began two days prior to the start of preseason. The official preseason began on Day 3 and concluded on day 16 as noted in Figure 1. Testing was completed on day 17, two days prior to the first game. Planned days off were observed on days 6, 11 and 15 to prevent cumulative fatigue.

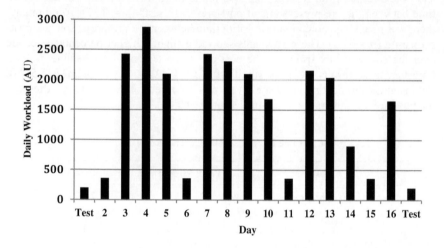

**Figure 1** Ratings of daily workload. Workload calculated by multiplying session RPE by the duration of the session in minutes. Days 1 and 17 were test days. Day 2 consisted of team meetings and equipment distribution. Preseason conditioning started on day 3 and concluded on day 16. Days 6, 11 and 15 were planned rest days.

## 4. DISCUSSION AND CONCLUSION

Power decrement in professional and youth soccer players persists following an intensive soccer game (Andersson *et al.*, 2008; Hoffman *et al.,* 2003) and is present during intensive preseason training without sufficient recovery. Since the collegiate soccer preseason lasts for only a brief period of two weeks, coaches try to maximize player development and enhance fitness by excessive loading. Preseason training for male collegiate soccer athletes in the United States typically consists of two practices per day for five to seven consecutive training days without a break. Our goal was to track how thoughtfully integrated recovery days would reduce or eliminate any potential power declines and cumulative fatigue that can result from repetitive hard training during preseason soccer training.

Our data show that lower extremity power and RSA neither improved nor declined during the preseason training period. This result may be surprising on the surface considering the expectation that preseason training should enhance performance leading up to the competitive season. No increase in performance may be explained by the fact that the collegiate preseason training period is too short and the physical load is quite high because of multiple and successive workout days. This typically results in an overreached training state leading to short-term performance decline (Coutts *et al.*, 2007). In addition, because the official preseason is short, athletes are expected to train on their own for up to four weeks leading up to the official preseason. Therefore, many of the athletes enter the official preseason training period in relatively good physical condition. This notion is supported as the values we report here are similar to those published from studies using well trained semi-professional youth in Europe (Tessitore *et al.*, 2007; Mujika *et al.*, 2009).

While we did not conduct a mid-preseason test, our athletes showed deep fatigue during the middle of the preseason period and likely would have showed performance decrements. Our results showing no difference in anaerobic power can only be considered in light of the preseason schedule. The 16-day schedule followed a general trend of three days of high total workload followed by a recovery day with little to no physical activity. Training began on day three and recovery days were introduced on days 6, 11 and 15. It is highly likely that two recovery days during the second week of preseason played a significant factor in restoring RSA and lower extremity power production, thus eliminating any short-term overreaching.

Using session RPE has been shown to be an effective way to monitor internal training loads (Impellizzeri *et al.*, 2004). This can be an easy and practical way for coaches to visualize and monitor training load during intense periods such as preseason.

Although aerobic testing may have proved valuable, we did not conduct any aerobic tests during, before, or after the preseason training period. Our primary reason was that the length and demands of most aerobic tests, such as the Yo-Yo intermittent tests, can add a significant physical and psychological load to the athletes already undergoing intensive physical training. We did not want to add to that load just prior to their first game.

In conclusion, short preseason training camps can exert a training load that, if unaccompanied by recovery days, could reduce lower extremity strength and power output. In our tracking study, we demonstrate that thoughtful incorporation of recovery days during a period of intensive training, particularly in the week directly leading up to the first competition, can help eliminate any performance decline from overreaching.

## Acknowledgments

The authors would like to thank the players, coaching and administrative staff of the University of Portland Men's Soccer Team for their participation.

## References

Andersson H. *et al.*, 2008, Neuromuscular fatigue and recovery in elite female soccer: Effects of active recovery. *Med Sci Sports Exerc*, **40**, 372–380.

Borg, G., 1998, *Borg's Perceived Exertion and Pain Scales*, Champaign, IL: Human Kinetics.

Coutts, A. *et al.*, 2007, Changes in selected biochemical, muscular strength, power, and endurance measures during deliberate overreaching and tapering in Rugby League players. *Int J Sports Med*, **28**, 116–124.

Day, M.L. *et al.*, 2004, Monitoring exercise intensity during resistance training using the session RPE scale. *J Strength Cond Res*, **18**, 353–358.

Foster, C. *et al.*, 2001, A new approach to monitoring exercise training. *J Strength Cond Res*, **18**, 109–115.

Hoffman, J.R. *et al.*, 2003, The effect of an intercollegiate soccer game on maximal power performance. *Can J Appl Physiol*, **28**, 807–817.

Impellizzeri, F.M. *et al.*, 2004, Use of RPE-based training load in soccer. *Med Sci Sports Exerc*, **36**, 1042–1047.

Mujika, I. *et al.*, 2009, Age-related differences in repeated-sprint ability in highly trained youth football players. *J Sports Sci*, **27**, 1581–1590.

Tessitore, A. *et al.*, 2007, Effects of different recovery interventions on anaerobic performances following preseason soccer training. *J Strength Cond Res*, **21**, 745–750.

Woods, C. R. *et al.*, 2002, The Football Association medical research programme. An audit of injuries in professional football: Analysis of preseason injuries. *Brit J Sports Med*, **36**, 436–441.

# CHAPTER NINETEEN

# Relationships between isokinetic knee strength, sprint and jump performance in young elite soccer players

T. Malý, F. Zahálka, L. Malá, P. Hráský, M. Buzek and T. Gryc

Faculty of P.E. and Sport, Charles University, Prague, Czech Republic

## 1. INTRODUCTION

Muscular strength is one of the most important components of physical performance in soccer, in terms of both high-level performance and injury occurrence. As a factor contributing to success, the quadriceps muscle plays a role in sprinting, jumping and ball-kicking; and the hamstrings contribute to knee flexion, which is a major factor in stride power (Lehance *et al.,* 2009). In soccer, the players are forced to switch between high demanding skills which require strength, power, coordination and agility, with these qualities being symmetrically distributed to the lower extremities for maximal body balance and skill efficiency (Fousekis *et al.,* 2010). Measurements of isokinetic muscle strength provides an objective approach to diagnostics and simpler quantification of muscle strength and its parameters in soccer players. Nevertheless, there are many gaps in this area dealing with its manifestation in young players (Weir, 2000).

The ability to perform high-speed running actions during a game is an important prerequisite for successful participation in soccer (Reilly *et al.,* 2000). According to Stølen *et al.* (2005) during a game, a sprint bout occurs approximately every 90s, each lasting an average of 2–4s. Sprinting constitutes 1–11% of the total distance covered during a game (Mohr *et al.,* 2003). The activity profile of an elite Italian soccer team revealed that 75.8% of high intensity sprinting ($>19$km.h$^{-1}$) is within the distance of 9m (Vigne *et al.,* 2010). Therefore, it is essential to investigate the relationships between the determining prerequisites for optimal player's performance followed by its transfer to sports training. Botek *et al.* (2010) state, that the traditional model of soccer training during the preparation phase (5 weeks, 35 training units, 13 primarily focused on development of strength and 11 on aerobic endurance development) does not lead to the desired changes in conditioning and somatic parameters in U18 soccer players. The aim of the study was to examine the relationships between knee extensors and flexors strength, linear sprint performance and jump performance in elite youth soccer players.

## 2. METHODS

### 2.1. Study sample

The monitoring was carried out on twenty-three Czech youth male soccer players, category U16 (age = 15.6±0.4 years, height = 177.7±6.9 cm, weight = 67.9±8.7 kg) at the national team training camp.

### 2.2. Assessment of strength and speed parameters

Maximum peak muscle torque of knee extensors ($PT_E$) and flexors ($PT_F$) on both legs (PL – preferred leg, NL – non-preferred leg) during concentric contraction in angular velocities (60, 120, 180, 240 and 300°·s⁻¹) were assessed by Cybex dynamometer (Cybex NORM®, Humac, CA, USA). Players completed a short warm-up of 4 min of jogging and dynamic half squats (2 sets/15 repetitions). The athlete's trunk and legs were fixed by means of fixing straps. The player held the side handles of the device. The testing protocol consisted of 5 maximum attempts at knee extension followed by knee flexion from the lowest to the highest velocity. The procedure from the lowest to the highest velocity has been standardized by Wilhite *et al.* (1992). Visual feedback and verbal stimulation were given during the testing. Acceleration sprint (5m, 10m) and maximal sprint (flying 20m) were assessed by photo cells (Brower Timing System). Vertical jumps (counter movement jump with free arms – $CMJ_{FA}$, counter movement jump – CMJ and squat jump – SJ) were assessed by force platform (Kistler Instrumente, Winterhur, Switzerland). Laboratory tests and field testing were carried out in the morning 24 hours apart.

### 2.3. Statistical analysis

Pearson correlation coefficients were used to determine the interrelationships between variables. A significant difference between PL and NL was at different tested velocities assessed by MANOVA. A level of p<0.05 was used for establishing statistical significance. Results of PT are presented in relative values as a ratio of PT and player's body weight.

## 3. RESULTS

Results of $PT_E$ and $PT_F$ are listed in Table 1 $PT_E$ and $PT_F$ were slightly higher in the preferred leg at each of the tested velocities. However, we have not found significant differences between the PL and NL at any of the monitored velocities (60°·s⁻¹: $F_{1,92}$ = 0.48; 120°·s⁻¹: $F_{1,92}$ = 0.09; 180°·s⁻¹: $F_{1,92}$ = 0.17; 240°·s⁻¹: $F_{1,92}$ = 0.19 and 300°·s⁻¹: $F_{1,92}$ = 0.19; p>0.05). Acceleration speed in sprint at 5m was 1.11±0.07s and in sprint at 10m it was 1.87±0.10s. In the test of the maximum running speed (flying 20m), the players achieved times of 2.45±0.12s. The assessment of power strength by means of jumps showed the following results: $CMJ_{FA}$ = 40.19±2.48cm; CMJ = 35.33±2.74cm and SJ = 33.22±3.30cm. PT at the lowest velocity did not correlate with any of the tests for the PL (Table 2) nor for the NL (Table 3). CMJ significantly correlated only with PL's flexors strength at the highest velocity (p<0.01). None of the examined isokinetic strength parameters has proved a significant correlation with the SJ test.

**Table 1** Peak muscle torque of knee extensors ($PT_E$) and knee flexors ($PT_F$) in relative values ($N \cdot m \cdot kg^{-1}$) in the PL and NL at different angular velocities ($° \cdot s^{-1}$).

|  | 60 ($° \cdot s^{-1}$) | 120 ($° \cdot s^{-1}$) | 180 ($° \cdot s^{-1}$) | 240 ($° \cdot s^{-1}$) | 300 ($° \cdot s^{-1}$) |
|---|---|---|---|---|---|
| **Preferred leg** | | | | | |
| $PT_E$ | 3.15±0.33 | 2.64±0.26 | 2.27±0.22 | 1.97±0.20 | 1.74±0.18 |
| $PT_F$ | 1.87±0.25 | 1.65±0.21 | 1.45±0.19 | 1.28±0.18 | 1.12±0.18 |
| **Non-preferred leg** | | | | | |
| $PT_E$ | 3.04±0.29 | 2.60±0.25 | 2.23±0.22 | 1.95±0.19 | 1.72±0.19 |
| $PT_F$ | 1.78±0.22 | 1.62±0.17 | 1.42±0.14 | 1.22±0.15 | 1.07±0.16 |

**Table 2** Correlations coefficient between strength, speed measures and power in PL.

|  | 5 m | 10 m | 20 m | $CMJ_{FA}$ | CMJ | SJ |
|---|---|---|---|---|---|---|
| $PT_{E60}$ | -0.405 | -0.214 | -0.170 | 0.163 | 0.045 | 0.112 |
| $PT_{E120}$ | -0.562** | -0.398 | -0.157 | 0.373 | 0.209 | 0.158 |
| $PT_{E180}$ | -0.519* | -0.476* | -0.185 | 0.449* | 0.270 | 0.218 |
| $PT_{E240}$ | -0.487* | -0.465* | -0.155 | 0.431* | 0.352 | 0.406 |
| $PT_{E300}$ | -0.647** | -0.558** | -0.250 | 0.501* | 0.347 | 0.377 |
| $PT_{F60}$ | -0.335 | -0.345 | -0.406 | 0.194 | 0.193 | 0.269 |
| $PT_{F120}$ | -0.543** | -0.556** | -0.529** | 0.537** | 0.402 | 0.386 |
| $PT_{F180}$ | -0.613** | -0.711** | -0.552** | 0.668** | 0.376 | 0.265 |
| $PT_{F240}$ | -0.543** | -0.609** | -0.393 | 0.600** | 0.269 | 0.126 |
| $PT_{F300}$ | -0.686** | -0.740** | -0.612** | 0.597** | 0.591** | 0.365 |

Legend: * p<0.05; ** p<0.01

**Table 3** Correlations coefficient between strength, speed measures and power in NL.

|  | 5 m | 10 m | 20 m | $CMJ_{FA}$ | CMJ | SJ |
|---|---|---|---|---|---|---|
| $PT_{E60}$ | -0.274 | -0.312 | -0.124 | 0.045 | 0.046 | 0.148 |
| $PT_{E120}$ | -0.538** | -0.503* | -0.190 | 0.257 | 0.331 | 0.292 |
| $PT_{E180}$ | -0.508* | -0.542** | -0.245 | 0.233 | 0.253 | 0.274 |
| $PT_{E240}$ | -0.500* | -0.552** | -0.337 | 0.367 | 0.332 | 0.374 |
| $PT_{E300}$ | -0.500* | -0.483* | -0.336 | 0.367 | 0.332 | 0.374 |
| $PT_{F60}$ | -0.201 | -0.220 | -0.298 | -0.165 | 0.046 | 0.181 |
| $PT_{F120}$ | -0.457* | -0.438* | -0.387 | 0.197 | 0.317 | 0.346 |
| $PT_{F180}$ | -0.368 | -0.287 | -0.434* | 0.306 | 0.258 | 0.368 |
| $PT_{F240}$ | -0.459* | -0.478* | -0.521* | 0.616** | 0.353 | 0.245 |
| $PT_{F300}$ | -0.537** | -0.435* | -0.487* | 0.459* | 0.325 | 0.170 |

Legend: * p<0.05; ** p<0.01

## 4. DISCUSSION

The results of the study did not reveal any significant differences in $PT_E$, or $PT_F$ between the preferred and non-preferred leg. No statistic significance between both legs has been found. This finding is consistent with the results of other studies (Fousekis *et al.*, 2010; Kellis *et al.*, 2001; Rahnama *et al.*, 2003). However, some studies indicate examples when soccer players reached higher values in the NL at least at one of the velocities (Lehance *et al.*, 2009; Mota *et al.*, 2010). $PT_E$ in both legs was higher in our players when compared to elite junior soccer players of the 1st Belgian league, U17 category (Lehance *et al.*, 2009). Values of $PT_F$ in our players were higher in comparison to the above stated study (PL: $PT_{F60}$ 4.1%; $PT_{F240}$ 6.6%; NL: $PT_{F60}$ 7.3%; $PT_{F240}$ 9.0%). Kellis *et al.* (2001) indicate values of $2.92 \pm 0.29$ $N \cdot m \cdot kg^{-1}$ at $60° \cdot s^{-1}$ angular velocity in young Greek players which is 7.3% lower when compared to our study. The level of muscle strength declined with increasing velocity in both legs. It is in line with results of other studies (Kellis *et al.*, 2001).

With increasing angular velocity, $PT_E$ decreased by 44.76% in PL and by 43.42% in the NL. In flexors, it was 40.32% in the PL and 39.88% in the NL. Wong and Wong (2009) indicate $PT_E$ decline in the preferred leg by 44.76% and $PT_F$ by 42% in young U17 Chinese national players. We found higher dependence between PT and acceleration speed (5m and 10m sprint) at higher angular velocities (240, $300° \cdot s^{-1}$). On the contrary, PT at the lowest velocity has not proved any significant relationship with any of the measured parameters (p>0.05). This fact could be explained as physical activity in sprints and jumps is performed in higher velocities with demands on high speed of contractions of particular muscle groups. Generally, the strength which the muscle is able to exert, decreases with increasing velocity of the movement in the concentric contraction. Maximum time available for the contact between actin and myosin filaments reduces with increasing velocity of concentric activity (Huxley model), thus duration of the contact phase reduces in the overall cycle. Cross-bridges have to be re-released shortly after their connection without sufficient time to produce power, so the share of combined bridges in the muscle declines and the produced strength is lower (Wirth and Schmidtbleicher, 2007).

Requena *et al.* (2009) indicate non-significant correlation between $PT_E$ at 60 and $180° \cdot s^{-1}$ and performance in 15m sprint in adult players. PT achieved at the lowest velocity ($60° \cdot s^{-1}$) did not correlate with the jump height in SJ and CMJ tests in the study, while we found a significant correlation (p<0.05) at higher velocity$180° \cdot s^{-1}$. Surprisingly, Lehance *et al.* (2009) mention higher dependence between 10m sprint and extensors strength achieved at $60° \cdot s^{-1}$ velocity (p<0.001) than at $240° \cdot s^{-1}$ (p<0.05). We found almost the same significant dependence in flexors at both velocities. Our results are also contrary to the study by Cometti *et al.* (2001) who did not find correlations between $PT_E$ values ($120–300° \cdot s^{-1}$) and 10- and 30 m sprint times in 95 French soccer players. Wong and Wong (2009) mentioned an average sprint time at 5m: $1.07\pm0.05$s, 10m: $1.81\pm0.05$s (on an athletics track) and jump height in CMJ: $39.33\pm4.82$cm in elite Chinese youth team players (U17 national players). Our players achieved worse results in comparison to that study at 5m sprint by 3.6%, 10m sprint by 3.3% and CMJ test by 10.2%.

Results of our study showed the highest correlations between PT at higher velocities (240, $300°·s^{-1}$) and jump height in the $CMJ_{FA}$ test. In the CMJ test, only $PT_F$ of the PL correlated significantly. Jump height in the SJ test did not correlate with any of the strength indicators at various velocities. It is in contrast to the study by Lehance *et al.* (2009), who mention dependence between SJ and $PT_E$ at $60°·s^{-1}$ velocity ($p<0.001$) and $PT_F$ ($p<0.001$). At higher velocity, $240°·s^{-1}$, $PT_E$ did not correlate with jump height, while $PT_F$ showed significant correlation ($p<0.05$).

Some results of our study are in accordance with results of other studies; however, some of them are in contrast. One of the possible reason could be the label 'elite soccer players' for different types of players' performance level (national level, 1st division players, professional players of the third league, participants of soccer academy or 'centre of talented players'). Another possible cause of divergent results could be differences in methods used for obtaining research data (warm-up procedures, testing on the isokinetic dynamometer with arms crossed on the chest or holding the handles, the surface on which acceleration and maximal speed are measured, equipment and calculation methods for determining jump height etc.).

The results of our study confirm a common basis for the performance level in the observed tests, apart from the SJ test, which starts with isometric contraction. Therefore, it is necessary to stimulate strength at high movement velocities with non-maximal resistance (plyometric exercises, the use of external supplementary resistance at specific movement, expanders, etc.).

## 5. CONCLUSION

Our players, despite higher production of muscle strength, produced worse results in motor tests than in other studies. Therefore, it is vital to address the issue of specificity in test selection and the transformation of muscle prerequisites into motor performance (connection of muscle strength production and neuromuscular coordination for motor performance of a player). We confirmed a common neuromuscular basis for muscle strength production at high velocities in $PT_E$ and $PT_F$, acceleration and maximal speed and explosive power of lower extremities ($CMJ_{FA}$). Significant correlation was reported between acceleration, maximum speed and PT at high velocities, which suggest that these indicators can be considered as a general measurement of quality in elite young soccer players.

### Acknowledgements

This project was supported by GACR P407/11/P784 and MSM 0021620864.

## References

Botek, Z. *et al.*, 2010, Conditioning and body constitution of soccer players in category U19 before and after completing a preparatory period. *Acta Universitatis Palackianae Olomucensis Gymnica*, **40**, 47–54.

Cometti, G. *et al.*, 2001, Isokinetic strength and anaerobic power of elite, subelite and amateur French soccer players. *Int J Sport Med*, **22**, 45–51.

Fousekis, K. *et al.*, 2010, Multivariate isokinetic strength asymmetries of the knee and ankle in professional soccer players. *J Sports Med Phys Fit*, **50**, 465–473.

Kellis, S. *et al.*, 2001, Bilateral isokinetic concentric and eccentric strength profiles of the knee extensor and flexors in young soccer players. *Isokin Exerc Sci*, **9**, 31–39.

Lehance, C. *et al.*, 2009, Muscular strength, functional performances and injury risk in professional and junior elite soccer players. *Scand J Med Sci Sports*, **19**, 243–251.

Mohr, M. *et al.*, 2003, Match performance of high-standard soccer players with special reference to development of fatigue. *J Sports Sci*, **21**, 519–528.

Mota, S. *et al.*, 2010, Variation of isokinetic strength and bone mineral density in youth Portuguese soccer players with age. *Open Sports Sci J*, **3**, 49–51.

Rahnama, N. *et al.*, 2003, Muscle fatigue induced by exercise simulating the work rate of competitive soccer. *J Sports Sci*, **21**, 933–942.

Reilly, T. *et al.*, 2000, Anthropometric and physiological predispositions for elite soccer. *J Sports Sci*, **18**, 669–683.

Requena, B. *et al.*, 2009, Functional performance, maximal strength, and dynamic characteristic in isometric and dynamic actions of lower extremities in soccer players. *J Strength Cond Res*, **23**, 1391–1401.

Stølen, T. *et al.*, 2005, Physiology of soccer: An update. *Sports Med*, **35**, 501–536.

Vigne, G. *et al.*, 2010, Activity profile in elite Italian soccer team. *Int J Sports Med*, **31**, 304–310.

Weir, J.P., 2000, Youth and isokinetic testing. In *Isokinetics in Human Performance*, Champaign: Human Kinetics, pp. 299–323.

Wilhite, M.R. *et al.*, 1992, Reliability of concentric and eccentric measurements of quadriceps performance using the KIN-COM dynamometer: The effect of testing order for three different speeds. *J Orth Sports Phys Ther*, **15**, 175–182.

Wirth, K. and Schmidtbleicher, D., 2007, Periodisierung im Schnellkrafttraining. *Leistungssport*, **1**, 35–40.

Wong, D.P. and Wong, S.H.S., 2009, Physiological profile of Asian elite youth soccer players. *J Strength Cond Res*, **23**, 1383–1390.

# CHAPTER TWENTY

# Validity of the Yo-Yo intermittent recovery test level 1 in assessing or estimating $\dot{V}O_{2max}$ among female soccer players

V. Martínez-Lagunas and U. Hartmann

Institute of Movement and Training Science, University of Leipzig, Germany

## 1. INTRODUCTION

The Yo-Yo Intermittent Recovery Test Level 1 (YYIR1) has gained large popularity in soccer to evaluate players' ability to perform repeated intense exercise (Bangsbo *et al.*, 2008; Krustrup *et al.*, 2003; Krustrup *et al.*, 2005). However, to date no study has simultaneously evaluated if maximal oxygen consumption ($\dot{V}O_{2max}$) could also be accurately assessed (via portable spirometry) or estimated (through an indirect formula based on distance covered) during the YYIR1 in a population of female soccer players. Therefore, a comparison of both direct and indirect $\dot{V}O_{2max}$ values attained during the YYIR1 with direct $\dot{V}O_{2max}$ measurements obtained during laboratory testing (gold standard) is still lacking.

The indirect $\dot{V}O_{2max}$ prediction from the YYIR1 has been performed to date using the general estimation formula recommended by Bangsbo *et al.* (2008), which is based on the total distance covered during this test. Unfortunately, the authors did not specify the gender and physical characteristics of the 141 subjects, from whom this prediction formula was derived. It is very likely that the majority, if not all of these subjects, were male players. Thus, it is still unknown if this formula will yield accurate results to predict the $\dot{V}O_{2max}$ of female soccer players. Additionally, it has been shown that gender distinct prediction equations provide a more accurate estimation of $\dot{V}O_{2max}$ when a similar field test (20-m shuttle run test) is used (Stickland *et al.*, 2003). Consequently, the purpose of the present study was to evaluate the validity of the YYIR1 in assessing or estimating $\dot{V}O_{2max}$ among female soccer players in comparison to a maximal laboratory treadmill test (LTT).

## 2. METHODS

Eighteen female soccer players (age, $21.5 \pm 3.4$ years; height, $165.6 \pm 7.5$ cm; body mass $63.3 \pm 7.4$ kg) competing in the $2^{nd}$ German National League participated in this study. They signed a written informed consent after receiving verbal and written explanation of the study procedures and its potential risks.

After test familiarization, the players randomly completed a LTT and a YYIR1 within one week during the second half of their competitive season. Players' $\dot{V}O_{2max}$ was directly measured during both tests using the same portable spirometry system (MetaMax3B, CORTEX Biophysik, Leipzig, Germany). The validity of this system was found to be satisfactory although it slightly overestimated $\dot{V}O_{2max}$ by 3–4%; its reliability was reported to be excellent, showing typical errors of only 2-3% (Vogler *et al.*, 2010). Before each test, proper pressure, volume and gas calibrations were conducted. Players performed both tests under similar environmental conditions, time of day, dietary and exercise state. They were also verbally encouraged to give their maximal effort.

Players' $\dot{V}O_{2max}$ during LTT and YYIR1 was individually determined from considering the attainment of at least two of the following criteria: a $\dot{V}O_{2max}$ plateau despite increasing speed, a respiratory exchange ratio (RER) > 1.15, an attainment of individual maximal heart rate (HR$_{max}$), and/or a peak blood lactate concentration of 8–10 mmol·l$^{-1}$ after maximal testing (McArdle *et al.*, 2001). Spirometry data were exported into 5-s intervals for determination of $\dot{V}O_{2max}$. During both tests, heart rate (HR) was monitored every 5 s with a HR monitor (Polar Team$^2$, Polar Electro Oy, Kempele, Finland). Blood samples were taken from the earlobe at rest, after the warm-up period, and at 1, 3, 5, 7, 10, and 12 min after each test. Blood lactate concentration was determined using the BIOSEN S_line lactate analyzer (EKF-diagnostic, Barleben, Germany).

In addition players' $\dot{V}O_{2max}$ was also indirectly estimated from their distance covered in YYIR1 using the formula recommended by Bangsbo *et al.* (2008) (YYIR1-est1) and from our own developed formula specific for female soccer players (YYIR1-est2). The latter formula was obtained through linear regression analysis from the relationship between players' distance covered in YYIR1 and their measured $\dot{V}O_{2max}$ in LTT in the present study.

$\dot{V}O_{2max}$ (ml·min$^{-1}$·kg$^{-1}$) = YYIR1 distance (m) x 0.0084 + 36.40     (YYIR1-est1)
$\dot{V}O_{2max}$ (ml·min$^{-1}$·kg$^{-1}$) = YYIR1 distance (m) x 0.0088 + 45.73     (YYIR1-est2)

The LTT was performed on a motorized treadmill (Bari-Mill, WOODWAY, Weil am Rhein, Germany) with an inclination of 1%. After a 10 min warm-up period at 8 km·h$^{-1}$, the test began at 12 km·h$^{-1}$. Subsequently, the speed was increased by 1 km·h$^{-1}$ every 30 s until players reached volitional exhaustion. The YYIR1 was performed indoors on a wooden sports floor according to the original tests procedures (Bangsbo, 2005). After completing a standardized warm-up for 10 min, the players performed the YYIR1, which consisted of 2 x 20 m shuttle-runs at progressive increasing speeds with a 10-s active recovery period in between runs (Bangsbo, 2005). The YYIR1 started at a speed of 10 km·h$^{-1}$. The speed was then increased by 2 and 1 km·h$^{-1}$ for the next two speed levels, respectively. Thereafter, the speed was increased by 0.5 km·h$^{-1}$ until players attained volitional exhaustion.

A table with a more detailed description of the YYIR1 protocol can be found in Castagna *et al.* (2006).

Descriptive statistics are presented as mean ± SD (range). Linear regression analysis, Pearson's product-moment correlations, and paired t-tests were conducted for data analysis. Additionally, Bland-Altman 95% limits of agreement were used to examine individual differences between the estimated (YYIR1-est1 and YYIR1-est2) and measured $\dot{V}O_{2max}$ values (Bland and Altman, 1986). Significance was set at $p < 0.05$.

## 3. RESULTS

Table 1 shows relevant test results from YYIR1 and LTT. The total test duration and distance covered during YYIR1 were significantly higher while YYIR1 peak velocity was slightly but significantly lower than during LTT ($p < 0.01$). Players attained similar $HR_{max}$ and peak post-lactate values in both tests with no statistically significant differences detected ($p > 0.05$).

**Table 1** Test results comparison between YYIR1 and LTT.

| Test | Duration (min) | Distance covered (m) | $\dot{V}_{max}$ (km·h⁻¹) | $HR_{max}$ (bpm) | Post-lactate$_{max}$ (mmol·l⁻¹) |
|------|------|------|------|------|------|
| **YYIR1** | 8.50 ± 3.17* (4.23-16.58) | 1051 ± 399* (520-2080) | 15.19 ± 0.67* (14.50-17.00) | 190 ± 7 (179-204) | 10.18 ± 2.53 (4.41-14.92) |
| **LTT** | 2.65 ± 0.37 (2.00-3.66) | 628 ± 106 (450-928) | 16.06 ± 0.80 (15.00-18.00) | 190 ± 6 (182-202) | 10.80 ± 2.10 (7.10-14.56) |

Results presented as mean ± SD. * significant at $p < 0.01$, n = 18. YYIR1: Yo-Yo Intermittent Recovery Test Level 1, LTT: maximal laboratory treadmill test, $\dot{V}_{max}$: peak velocity, $HR_{max}$: maximal heart rate, Post-lactate$_{max}$: peak blood lactate concentration after each test.

Large correlation coefficients (r > 0.50, Cohen, 1988) were found between the measured $\dot{V}O_{2max}$ in YYIR1 and LTT, and between YYIR1-est1 or YYIR1-est2 and the measured $\dot{V}O_{2max}$ in LTT ($p < 0.01$). The $\dot{V}O_{2max}$ mean difference between measured $\dot{V}O_{2max}$ in YYIR1 and LTT, and between estimated $\dot{V}O_{2max}$ from YYIR1-est1 and measured $\dot{V}O_{2max}$ in LTT, was statistically significant ($p < 0.01$). In contrast, the $\dot{V}O_{2max}$ mean difference between YYIR1-est2 and LTT did not differ significantly ($p > 0.05$) (Table 2). In general, the measured and estimated $\dot{V}O_{2max}$ values obtained in YYIR1 were lower than those obtained in LTT. The Bland-Altman 95% limits of agreement revealed large individual differences between the estimated and measured $\dot{V}O_{2max}$ values (Table 2). The individual relationship between distance covered in YYIR1 and the $\dot{V}O_{2max}$ measured in LTT is illustrated in Figure 1. The regression lines and equations of YYIR1-est1 and YYIR1-est2 are also included. Players with a similar $\dot{V}O_{2max}$ showed a large variation in distance covered during the YYIR1.

**Table 2** Measured and estimated $\dot{V}O_{2max}$ from YYIR1 and LTT.

| Test Pair | $\dot{V}O_{2max}$ (ml·min$^{-1}$·kg$^{-1}$) | r | Difference (ml·min$^{-1}$·kg$^{-1}$) | B-A 95% LA (ml·min$^{-1}$·kg$^{-1}$) |
|---|---|---|---|---|
| YYIR1 LTT | 49.87 ± 4.88 (40.98-57.32) 55.02 ± 5.28 (45.88-67.05) | .83* | -5.15 ± 3.00* (-9.36 %) | -10.98 to 0.78 (-19.96 to 1.42 %) |
| YYIR1-est1 LTT | 45.23 ± 3.36 (40.77-53.87) 55.02 ± 5.28 (45.88-67.05) | .67* | -9.79 ± 3.92* (-17.79 %) | -17.48 to -2.09 (-31.78 to -3.81 %) |
| YYIR1-est2 LTT | 54.98 ± 3.52 (50.31-60.16) 55.02 ± 5.28 (45.88-67.05) | .67* | -0.04 ± 3.92 (-0.07 %) | -7.94 to 7.74 (-14.44 to 14.07 %) |

Results presented as mean ± SD. * significant at *p < 0.01*, n = 18. YYIR1: Yo-Yo Intermittent Recovery Test Level 1, LTT: maximal laboratory treadmill test, YYIR1-est1: $\dot{V}O_{2max}$ estimation formula recommended by Bangsbo *et al.* (2008), YYIR1-est2: $\dot{V}O_{2max}$ estimation formula obtained from our own data, $\dot{V}O_{2max}$: maximal oxygen consumption, r: Pearson's correlation coefficient, B-A 95% LA: Bland-Altman 95% limits of agreement.

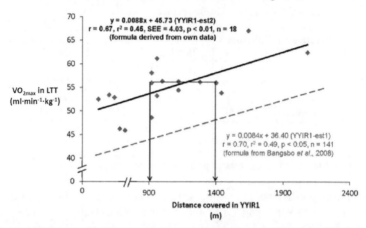

**Figure 1** Individual relationship between distance covered in the Yo-Yo Intermittent Recovery Test Level 1 (YYIR1) and measured $\dot{V}O_{2max}$ during the maximal laboratory treadmill test (LTT). This figure also shows the regression lines of the $\dot{V}O_{2max}$ estimation formulas derived from our own data (YYIR1-est2) and from Bangsbo *et al.*, 2008 (YYIR1-est1). The vertical lines indicate the variation of the distance covered in YYIR1 (920–1400 m) for a given $\dot{V}O_{2max}$ of 56 ml·min$^{-1}$·kg$^{-1}$. SEE: standard error of the estimate, $r^2$: coefficient of determination.

## 4. DISCUSSION AND CONCLUSION

The primary objective of the present study was to evaluate the validity of the YYIR1 in assessing or estimating $\dot{V}O_{2max}$ among female soccer players compared to a LTT. To our knowledge, no other study has previously included direct $\dot{V}O_{2max}$

measurement during the YYIR1. Most studies have mainly evaluated the relationship between YYIR1 performance (distance covered) and $\dot{V}O_{2max}$ assessed during laboratory testing (Bangsbo *et al.*, 2008; Krustrup *et al.*, 2003; Krustrup *et al.*, 2005). Only the latter study examined this relationship among female soccer players but no linear regression equation was reported. The results of the present study showed that the YYIR1 did not provide an accurate measure or prediction of $\dot{V}O_{2max}$ which was supported by significant mean differences (up to −18%) between measured and estimated values in YYIR1 and LTT and large 95% limits of agreement (−32 to 14%) obtained by the Bland-Altman approach to compare two methods of measurement (Bland and Altman, 1986).

Possible reasons that may explain these findings include the intermittent nature and longer duration, the skill and energy cost required for the constant changes of direction and the anaerobic demands of the YYIR1 compared to LTT. The absence of gender-specific formulas for $\dot{V}O_{2max}$ prediction may also play a role in justifying these findings. Field tests with a continuous exercise protocol, such as the 20-m Shuttle Run Test (Leger and Gadoury, 1989) and the Yo-Yo Endurance Test (Bangsbo, 2005) might be better alternatives to predict $\dot{V}O_{2max}$ among female soccer players. However, further research is required in this area.

Despite the lack of precision of the YYIR1 to accurately assess or estimate $\dot{V}O_{2max}$ among female soccer players, this test might have other relevant practical applications in women's soccer. For instance, the fact that players achieved very similar $HR_{max}$ values during the YYIR1 and LTT, suggests that the YYIR1 can be used to determine $HR_{max}$ among female soccer players in a practical and inexpensive way. Additionally, distance covered in YYIR1 has been reported to be a good indicator of physical match performance among female players because it is highly related to the amount of high-intensity running covered during match-play, and it may provide a more sensitive measure to detect differences among competition levels, playing positions, and seasonal changes in performance (Bangsbo *et al.*, 2008; Krustrup *et al.*, 2005). Moreover, $\dot{V}O_{2max}$ is not the only physiological determinant of endurance performance, other factors such as lactate threshold, running economy and morphological components (e.g., muscle capillary density, muscle fiber type, etc.) also play an important role (Coyle, 1999).

In summary, although the direct and indirect $\dot{V}O_{2max}$ values were significantly related, the YYIR1 significantly underestimated $\dot{V}O_{2max}$ among female soccer players compared to LTT (gold standard). Up to 9% or 18% underestimation resulted when player's $\dot{V}O_{2max}$ was directly assessed by portable spirometry in YYIR1 or indirectly estimated from YYIT1-est1 (Bangsbo *et al.*, 2008), respectively. The estimation formula derived from our own data (YYIR1-est2) yielded closer results to the real $\dot{V}O_{2max}$ values obtained in LTT. However, further studies including a larger number of female soccer players should verify these results.

## Acknowledgements

The authors would like to thank the players, coaching and administrative staff of the women's soccer club '1. FC Lokomotive Leipzig' for their participation.

## References

Bangsbo, J., 2005, *The Yo Yo Tests*. Espergaerde: Bangsbosport.com.

Bangsbo, J. *et al.*, 2008, The Yo-Yo intermittent recovery test: A useful tool for evaluation of physical performance in intermittent sports. *Sports Med*, **38**, 37–51.

Bland, J.M. and Altman, D.G., 1986, Statistical methods for assessing agreement between two methods of clinical measurement. *Lancet*, **i**, 307–310.

Castagna, C. *et al.*, 2006, Aerobic fitness and Yo-Yo continuous and intermittent tests performances in soccer players: a correlation study. *J Strength Cond Res*, **20**, 320–352.

Cohen, J., 1988, *Statistical Power Analysis for the Behavioral Sciences*. 2nd ed., New Jersey: Lawrence Erlbaum.

Coyle, E., 1999, Physiological detrminants of endurance performance. *J Sci Med Sport*, **2**, 181–189.

Krustrup, P. *et al.*, 2003, The Yo-Yo intermittent recovery test: physiological response, reliability and validity. *Med Sci Sport Exerc*, **35**, 697–705.

Krustrup, P. *et al.*, 2005, Physical demands during an elite female soccer game: importance of training status. *Med Sci Sport Exerc*, **37**, 1242–1248.

Leger, L.A. and Gadoury, C., 1989, Validity of the 20 m shuttle run test with 1 min stages to predict $\dot{V}O_{2max}$ in adults. *Can J Sports Sci*, **14**, 21–26.

McArdle, W.D. *et al.*, 2001, *Exercise Physiology: Energy, Nutrition, and Human Performance*. Philadelphia: Lippincott Williams and Wilkins.

Stickland, M.K. *et al.*, 2003, Prediction of maximal aerobic power from the 20-m multi-stage shuttle run test. *Can J Appl Physiology*, **28**, 272–282.

Vogler, A.J. *et al.*, 2010, Validity and reliability of the Cortex MetaMax3B portable metabolic system. *J Sports Sci*, **28**, 733–742.

# CHAPTER TWENTY-ONE

# Physiological and anthropometric characteristics of elite women's rugby union players

S. Pogliaghi, G. Da Lozzo, V. Ceradini and G. F. De Roia

Faculty of Human Movement Sciences, University of Verona, Italy

## 1. INTRODUCTION

Rugby union is a collision team sport, classified as an interval aerobic-anaerobic activity involving great strength and power of the upper and lower extremities (Duthie *et al.*, 2003). Since the first World Cup open to woman in 1991, this traditional male sport is increasingly practiced, non-professionally, by female athletes. Game analysis (Duthie *et al.*, 2003; 2005; Deutsch *et al.*, 2007) and functional evaluation (Scott *et al.*, 2003; Duthie *et al.*, 2003) of players of different skill, gender and/or age are classical approaches to the understanding of the physical demands of rugby (Reilly and Gilbourne, 2003). However there appears to be limited scientific papers examining women's rugby at the elite level. A recent paper has been published on women's rugby league (Gabbett, 2007), which is a similar but distinct sport from rugby union. The only specific reference that we are aware of is a fifteen years old congress proceeding (Kirby and Reilly, 1993). Therefore, due to the specificity of rugby codes and to the evolution of rugby union in recent years (Duthie *et al.*, 2003), the data that are currently available on women's rugby union may not reflect the current game.

This descriptive study was aimed to provide normative data on laboratory-based, physiological and anthropometric variables of elite women players from the northern hemisphere. These parameters can be useful to establish the physical requirements of female players, and to identify role differences while informing training decisions. It is also hoped that this study will stimulate further research in the field of women's rugby union.

## 2. METHODS

This sample consisted of 22 female players (11 forwards (FW), 11 backs (BK)) from the Italian National rugby union senior team. During the competitive season the athletes played ~1 match/week with their club and had three 1.5-hour field and two 1-hour weight training sessions each week. Tests were performed in the one testing session in March 2007, after the Six Nations championship. Body mass (digital scale, Seca 877, Seca, Leicester, UK) and stature (vertical stadiometer, Seca, Leicester, UK) were determined to the nearest 0.1 kg and 0.5 cm. Skinfolds thickness was measured, in triplicate, by a single skilled investigator using a pincer type caliper (Holtain T/W skinfold caliper, Holtain limited, UK). For each skinfold (scapular, triceps, iliac, abdominal and thigh), an average value was calculated and body fat percentage was estimated based on the sum of the 5 skin fold thicknesses (SS, in mm) with the following formula (Golding *et al.*, 1982):

$$\% \text{ body fat} = (0.3 * (SS)) - (0.0005 * SS^2) + (0.03 * age) - 0.6$$

and lean body mass (LBM) was calculated as:

$$LBM = \text{body mass (body mass} * \% \text{ body fat)}.$$

Next athletes underwent an incremental test to exhaustion on a magnetically braked cycle ergometer (3-min warm up at 50 watt +20 watt/min until voluntary exhaustion, at 60-70 revolutions per minute). During the test, ventilatory parameters were measured breath by breath (Quark $b^2$ Cosmed, Italy) and $VO_2max$ was calculated as the average of the last 10 seconds of exercise prior to exhaustion if one of the following criteria was met: i) $VO_2$ plateau ($VO_2$ increase < 50% of the expected based on work load increment); ii) respiratory exchange ratio (R) > 1.15; iii) heart rate (HR) upon exhaustion > 90% of age predicted maximal HR (Tanaka *et al.*, 2001).

Thirty minutes after the cycling test, athletes performed a total of 6 single jumps (3 squat jumps, SJ, and 3 counter movement jumps, CMJ), separated by 2-min resting intervals to determine leg power. The height of jumps was assessed based on flight time (t) (Optojump, Microgate, Italy). Descriptive statistics (mean and standard deviation (SD) were calculated for forwards (FW) and backs (BK) as well as the following positional subgroups: *Front row forwards*: props and locks; *Back row forwards*: flankers, number eight and hooker; *Inside backs*: fly-half and centres; *Outside backs*: wings and full back (Deutsch *et al.*, 2007). The scrum half was not included in the above subgroups due to its unique role. Groups were compared using un-paired *t*-test followed by Bonferroni correction and the significant level was set at < 0.05.

## 3. RESULTS

Athletes were 24±4 years old, with an average playing experience of 9 years (SD=6 years). Table 1 indicates that FW were significantly heavier and taller compared to BK and had a larger fat free mass. No difference in body fat percentage was detected between the groups. Front row FW were significantly heavier and taller and had a larger body fat percentage and fat free mass than back row FW. On the contrary, no difference was found within BKs. All the athletes completed the incremental test to exhaustion meeting the criteria for definition of maximal effort. Average $HR_{max}$ was 93±6% of predicted maximal (Tanaka *et al.*,

2001), while R was 1.12±0.02 for all playing group. The FW recorded significantly larger absolute VO$_{2max}$ compared to BK (Table 2). However, this difference disappeared when data were expressed relative to body mass.

With regard to leg power FW performed significantly higher squat jumps compared to BK. However, counter movement jump height was not significantly different between FW and BK and there was no difference in leg power between the FW and BK subgroups.

**Table 1** Antropometric characteristics (mean ± SD) of forwards (FW) and backs (BK) and subgroups.

| group | N | mass (kg) | stature (m) | fat (%) | lean mass (kg) |
|-------|---|-----------|-------------|---------|----------------|
| FW | 11 | 71.2±11.6* | 1.68±0.1* | 24.4±5.5 | 53.3±4.5* |
| BK | 11 | 62.5±5.7 | 1.63±0.1 | 24.3±4.0 | 47.2±3.8 |
| FR FW | 5 | 78.8±13.5§ | 1.71±0.1§ | 27.8±6.4§ | 56.2±4.6§ |
| BR FW | 6 | 65.0±4.5 | 1.64±0.0 | 21.6±2.6 | 50.9±2.9 |
| I BK | 6 | 64.0±5.6 | 1.63±0.1 | 25.8±3.6 | 47.4±3.2 |
| O BK | 4 | 61.0±6.5 | 1.63±0.1 | 22.0±4.1 | 47.5±5.3 |

\* and § indicate a significant difference from BK and within positional subgroups.

**Table 2** Functional data of forwards (FW) and backs (BK) and subgroups (mean±SD).

| group | N | VO$_{2max}$ (l*min$^{-1}$) | VO$_{2max}$ (ml*kg$^{-1}$*min$^{-1}$) | SJ (cm) | CMJ (cm) |
|-------|---|----------------------------|----------------------------------------|---------|----------|
| FW | 11 | 3.0±0.4* | 42.6±5.3 | 26.4±4.3* | 29.2±3.3 |
| BK | 11 | 2.7±0.5 | 43.1±5.3 | 23.8±2.9 | 28.5±3.5 |
| FR FW | 5 | 3.1±0.3 | 40.7±5.9 | 25.4±2.3 | 28.0±1.9 |
| BR FW | 6 | 2.9±0.4 | 44.3±4.7 | 27.3±5.5 | 30.2±4.0 |
| I BK | 6 | 2.8±0.5 | 42.7±6.6 | 23.6±2.7 | 28.7±3.0 |
| O BK | 4 | 2.6±0.3 | 42.4±1.8 | 24.0±3.6 | 28.8±4.6 |

\* indicates a significant difference from BK. No difference was detected within positional subgroups.

## 4. DISCUSSION

This descriptive study provides normative data on laboratory-based physiological and anthropometric variables in elite European women rugby union players, with special reference to positional groups. In accordance with male studies, significant role differences in the majority of the measured parameters were detected between forwards and backs and between FW subgroups and no differences were detected in either anthropometric or physiological parameters within BK positional subgroups. This suggests that specificity in the physical requirements of rugby union in individual playing positions is present in women as well as in males playing at the international level.

The national athletes in this study were of a similar age and playing experience as reported by Kirby and Reilly (1993). Interestingly, while the stature and fat free mass of the forwards and backs were comparable to those in the Kirby and Reilly study, they recorded higher levels of body fat (i.e. 3.5–4% of body fat) compared to their British colleagues. A high percent body fat can provide protection against physical collision and represents a static advantage over opponents in scrums. However, it also increases the physiological demands of playing during both training and matches. It could be speculated that the high body fat may reflect a low training volume in these athletes.

Functional evaluation of aerobic performance was also performed in our study. Compared to different field-based team sports our data are comparable with those of college level lacrosse and soccer athletes (Enemark-Miller *et al.*, 2009), yet lower than those of international level soccer (-15%) (Krustrup *et al.*, 2005) and field hockey (-7%) (Hinrichs *et al.*, 2010) athletes. In these sports, a high $VO_{2max}$ facilitates the repetition of and the recovery from high intensity anaerobic efforts inherent to both training and competition. Furthermore, in rugby league, $VO_{2max}$ has been demonstrated to be positively related to different indexes of players' performance during the actual game and to be associated with lower injury rates (Gabbett, 2007). Yet, $VO_{2max}$ is only one component of the several requirements of the overall fitness profile and rugby union players normally do not include specific sessions to develop $VO_{2max}$ in their training regimen. Therefore, the relatively low $VO_{2max}$ observed in our study could be ascribed to both a low exercise volume and to the fact that training is normally not addressed at improving this functional parameter, despite its potential importance for fatigue resistance and injury prevention.

Rugby performance requires high levels of muscular strength and power for success, with the forwards requiring more strength and the backs requiring more speed (Duthie *et al.*, 2003). The force produced during a vertical jump has been shown to be related to scrum force (Duthie *et al.*, 2003). Direct comparison of studies is difficult due to difference in test protocols and to the rapid evolution of the game, especially over the last decade; yet, our subjects appear to have a lower level of muscular power compared to international level athletes of different team sports (Enemark-Miller *et al.*, 2009).

Collectively these results suggest that, although the women rugby players in this study had adequate playing performance to warrant selection into the national team, they are nonetheless characterized by fitness levels that are lower than those reported in the literature for team sports. Furthermore, FW and BK appear to be less differentiated compared to male rugby players. This may be influenced by the following factors: i) the recent exposure to high level international competition; ii) suboptimal training regimens in terms of training volume and specificity in these non-professional athletes; iii) less competition for selection based on lower participant numbers. Furthermore, due to a less organized team structure and a smaller playing population compared to professional male rugby, the role assignment in Italian women's rugby is quite diverse. It is common for a player to have a different role when competing in international competitions compared to national club competitions. Consequently female players are less likely than male players to conform to the physical requirements of specific roles. It must be noted, however, that our small sample size and the high between-subject variability of our group, may reduce the likelihood to identify significant differences among positional subgroups.

## 5. CONCLUSION

In conclusion, this study provides physiological and anthropometric data for elite women rugby union players. Only by increasing the number of published studies can we gain a better understanding of this specific athletic population. These findings may assist in talent selection, addressing individual athletes to the role for which they are more suited and guide individualized training to match the demands of the game. Finally, we hope to stimulate further research in this rather unexplored field.

### References

Deutsch, M.U. *et al.*, 2007, Time-motion analysis of professional rugby union players during match-play. *J Sports Sci*, **25**, 461–472.

Duthie, G. *et al.*, 2003, Applied physiology and game analysis of rugby union. *Sports Medicine*, **33**, 973–991.

Duthie, G. *et al.*, 2005, Time motion analysis of 2001 and 2002 super 12 rugby. *J Sports Sci*, **23**, 523–530.

Enemark-Miller, E.A. *et al.*, 2009, Physiological profile of women's lacross players. *J Strength Cond Res*, **23**, 39–43.

Gabbett, T.J., 2007, Physiological and anthropometric characteristics of elite women rugby league players. *J Strength Cond Res*, **21**, 875–881.

Golding, L. *et al.*, 1982, *The Y's Way to Physical Fitness*. Rosemont, IL: National Board of the YMCA.

Hinrichs, T. *et al.*, 2010, Total hemoglobin mass, iron status, and endurance capacity in elite field hockey players. *J Strength Cond Res*, **24**. 629–638.

Kirby, W.J. and Reilly, T., 1993, Anthropometric and fitness profiles of elite female rugby union players. In: *Science and Football II*, London: Routledge, pp. 27–30.

Krustrup, P. *et al.*, 2005, Physical demands during an elite female soccer game: importance of training status. *Med Sci Sports Exerc*, **37**, 1242–1248.

Reilly, T. and Gilbourne, D., 2003, Science and football: A review of applied research in the football codes. *J Sports Sci*, **21**, 693–705.

Scott, A.C. *et al.*, 2003, Aerobic exercise physiology in a professional rugby union team. *Int J Cardiol*, **87**, 173–177.

Tanaka, H. *et al.*, 2001, Age-predicted maximal heart rate revised. *J Am Coll Cardiol*, **37**, 153–156.

# Part III

# Match analysis

# CHAPTER TWENTY-TWO

# 'Temporary fatigue' is not apparent in elite youth soccer players

R. Lovell[1,2], S. Barrett[1,3] and G. Abt[1]

[1]Department of Sport, Health and Exercise Science, The University of Hull, UK,
[2]School of Science and Health, University of Western Sydney, Australia,
[3]Perform Better, Warwickshire, UK

## 1. INTRODUCTION

Recent time-motion analyses have identified and described the phenomenon of 'temporary fatigue' in elite-level soccer match-play (Mohr *et al.*, 2003, 2008), whereby the players' work-rate is temporarily decreased after intense period of play. The approach typically adopted to detect this phenomenon involves categorising time-motion data into pre-determined 5-min periods, with 'temporary fatigue' denoted as a marked reduction in the players' high-speed running distance ($\geq$15 km·h$^{-1}$; HSR) in the 5-min period immediately subsequent to the 5-min period in which the most HSR is observed. 'Temporary fatigue' is said to be evident where the HSR in the subsequent 5-min pre-determined period is lower than the average 5-min match period (Mohr *et al.*, 2003, 2008).

However, the use of velocity bands to characterise 'temporary fatigue' is a technique that might be insensitive to some high-intensity activities, which may cause transient fatigue through neuromuscular or metabolic pathways. High-intensity actions such as collisions, accelerations, decelerations, unorthodox running and turns often occur at velocities below 15 km·h$^{-1}$, but these activities are metabolically taxing (Osgnach *et al.*, 2010; Reilly and Bowen, 1984). The advancement of micro-sensor technology now enables practitioners in team sports settings to measure the frequency and magnitude of instantaneous accelerations in the anterior-posterior, medio-lateral, and longitudinal planes. The tri-axial accelerometer is typically used for estimates of physical activity and energy expenditure, therefore powerful movements and accelerations, which are absent from traditional time-motion techniques, can now be quantified during match-play in field-based settings. We postulated that the use of tri-axial accelerometer data might be a more sensitive tool to detect 'temporary fatigue'.

Whilst the 'temporary fatigue' phenomenon has been demonstrated in 'top-class' male (Mohr *et al.*, 2003) and female players (Mohr *et al.*, 2008), it is presently unclear if the same pattern is evident in youth players. There is a growing body of work in the literature researching the match-play demands of elite youth soccer (Buchheit *et al.*, 2010a, 2010b; Harley *et al.*, 2010) and players' physical and physiological capacities (Buchheit *et al.*, 2010b) in an attempt to improve talent identification and training processes. The demands of youth soccer match-play, in particular the distances covered in different locomotor categories have been reported between the ages of 12–18 (Buchheit *et al.*, 2010b; Harley *et al.*, 2010). However, in this population little is known about the changes in work-rate over the course of the match, which may provide information regarding the development of fatigue as a consequence of intense match periods. There is evidence to suggest that the fatiguing patterns may have different characteristics to those observed in the elite adult player, as adolescents are able to resist fatigue during repeated maximal exercise to a better extent that adults (Beneke *et al.*, 2005). Therefore we hypothesised that 'temporary fatigue' as defined in the literature (Mohr *et al.*, 2003, 2008) may not be evident in elite youth players.

Therefore the aim of this study was to examine whether 'temporary fatigue' exists in elite youth players. We also aimed to compare methods for identifying this transient fatigue development, using both arbitrary velocity thresholds from GPS data, and a tri-axial accelerometer that resides inside the GPS unit.

## 2. METHODS

Twenty elite male youth soccer players (Age: $17 \pm 1$ yrs; VO$_2$max: $61 \pm 6$ ml·kg$^{-1}$·min$^{-1}$) participated in this study, which attained a priori ethical approval and informed consent. Each player was post-adolescent with a mean of 3.2 ($\pm$ 0.4) years after peak height velocity. Players trained on a 'full-time' professional basis for 13.5 hrs per week, which included specific technical and conditioning sessions, and one competitive fixture each week.

Players were harnessed with a 5 Hz GPS (MinimaxX, Catapult, Australia) unit during 21 competitive league fixtures ($5 \pm 3$ matches per player) during the 2008/09 and 2009/10 seasons. Injury time was excluded in this study, as were any incidences where the player did not complete the full game or changed tactical position during match-play, resulting in 111 match observations. Locomotor activities in arbitrary velocity bands, and tri-axial accelerometer data (Player Load$^{TM}$–PL) were derived from the GPS system and classified into pre-defined 5-min periods. High speed running was reported as the distance covered at $\geq 15$ km·h$^{-1}$. Peak HSR distance represented the greatest distance covered in a 5-min period specific to each match instance. The HSR performed in the subsequent 5-min interval, and the mean of the remaining 5-min periods were compared as in previous research. However, we also ranked each 5-min epoch (1-18; where 1 = peak HSR period) to facilitate contextualisation of the 'temporary fatigue' phenomena in relation to other match-periods characterised by a reduced work-rate.

The peak PL was compared to both the subsequent and mean values as described above. The PL in each 5-min epoch was also ranked (1-18; where 1 = peak PL period). The PL was reported as a vector magnitude, which sums the frequency and magnitude of accelerations in all axial planes and is the most common algorithm reported in studies using this technology. Whilst accelerometer measures in sport and exercise settings are in their infancy, the between-unit variability is low during team-sport activity (~2 % CV; Boyd *et al.*, 2011) and they may provide a more rigorous assessment of the players' external load than the traditional time-motion metrics. Paired-samples T-tests were used for pairwise comparisons. Significance was accepted at p < 0.05. Data are presented as mean ± SD.

## 3. RESULTS

### High-speed running

12.2% of match observations were ineligible for this temporary fatigue analysis as the peak HSR was observed in the final 5 min periods of the first (4.7%) and second halves (7.5%). 60% of peak HSR incidences occurred during the first half, with 43% observed within the first 25 min period of match-play (see Figure 1). The mean rank of the subsequent 5-min period was 9.8 ± 4.4. The HSR distance covered in the peak 5-min periods was 178 ± 42 m (see Figure 2), with a 47 ± 23% decrease observed in the subsequent interval (94 ± 46 m). However, there was no significant difference between the HSR in the subsequent and mean (88 ± 25 m) 5-min epochs. The corresponding PL at the HSR peak (83.5 ± 20.2 au) was greater than the subsequent (70.9 ± 19.6 au) and mean (69.0 ± 15.0 au) periods, with no difference subsequent and mean values.

### Player Load[TM]

12.4% of peak PL cases were ineligible for the analysis as the peak was observed in the final 5 min-periods of the first (4.8%) and second halves (7.6%). The 5-min periods were ranked for PL, and the mean rank of the subsequent 5-min period was 8.5 ± 4.5. The peak PL was 92.0 ± 18.7 au, with a 22 ± 12% decrease observed in the subsequent interval (71.7 ± 17.4 au), and a significant difference between the HSR in the subsequent and mean (67.8 ± 13.6 au) 5-min epochs (See Figure 2).

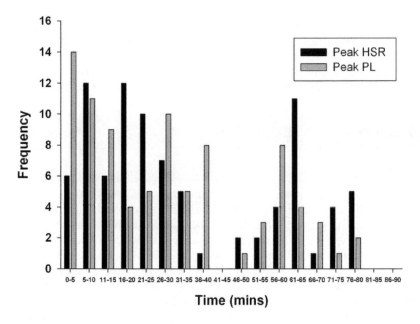

**Figure 1** Distribution of peak HSR and PL according to the pre-determined match period in which they occurred.  HSR = High speed running ($\geq$ 15 km·h⁻¹); PL = Player load™.

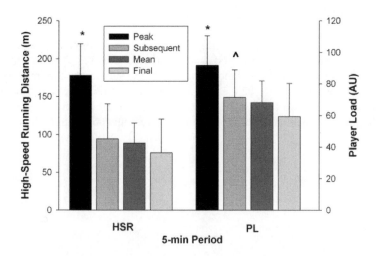

**Figure 2** Peak high-speed running and peak player load in a 5-min period, subsequent 5-min, final 5-min (85–90 min) and mean values of all other 5-min periods. * Denotes peak greater than all other 5-min periods (P<0.001). ^ Denotes greater than mean and subsequent 5-min periods (P<0.01). HSR = High speed running ($\geq$ 15 km·h⁻¹); PL = Player load™.

## 4. DISCUSSION

The aim of the current study was to determine if 'temporary fatigue' is evident in elite youth players, using the approach employed previously (Mohr *et al.*, 2003, 2008) and a novel technique, which used tri-axial accelerometer data to incorporate high intensity actions that occur below 15 km·h⁻¹. We hypothesised that: 1) PL would be a more sensitive measure of transient fatigue and; 2) using the pre-determined 5-min match periods, 'temporary fatigue' would not be observed in our sample population.

The data collected in this study suggests that the latter hypothesis can be accepted, since the subsequent 5-min periods to both the peak HSR and PL epochs were not lower than the 5-min mean. The magnitude of the peak HSR distance was somewhat lower than that observed in 'top-class' male players (Mohr *et al.*, 2003), but not dissimilar to 'moderate-standard' male (Mohr *et al.*, 2003) and 'top-class' female adult players (Mohr *et al.*, 2008). The subsequent decrement in HSR during the following pre-determined 5-min period was ~47%, which is of a similar magnitude to that reported for elite male players (Mohr *et al.*, 2003). However, the HSR and PL values observed in the subsequent 5-min period were not lower than the match mean. Furthermore, the subsequent 5-min period was ranked moderately for both HSR and PL. This data suggests that temporary fatigue is not observed in elite youth players when quantified using either HSR or PL with pre-determined 5-min periods.

The absence of 'temporary fatigue' with HSR data in the current investigation is in contrast to other studies in elite senior players (Mohr *et al.*, 2003, 2008). However, the current study is not the first observation of its kind, as the subsequent period was not significantly different to the match mean in lower ranked male (Mohr *et al.*, 2003) and female (Mohr *et al.*, 2008) senior players. The reason for this discrepancy has not been identified in the literature. However, the current data may be indicative of a pacing strategy adopted by the elite youth players, to attenuate fatiguing symptoms both immediately after an intense match period, and in the latter stages of match-play. Since elite players have greater *a priori* experience of the demands of soccer match-play, they may employ a different pacing approach (Edwards and Noakes, 2009), which may partly explain the lack of transient fatigue denoted in both the elite youth players, and in lower ranked male (Mohr *et al.*, 2003) and female (Mohr *et al.*, 2008) players.

An alternative explanation for the current results is that players of this age may be able to resist fatigue during repeated bouts of supra-maximal intensity exercise better than their adult counterparts (Beneke *et al.*, 2005). Glenmark *et al.* (1994) observed a greater proportion of oxidative muscle fibres and fewer type IIa and b fibres in 16 year-old males versus adults. Hence during an intense bout of match-play, younger players may rely more on oxidative metabolism, reducing the accumulation of glycolytic bi-products and enabling them to resist 'temporary fatigue'.

The common approach used here to determine 'temporary fatigue' may be limited by the use the use of pre-determined 5-min periods and its criteria. Pre-determined 5-min periods may not be sensitive enough to detect transient fatigue, since an intense bout may cross the boundaries of adjacent match periods. The 5-min epochs may also be too long to detect the intricacies of repeated or prolonged high intensity bouts. Therefore the challenge for researchers is to develop alternative techniques (i.e. Buchheit *et al.*, 2010a) to monitor intense passages of play, which may include rolling time-periods and/or shorter sampling periods (i.e. < 60-s). Moreover, it is unclear whether a decrease in HSR or PL after the most intense period is practically relevant or represents an analytical artefact.

We also hypothesised that player load would be more sensitive to denote subsequent fatigue since it incorporates utility movements and accelerations with a high energy cost. However, this parameter was less sensitive to 'temporary fatigue' than HSR, with only a ~22% decline denoted in the following period. As the accelerometer adopted in this study measured instantaneous accelerations in all three planes, our data may be explained by the large contribution of the vertical axis to this vector magnitude, which is active during any type of gait. Therefore, PL may also accumulate during periods of low activity such as walking and jogging, which are the most prevalent activities during soccer match-play (Mohr *et al.*, 2003). Therefore, future work might attempt to determine the contribution of locomotor activities to the PL algorithm. While the use of tri-axial accelerometer algorithms is becoming more prevalent in sports performance settings, there is a dearth of empirical data available to assess the validity of this technique and further work is warranted.

In summary, elite youth players did not demonstrate the phenomenon of 'temporary fatigue' using the method established in the literature (Mohr *et al.*, 2003; 2008). There are a number of reasons that might explain our results: 1) pre-determined 5-min match periods may be an insensitive approach; 2) younger players may be better able to perform repeated bouts of maximal exercise (Beneke *et al.*, 2005); and 3) elite youth players may adopt a different pacing strategy than 'top class' adult players due to lower levels of physical fitness and match experience (Edwards and Noakes, 2009). Further work is required to examine if the temporary fatigue phenomenon is dependent upon playing position, and to determine if the transient reduction in performance is caused by fatigue or the match tempo.

# References

Beneke, R. *et al.*, 2005, Modeling the blood lactate kinetics at maximal short-term exercise conditions in children, adolescents, and adults. *J Appl Physiol*, **99**, 499–504.

Boyd, L.J. *et al.*, 2011, The reliability of MinimaxX accelerometers for measuring physical activity in Australian football. *Int J Sports Physiol Perf*, **6**, 311–321.

Buchheit, M. *et al.*, 2010a, Repeated-sprint sequences during youth soccer matches. *Int J Sports Med*, **31**, 709–716.

Buchheit, M. *et al.*, 2010b, Match running performance and fitness in youth soccer. *Int J Sports Med*, **31**, 818–825.

Edwards, A.M. and Noakes, T.D., 2009, Dehydration: causes of fatigue or sign of pacing in elite soccer? *Sports Medicine*, **39**, 1–13.

Glenmark, B. *et al.*, 1994, Muscle strength from aldolescence to adulthood-relationship to muscle fibre types, *Eur J Appl Physiol Occup Physiol*, **68**, 9–19.

Harley, J.A. *et al.*, 2010, Motion characteristics of elite 12–16 year old soccer match play. *J Sports Sci*, **28**, 1391–1397.

Mohr, M. *et al.*, 2003, Match performance of high-standard soccer players with special reference to development of fatigue. *J Sports Sci*, **21**, 439–449.

Mohr, M. *et al.*, 2008, Match activities of elite women soccer players at different performance levels. *J Strength Cond Res*, **22**, 341–349.

Osgnach, C. *et al.*, 2010, Energy cost and metabolic power in elite soccer: a new match analysis approach. *Med Sci Sports Exerc*, **42**, 170–178.

Reilly, T. and Bowen, T., 1984, Exertional costs of changes in directional modes of running, *Percept Motor Skills*, **58**, 149–150.

# CHAPTER TWENTY-THREE

# Evolution of rule changes and coaching tactics in Australian Football: impact on game speed, structure and injury patterns

K. Norton

University of South Australia, Australia

## 1. INTRODUCTION

Australian football was codified in 1859 as a set of 10 rules. Today the Australian Football League (AFL) rule set includes over 360 laws contained in a 100-page book and is updated annually. The evolution of AF extends to the way the game is played, how it looks and the tactics employed by the teams and coaches (Norton *et al.* 1999). The players became full-time professionals in the 1990s and this led to rapid developments in player fitness, skills and size (Norton *et al.* 1999). AF is a fast-paced, contact sport with little protective equipment that results in one of the highest injury incidence rates among team sports (Orchard and Seward, 2011). Injury levels rose rapidly as the players became more professional and there has been focused attention on understanding the development of these injuries and on how to reduce the number and severity of injuries at all levels of the game (Norton *et al.* 2001; Orchard and Seward, 2011). In the most recent decade a large number of rule and umpire-interpretation changes have been introduced, ostensibly to control the injury risk and increase player welfare in the short and long term. This chapter sheds light on why these changes to rules and interpretations have been made, why they are necessary and why there is still the need to continually work towards making the game safer to play.

## 2. METHODS

Understanding how Australian football has evolved requires reviewing the highest quality games that are available; namely the AFL and the highest antecedent competition, the VFL. Since past games can only be reviewed using video analysis this restricts both the type of analysis that can be done as well as the range of years available. Specially designed computer-based tracking software has been developed to quantify elements of the game to provide information on game trends across decades of competition (Edgecomb and Norton, 2006). The variables that can be quantified from past games include ball speed (also referred to as game speed) since the camera almost invariably follows the ball, 'player density' around the ball, and times associated with play and stop periods within the game. The ball speed is defined as the speed of the ball (m/s) when the ball is in play, that is, not including any stoppage time. Player density was measured as the number of players within a 5 m radius of the ball measured after stopping the video and counting at 15 s intervals throughout the play periods of the game. Play and stop periods were timed when the umpire started and stopped play for specific rule infringements, when the ball left the playing area or when other specific game events took place.

Video recordings of VFL/AFL games were obtained from 1961 to the 2010 premiership season. A series of both finals games [n=9] and premiership season games [n=129] were reviewed, most covering the period 2000–2010. Information on AFL injury rates were obtained from annually published injury reports produced by the AFL Medical Officer's Association (Orchard and Seward, 2011). These have been produced every year for the past 19 years. A third independent dataset was also used (Wisbey *et al.*, 2010). This dataset on player movement is based on GPS-tracking and contains six years of data collection. Annual reports are published providing information on player distances, speed breakdowns and time on the field. Other statistical information has also been gathered from Champion Data (www.championdata.com), the official statistician of the AFL.

## 3. RESULTS

### 3.1 Game speed

There has been a significant increase in play speed in the AFL over recent decades as illustrated in Figure 1. Since 1961 play speed has approximately doubled.

### 3.2 Play time

Play time is the proportion of the game that involves players competing for the ball. That is, when the umpire has not called a stoppage period. The percentage of the game that was coded as play time across the period 1961–2010 is illustrated in Figure 2. It is clear that the general trend for AF is a decrease across the period up to the early 2000s. In more recent seasons there has been an obvious and dramatic increase in the proportion of play time for AFL.

### 3.3 Play and stop periods

Figure 3 shows play period durations were gradually decreasing over the period 1961–1999. Since that time, play period duration has been increasing. The average stop period duration increased up to about 2005 and then declined dramatically thereafter. Interchange rates increased in an accelerated pattern from the early 2000s, as shown in Figure 4. From the first year that interchanging players was allowed in 1978, the use of the interchange as a coaching tactic was rare and interchange rates remained low for over two decades.

## 3.4 Player density

Player density or congestion around the ball in Australian football has increased significantly over the period 2001–2010 (r=0.48; p<0.05). Player density in AFL reached 2.3 in 2010 up from less than 2 in 2006 (Norton, 2010).

## 3.5 Injury and speed patterns

The injury incidence for the AFL over the last 14 years (when all clubs contributed to the national injury database) is illustrated below in Figure 5 (Orchard and Seward, 2011). The figure also shows both the speed of the ball across the same period and, in the last six years GPS-derived player movement speeds (Wisbey *et al.* 2010).

## 4. DISCUSSION

This study reviewed games of elite AF to determine patterns of evolutionary changes in variables linked to game speed and structure. It also used published reports on AF injury statistics and GPS-based player movement patterns to hypothesise a link among these variables. The data collected show patterns of changes across the time period assessed. It is clear that AF game speed has steadily increased over time. The ball speed is more than twice as fast today than in the 1960s. This may be due to many game elements, including greater skills in passing the ball, increased running speed of players, changes in the pattern (time and number) of stoppages, officiating decisions or a combination of these and other factors. The GPS data collected in the most recent seasons show players are moving faster during games, although this data has only been collected since 2005.

The natural progression in many field sports is for play time to decrease (Figure 2) as the ball moves faster around the ground, increasing the potential for a stoppage to occur. At the same time the increased speed and corresponding physical demands increase the requirement for players to recover quickly. This results in a gradual increase in the duration of the stop periods as shown in Figure 3. However, the longer stoppages and more complete recovery support high-intensity play when the game re-starts. The AFL rules committee released action items for the period 2002–2009 with a primary focus to 'trend the game back to more continuous play, decrease player density around the ball, and reduce high impact collisions associated with high-speed running' (www.afl.com). Most notable were rules allowing play to re-start faster by both the players and the umpires, reversing the patterns seen in Figures 2 and 3. The unexpected outcome of this was a coaching tactic of rotating fresh players for fatigued players more frequently, as illustrated in Figure 4. The rate of change was unprecedented, to the point where additional officials were required to monitor the changes, new rules were established to prevent too many players on the field at once, and penalties introduced for teams that couldn't correctly regulate this escalating trend. GPS data found that players were spending less time on the field but that the intensity of effort once back on the field was increasing (Wisbey *et al.* 2010).

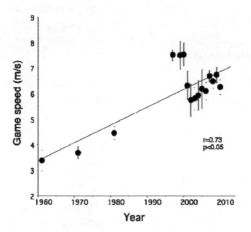

**Figure 1** Trends in average (±SE) game speed for AFL/VFL games. Regression analysis shows it is highly significant (p<0.05).

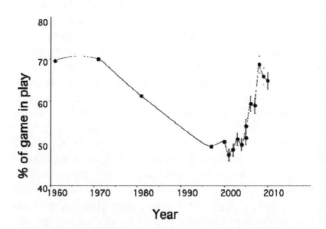

**Figure 2** Average (±SD) proportion of game time in AF categorised as play time. Play time is when the players can compete for the ball and the umpires have not stopped play. A computer-derived interpolation line is shown.

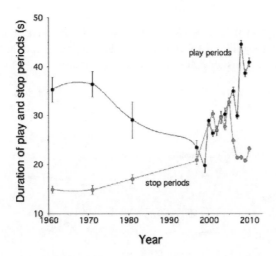

**Figure 3** Trends in both play period and stop period durations in AFL/VFL since 1961. Interpolation lines have been computer-derived to show the patterns.

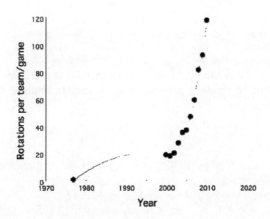

**Figure 4** Trends in the average number of interchange rotations made per team per game in seasons from 1978 for AFL/VFL games. Data are from Champion data. A computer-derived interpolation line has been included.

The injury patterns, which had been controlled to a certain extent following the peaks in the late 1990s, were now rising again (Orchard and Seward, 2011) despite improved injury and rehabilitation treatment programs. Player density levels were increasing, which were also associated with increasing contested play and tackle rates (www.championdata.com) and were possibly contributing to the increasing injury statistics. Figure 5 suggests a potential explanation. It shows a graphical and statistical association that supports a link between interchange rotations allowing faster play, the GPS and ball speed data both demonstrating a trend towards faster play, and the injury statistics that mirror these other trends.

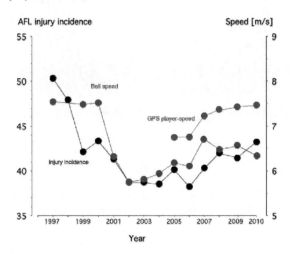

**Figure 5** AFL trends in the average injury incidence (Orchard and Seward, 2011), GPS player movement speed (Wisbey *et al.* 2010) and game speed.

The interaction among the speed, game structure and injury elements in AF is a developing case study in the evolution of elite sport. It is a delicate process that is constantly challenging coaches, players, sports scientists, medical officers and the AFL administration.

**References**

Edgecombe, S.J. and Norton, K.I., 2006, Comparison of global positioning and computer-based tracking systems for measuring player movement distance during Australian Football. *J Sci Med Sport*, **9**, 25–32.

Norton, K.I. *et al.*, 1999, Evolution of Australian football. *J Sci Med Sport*, **2**, 389–404.

Norton, K. *et al.*, 2001, Evidence for the aetiology of injuries in Australian football. *Brit J Sports Med*, **35**, 418–423.

Norton, K., 2010, Player density trends in the AFL 2001–2010. *AFL Research Report*, TrakPerformance Pty Ltd, Adelaide, SA.

Orchard, J. and Seward, H., 2011, 2010 Injury report, Australian Football League. *AFL Research Report,* Australian Football League, Melbourne, Vic.

Wisbey, B. *et al.*, 2010, Quantifying changes in AFL player game demands using GPS tracking, 2010 AFL season. In *AFL Research Report*, FitSense, Canberra, ACT.

# CHAPTER TWENTY-FOUR

# Match analysis in AFL, Soccer and Rugby Union: patterns, trends and similarities

K. Norton

University of South Australia, Australia

## 1. INTRODUCTION

All sports evolve over time. Even sports that may appear to be very stable or consistent are regularly changing. For example, golf began in 1744 with a simple set of 13 rules but the most recent edition of the rulebook was 208 pages, outlining literally hundreds of rules (www.randa.org). Australian Football (AF) was codified in 1857 with 10 rules and now has in excess of 360 (www.AFL.com.au). However, it is more than just rule changes that contribute to the evolution of a sport, it is also the skills and abilities of the players, game tactics employed by coaches and, in field and court-based sports, the speed and style in which the game is played. This paper reviews the evolution of three football codes: AF, Association Football (soccer) and Rugby Union. Specifically, the aim was to determine if there are any consistent patterns of evolutionary changes common to these field sports that may help to understand forces associated with game structure or tactics that might influence the way these sports change over time.

## 2. METHODOLOGY

Understanding how sports evolve typically requires reviewing the highest quality athletes involved in the sport. This means the national football league in AF (AFL), and World Cup matches in both soccer and Rugby Union. Through necessity this also means past games can only be reviewed using video analysis. Specially designed computer-based tracking software has recently been developed to quantify elements of the game that, theoretically, could provide information on game trends across decades of competition (Edgecombe and Norton, 2006).

The main features that are quantified from past games include ball speed (also referred to as game speed) since the camera almost invariably follows the ball, 'player density' around the ball, physical elements such as tackles and collisions, and times associated with play and stop periods within the game. The ball speed is defined as the speed of the ball (m/s) when the ball is in play, that is, not including any stoppage time. Player density was measured as the number of players within a 5 m radius of the ball measured after stopping the video and counting at 15 s intervals throughout the play periods of the game. Play and stop periods were timed when the referee started and stopped play for specific rule infringements, when the ball left the playing area or when other specific game events took place. Tackles and collisions were obtained from either official statistician reports (Champion data in the AFL: www.championdata.com) or determined manually by reviewing the videos and using a standardised reference template to categorise collisions (Norton *et al.*, 2001). A 'physicality' metric was estimated in Rugby Union by multiplying the number of players involved in the tackle/collision by a weighted 'intensity' of the tackle/collision. Intensity ratings were either 1 (lowest intensity), 2 or 3 (highest intensity) and were based on a previous reference system that effectively assesses the probability of injury to players involved in the impact (Norton *et al.*, 2001). Some or all of these variables were measured across each of the three sports. In Australian Football video recordings from 1961 to 2010 season games [n=138] were used. In soccer, the World Cup soccer finals from 1966 to 2010 were used [n=12] and in Rugby Union the World Cup finals from 1987–2007 were used [n=6], as well as other segments from international games.

## 3. RESULTS

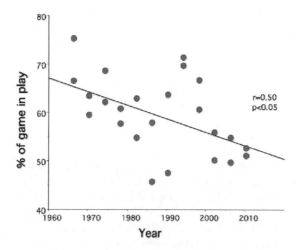

**Figure 1** The proportion of the game time within each half of the soccer World Cup final that is categorised as play time. Play time is when the players can compete for the ball and the referees have not stopped play. A line of best fit is shown.

## Play time

The fraction of the game that involves 'play time' is illustrated for soccer in Figure 1. There was a significant decrease in play time across the five decades of World Cup tournaments. Similarly, AF games have also shown decreased play time from the earliest games analysed in 1961 through to about 2000 when rule changes were introduced to reverse this significant decrease. A combination of a reduced number of stoppages and shorter average stoppage duration in Rugby Union has had the opposite effect, as total play time has increased. Figure 2 shows the time taken for key stoppage events in soccer. All these events are increasing in duration over time. This pattern was also observed in AF games up until about 2000 when strategic measures were introduced to minimise stoppage duration. These included instructions to umpires to re-start play faster, restricting players in the time they could take to have set shots for goals, and allowing players to play on (if they perceived an advantage) despite an infringement being called.

## Game speed

There have been significant increases in play speed in both AF ($r=0.95$; $p<0.05$) and soccer ($r=0.80$; $p<0.05$) over recent decades. For example, in AF the speed has doubled from about 3.4 m/s in 1961 to approximately 6.7 m/s in 2010. Soccer game speed has increased by about 15% over a similar time period from 8.0 m/s to 9.2 m/s. Rugby Union has had a 21% decrease in ball speed from 5.7 m/s in the first World Cup in 1987 to 4.5 m/s in 2007 ($r=0.95$; $p<0.05$).

## Player density

Player density in AF has increased significantly over the period 2001–2010 ($r=0.48$; $p<0.05$) and also in Rugby Union since 1987 ($r=0.83$; $p<0.05$). Player density in AF reached 2.3 in 2010, whereas in the 2007 Rugby Union World Cup final it was 6.1 players (Figure 3). Soccer player density was relatively stable for much of the period reviewed, but has increased slightly and significantly over the course of the last 3 World Cup finals to average 1.9 players in 2010.

## Tackles and collisions

Both tackles and collisions have changed in AF over the last five decades. Collision rates measured in the present study increased steadily from 1961 up to about 2000 and have since decreased (Norton *et al.*, 2001; Norton, 2010a). On the other hand, tackles have only been reported over the nine most recent seasons and have increased significantly from 42 to 68 per team/game, in an accelerated pattern (www.championdata.com). In Rugby Union the 'physicality' score was found to have increased significantly by approximately three-fold in a near linear fashion over the six World Cups. No measures were made for soccer games.

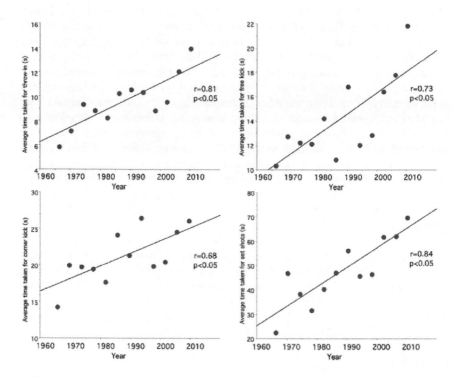

**Figure 2** Trends in soccer game events involving stoppage time for World Cup finals games. The regression lines for each stoppage graph (throw-ins, free kick, corner kick, set shot for goal) are significant (p<0.05).

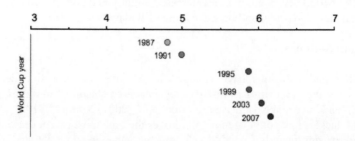

**Figure 3** Trends in average player density in World Cup Rugby Union finals.

## Play and stop periods

Play period durations are, in general, getting longer in both the AF and Rugby Union codes. In soccer the play period duration has been relatively constant, ranging between approximately 20–30 seconds across the World Cup finals. The average play period in AF decreased from about 35s in 1961 to 21s in 2000. It then rose relatively linearly to reach over 40s by 2010. In Rugby Union the average play period in 1987 was approximately half of that found in 2007 (Figure 4). The stop period durations have been increasing in soccer as illustrated in Figure 2, as has the total stoppage time in the games. In AF the stop period duration has decreased in the last decade as it has in the most recent Rugby Union World Cup games.

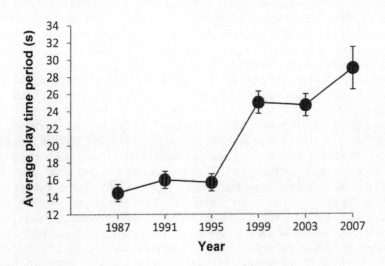

**Figure 4** Trends in the average (±SD) play period duration during the World Cup Rugby Union finals.

## 4. DISCUSSION

The data collected show patterns of changes across the various football codes that are unlikely to occur by chance. There are forces operating that drive play styles and elements of game structure in consistent ways. These forces are not only physical and may sometimes differ among the codes. For example, the AFL, made a strategic decision in the early 2000s to increase the play period duration and shorten stoppage time in order to attenuate the rising speed of both player and ball movement. The rationale was to minimize the potential for collision-related injuries. In Rugby Union there has been a very dramatic shift from the kick-for-touch strategy used up until the mid-1990s to one of maintaining possession at all costs in a running-focused game style. One consequence has been an impressive increase in the body mass index levels of the elite players (Old, 2001). Soccer has permitted increases in the drama of the set shot for goal, which now takes an average of about 70s.

One conclusion that can be drawn from the results of this study is that there is a general trend towards faster game speed in both soccer and AF. While the same was not found in Rugby Union, there was a very large increase in the physicality measure in this code across the six World Cup events. Additionally, Rugby Union also had a combination of increasing play period duration and decreasing stop time. Together, these all point towards a much more intense and physical game for rugby players, since reduced work-to-rest ratios and increased physical contact elevate game demands. Similarly, in AF over the most recent decade play duration has increased substantially and total stoppage time has decreased. Although collision rates have decreased, tackling rates have accelerated. Overall, the faster game speed combined with shorter work-to-rest ratios also increase player demands. Soccer, on the other hand, has evolved towards a faster game with longer average stoppage duration, with a relatively constant play period time. The stoppages are particularly long when the stakes are elevated, for example, during set shots for goal where there is an increased probability of scoring (Yiannakos and Armatas, 2006).

Speed of movement, both by the players and of the ball, confers an advantage. However, moving at speed also requires fitness, or more specifically in a game, 'freshness'. When left untouched by coaching tactics and rule changes field games such as the soccer and Australian football codes show an evolving pattern that can be characterised by shorter, faster play periods interspersed by longer periods for recovery. If left to the players this is a natural decision, that is, play intensely and with speed, then rest for longer to recover so that it can be repeated. In collision-based sports the 'freshness' leads to higher collision and tackling intensities and justifies rule changes in AF making the game more continuous with less recovery time. This is probably one reason why many of these sports are reporting rising rates of player injuries, even in the face of better medical and rehabilitation procedures (O'Connor, 2011; Orchard and Seward, 2011).

All codes showed increases in the number of players in close proximity to the ball. Raising player density leads to elevated levels of skill, speed and precision required to move through the player 'traffic', and increases the number of variables included in decision-making, while at the same time forcing players to hurry selections. Decreasing player density allows players more time and space and it has been shown that the probability of scoring in soccer doubles for every metre of free space around the kicker when shooting for goal (Pollard *et al.*, 2004).

# References

Edgecombe, S.J. and Norton, K.I., 2006, Comparison of global positioning and computer-based tracking systems for measuring player movement distance during Australian Football. *J Sci Med Sport*, **9**, 25–32.

Norton, K.I. *et al.*, 1999, Evolution of Australian football. *J Sci Med Sport*, **2**, 389–404.

Norton, K. *et al.*, 2001, Evidence for the aetiology of injuries in AFL. *Brit J Sports Med*, **35**, 418–423.

Norton, K., 2010a, AFL and NAB Cup annual reports 2010. *AFL Research Report*, TrakPerformance Pty Ltd, Adelaide, SA.

Norton, K., 2010b, Player density trends in the AFL 2001–2010. *AFL Research Report*, TrakPerformance Pty Ltd, Adelaide, SA.

O'Connor, D., 2011, NRL injury report 2010. *Sport Health*, **29**, 17–26.

Olds, T., 2001, The evolution of physique in male rugby union players in the twentieth century. *J Sports Sci*, **19**, 253–262.

Orchard, J. and Seward, H., 2011, 2010 Injury report, Australian Football League. *AFL Research Report*, Australian Football League, Melbourne, Vic.

Pollard, R. *et al.*, 2004, Estimating the probability of a shot resulting in a goal: the effects of distance, angle and space. *Int J Soccer Sci*, **2**, 50–55.

Yiannakos, A. and Armatas, V., 2006, Evaluation of the goal scoring patterns in European Championship in Portugal 2004. *Int J Perf Analysis Sport*, **6**, 178–188.

# CHAPTER TWENTY-FIVE

# Spatial strategy used by the world champion in South Africa 2010

F. Robles[1], J. Castellano[2], A. Perea[3], R. Martínez-Santos[2] and D. Casamichana[2]

[1]University of Malaga, Spain, [2]University of the Basque Country (UPV-EHU), Spain, [3]Turnverein Cannstatt 1846 e. V. , Stuttgart, Germany

## 1. INTRODUCTION

Match analysis is commonly used in many sports as a tool that allows coaches to collect objective information that can be used to provide feedback on performance (Carling *et al.*, 2005). Coaches are turning increasingly to match analysis as a way for optimizing the training process of their players and teams (Hughes and Franks, 2004), with the main aim of match analysis to identify the strengths and weaknesses of the team (Carling *et al.*, 2008). The same as any other invasion game, soccer is a battle for space and position and the description of play events in relation to their spatial and chronological order of appearance is the first step for understanding the nature of this game. The playing action in soccer is built up collectively, which means that players' placements and movements can be considered a major factor of the team's strategy.

Polar coordinate analysis is a suitable technique to analyse the dynamic interrelations among different uses of the interaction. This analysis is a double data reduction strategy providing a vector representation of the complex network of interrelations among the different behavioural categories of an ad hoc system (Bakeman and Quera, 1995). Several studies have tried to explain the complex relations in soccer producing inter-relational maps and identifying stable patterns considering the used space (Alday *et al.*, 2008), the relations among players (Lago and Anguera, 2002) and spatial-interactional context (Castellano, 2000; Castellano and Hernandez-Mendo, 2003; Perea, 2008).

The objective of this study is to describe and understand the spatial strategy, interaction contexts (IC) performed during the games played by the Spanish national team and their opponents in the World Championship in South Africa 2010.

## 2. METHODS

### Sample

The seven games played by the Spanish team in the final phase of South Africa 2010 World Cup were analyzed by means of an *ad hoc* taxonomic system.

### Taxonomic system

The present investigation used the System for Observing Play in Soccer (SOCCAF; Castellano, 2000), which has already been employed in previous studies (Castellano *et al.*, 2007a, 2007b and 2009; Jonsson *et al.*, 2006). This tool is based in the definition of effective space covered from previous studies (Gréhaigne, 1992) and is similar to later works (Seabra and Dantas, 2006) but allows to differ between defence, midfield and attacking areas of each team and it is able to determine in broad terms the development of play among twenty-two players. The relation between the areas or sectors of both teams (Figure 1) determines the current interaction contexts (IC) (e.g.: AR context means that the ball is between A area from one team and R area for the other team). In total, there are nine ICs: *RM, RA, MR, MM, MA, AR, AM, ER* and *AO* (definitions are in Table 1).

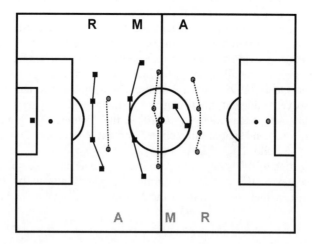

**Figure 1** Example of defence, midfield and attacking areas or sectors for the observed team (in black) and the opponent team (in grey). A is attack area, M is middle area and R is rear or back area of the each team.

## Analysis of data quality

The estimated values for within- and between-observer reliability (Cohen's kappa) may be considered as optimum, since in all cases the values obtained were above 0.75 (Castellano, 2000; Perea, 2008).

## Software

Data collection was performed using *MOTS* (Castellano *et al.*, 2008). Once the adjusted residuals of the sequential analysis was obtained via *SDIS-GSEQ* 5.0 (Bakeman and Quera, 1995, http://www2.gsu.edu/~psyrab/gseq/index.html), a polar coordinate analysis was performed. For this, a software application called CoordenadasPolares.m was developed (Perea *et al.*, 2011 in press), being this a m-file for execution in MatLab (The MathWorks, Inc. http://www.mathworks.com/), which performs the polar coordinates analysis of the data for a given category and represents the relations of activation and inhibition between the behaviours on a vector map. The discriminant analysis was performed using SPSS 16.0 for Windows.

## Statistical analysis

Firstly, the homogeneity of variances was analyzed by means of Levene's and Kolmogorov-Smirnov tests and with the objective of verifying the normality. Secondly, a discriminant analysis was performed in order to identify the variables which best discriminated between Spain and the opponent teams (Ntoumanis, 2001). This was done by calculating the structural coefficients (SC), being the obtained values >0.30 regarded as significant (Tabachnick and Fidell, 2007). All the statistical analyses were performed using a significance set at $p<0.05$. Finally, the polar coordinate analysis was performed. We applied this analysis to one IC (MM) to compare Spain and the opponent teams in South Africa 2010. The analysis combines simultaneously in a single diagram a diachronic perspective (forward in time) with a retrospective one (back in time). It represents a system, which is able to maintain without distortion a large amount of information about the way in which the teams tend to develop their play.

## 3. RESULTS AND DISCUSSION

Table 1 shows the results of the discriminant analysis for the last World Cup from Spain and their opponents. The discriminant functions classified correctly 100% of Spain and opponent teams and the discriminant function obtained was significant ($p<0.05$). Only one variable had discriminatory power in the discriminant function: it was the MM interaction context (SC = 0.301), that is, when the ball was located between the middle area of the observed team and the middle area of the other team.

**Table 1** Standardized coefficients from the discriminant analysis of the game statistics in the interaction context (IC) between Spain and the opponent teams from the games in South Africa 2010.

| IC definition: when the ball is located between... | IC | Function 1 |
|---|---|---|
| the *middle* area of the observed team and the *middle* area of the other team | **MM\*** | **0.301** |
| the *forward* area of the observed team and the *rear* area of the other team | AR | 0.246 |
| the *middle* area of the observed team and the *forward* area of the other team | MA | 0.121 |
| the *forward* and *external* area of the observed team and the *rear* area of the other team | ER | 0.120 |
| the *middle* area of the observed team and the *rear* area of the other team | MR | 0.107 |
| the *rear* area of the observed team and the *forward* area of the other team | RA | 0.085 |
| the *forward* area of the observed team and the *empty* area of the other team | AO | -0.034 |
| the *forward* area of the observed team and the *middle* of the other team | AM | 0.016 |
| the *rear* area of the observed team and the *middle* area of the other team | RM | -0.005 |

Note. *SC discriminant value $\geq |.30|$. *Eigen value = 53.37, Wilks' Lambda = 0.02, Canonical Correlation= 0.99, Chi-squared =29.9, Significance = 0.001, % of variante = 100%.*

As in previous studies about World Cups (Castellano and Hernandez-Mendo, 2003; Perea, 2008), the MM interaction context has elicited specific relationships with other contexts, which is a very meaningful indicator about how teams build their attacking phases.

As far as the South Africa 2010 World Cup is concerned, the IC activated or inhibited by the focal category MM were different for the Spanish squad in comparison to the rest of the teams (Figures 2a and 2b). This indicates that the spatial strategy employed by Spain to progress in possession of the ball was unique. Furthermore, we would like to highlight the following aspects of these differences: 1) The association of MM with itself both on prospective and retrospective planes (quadrant I) is stronger for the Spanish (25.1) than for the rivals (10.4) which indicates the Spanish offensive superiority in the centre of the field; 2) AM category is not prospectively activated by MM in Spain (quadrant IV) as it is in the rivals play action: opponent teams playing against Spain needed to bring their forwards closer down to the midfield to keep possession; 3) RM is located in quadrant II for Spain (4.1) whereas it is in quadrant I (2.3) for the rivals: this IC is only activated retrospectively for Spain and in both senses for the other teams; 4) Finally, it is worth mentioning that Spain activated MR (4.2) and AR (8.8) in quadrant IV more strongly than its opponents (2.9 and 3.5 respectively) which leads to pay attention to the greater ability of the Spanish team for taking the ball closer to the goal.

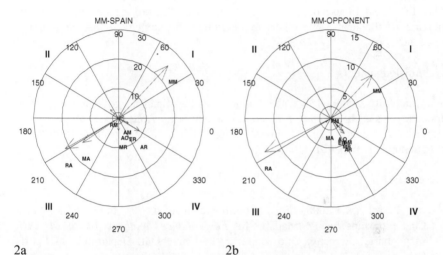

| MM | | RA | RM | MA | MM | MR | AM | AR | ER | AO |
|---|---|---|---|---|---|---|---|---|---|---|
| | Quadrant | III | II | III | I | IV | I | IV | IV | IV |
| Spain | Ratio | 21.5 | 4.1 | 15.2 | 25.1 | 4.2 | 1,8 | 8.8 | 4.0 | 1.3 |
| | Angle | 208.9 | 133.3 | 212.8 | 45 | 272.0 | 15.6 | 330.5 | 336.2 | 307.3 |
| | Quadrant | III | I | III | I | IV | IV | IV | IV | IV |
| Opponent | Ratio | 13.0 | 2.3 | 1.1 | 10.4 | 2.9 | 2.7 | 3.5 | 1.9 | 1.7 |
| | Angle | 206.2 | 89.4 | 215.2 | 45 | 315.2 | 330.1 | 313.0 | 313.7 | 330.7 |

**Figure 2** Representation of the vector plane when taking the category MM as the criterion behaviour: 2a from Spain and 2b from their opponents.

## 4. CONCLUSION

The results obtained from the polar coordinate analysis help us describe the game action in soccer taking into account the diachronic dimension of the events and combining the prospective and retrospective perspectives. The polar coordinates technique has enabled us to produce a conceptual map of the relations between the interaction contexts (IC). The opportunity for representing the relations among ICs taken as the focal behaviour and the rest of the ICs in the same conceptual map makes it clear that action in soccer is not built up statically. This study reveals some key aspects underlying the complex game of soccer.

The practical application carried out in the context of soccer enabled us to derive a vector plane of the relations between the IC used by the Spanish team as the matches unfold. The depiction of the relations between ICs, being these considered as focal behaviours, revealed the different routes used by the World Champion in its attempt to score. At the highest levels of competitive soccer, teams are similar in ability. Therefore, knowing their 'preferred routes' and the patterns of play they tend to use during a match facilitates the preparation and decision-making of the team, as well as to determine the strategy to use in a future encounter.

## Acknowledgements

We gratefully acknowledge the support of the Spanish government project Innovaciones en la evaluación de contextos naturales: Aplicaciones al ámbito del deporte (Dirección General de Investigación, Ministerio de Ciencia y Tecnología) [Grant number BSO2001-3368].

## References

Alday, L. *et al.*, 2008, Polar coordinate analysis of the soccer World Championships using Matlab. In *Performance Analysis of Sport VIII*, Magdeburg, Germany: Otto-von-Guericke-Universität, Department of Sports Science, pp. 152–160.

Bakeman, R. and Quera, V., 1995, *Analyzing Interaction: Sequential Analysis with SDIS and GSEQ.* Cambridge, UK: Cambridge University Press.

Carling, C. *et al.*, 2008, The role of motion analysis in elite soccer. *Sports Med*, **38**, 839–862.

Carling, C. *et al.*, 2005, *Handbook of Soccer Match Analysis.* London: Routledge.

Castellano, J., 2000, *Observación y análisis de la acción de juego en fútbol.* Doctoral thesis. San Sebastian: Universidad del País Vasco.

Castellano, J. and Hernandez-Mendo, A., 2003, El análisis de coordenadas polares para la estimación de relaciones en la interacción motriz en fútbol. *Psicothema*, **15**, 569–574.

Castellano, J. *et al.*, 2007a, Optimising a probabilistic model of the development of play in soccer. *Quality and Quantity*, **41**, 93–104.

Castellano, J., *et al.*, 2007b, Diachronic analysis of interaction context in '06 World Championship. *J Sports Sci Med*, **6**, 200–201.

Castellano, J. *et al.*, 2008, Measuring and observation tool in sports. *Behavior Research Methods*, **40**, 898–903.

Castellano, J. *et al.*, 2009, Has soccer changed in the last three World Championships? In *Science and Football VI*, London: Routledge, pp. 167–170.

Grèhaigne, J-F., 1992, In *L'organisation du jeu en Football.* Paris: Actio.

Hughes, M. and Franks, I. M., 2004, *Notational Analysis of Sport Systems for Better Coaching and Performance in Sport*. London: Routledge.

Jonsson, G.K. *et al.*, 2006, Hidden patterns of play interaction in football using SOFT-CODER. *Behav Res Method Instrum Comp*, **38**, 372–381.

Lago, C. and Anguera, M.T., 2002, Use of the polar coordinates technique to study interactions among professional soccer players, *Revista Portuguesa de Ciências do Desporto*, **2**, 21–40.

Ntoumanis N., 2001, *A Step-by-Step Guide to SPSS for Sport and Exercise Studies*. London: Routledge.

Perea, A., 2008, Análisis de las acciones colectivas en el fútbol de rendimiento. Unpublished doctoral thesis: Universidad del País Vasco.

Perea, A. *et al.*, 2011 (in press), Analysis of behaviour in sports through Polar Coordinate Analysis with MATLAB®. *Quality and Quantity*.

Seabra, F. and Dantas, L.E.P.B.T., 2006, Space definition for match analysis in soccer. *Int J Perf Analysis Sports*, **6**, 97–113.

Tabachnick, B.G. and Fidell, L.S., 2007, *Using Multivariate Statistics*. 3rd edition, New York: Harper Collins.

# CHAPTER TWENTY-SIX

# Ball dynamics constrain interpersonal coordination in futsal

B. Travassos[1,2], D. Araújo[3], R. Duarte[3] and T. McGarry[4]

[1]Department of Sport Sciences, University of Beira Interior, Portugal,
[2]CIDESD, Research Centre in Sports, Health Sciences and Human Development,
Portugal, [3]Faculty of Human Kinetics, Technical University of Lisbon, Portugal,
[4]Faculty of Kinesiology, University of New Brunswick, Canada

## 1. INTRODUCTION

Patterns of interpersonal coordination in game competition such as football and futsal emerge under the competing and cooperating aims of the two teams. In this context, the sports behaviours that characterize these types of games are proposed to result from spontaneous, self-organizing, localized, dynamical interactions operating under a variety of individual, task, and environmental constraints (Araújo et al., 2006; Passos et al., 2008). In team sports the behavioural patterns that emerge during performance may be investigated at different levels of analysis, from interactions between individual players (Travassos et al., 2011) to interactions between teams (Frencken and Lemmink, 2008; Travassos et al., in press). These studies reported general tendencies of synchronized displacements of players and teams in both lateral (i.e., side-to-side) and longitudinal (i.e., forward-backward) directions, particularly the latter direction. Furthermore, singular moments of the game such as changes in ball possession, or goal-scoring opportunities, revealed specific patterns between teams in terms of phase stabilities and/or phase transitions (Bourbousson et al., 2010; Frencken and Lemmink, 2008).

While ball kinematics are thought to constitute an important informational constraint on game behaviour in team sports (Davids et al., 2008; McGarry, 2009) they remain uninvestigated to date. Thus, a need exists to understand how ball dynamics constrain spatial-temporal behaviours of players, from consideration of the individual (player) through to the collective (team). This investigation addresses this issue of ball dynamics as a constraint on game behaviour by analyzing space-time relations between ball, players and teams kinematics.

## 2. METHODS

Fifteen male senior players of the National Futsal University Team in Portugal participated in this study ($M$ = 23.3 years, $sd$ = 2.0 years and $M$ = 11.5 years of practice, *sd* = 1.3 years of practice), with each player giving informed consent before data collection. Participants were grouped into three teams of five players each. Futsal is a 5-a-side indoor soccer game that is played on a pitch of 40m length x 20m width. In this study, we investigated a particular sub-phase of a futsal game whereupon the goalkeeper of the trailing team is substituted late in the game for an extra outfield player with a view to increasing the chances of scoring a goal. Strategic goalkeeper substitution for the trailing team is commonly used by coaches during competitions. For instance, in the final four of the UEFA Futsal Cup in Lisbon, 2010, half of the goals that occurred in the last five minutes were scored using strategic goalkeeper substitution. We will refer to this futsal game condition as 5-v-4+GK.

The movements of ball and players, in nine 5-v-4+GK game practice sessions, were video recorded at 25 Hz using a digital camera placed in the superior plane. For purposes of data analysis, all players were assigned a unique identifier by virtue of their membership to the attacking (A) or defending (D) team, as well as their starting position at the onset of the practice session.

From the available data, the movement trajectories of ball and players from 21 trial sequences ending with a shot at goal were digitized in slow video by the first author using TACTO 8.0 software (see Fernandes *et al.*, 2010). The virtual coordinates obtained from the digitization were transformed to pitch coordinates using a bi-dimensional direct linear transformation method (2D-DLT) (see Duarte *et al.*, 2010; Fernandes *et al.*, 2010), before being subjected to a 6 Hz low pass filter (Winter, 2005). Two time series were obtained for the ball, for the individual players, and for the geometric centre of both teams, that data being the lateral (i.e. side-to-side) and longitudinal (i.e. forward-backward) displacements on the pitch.

The geometric centre of both teams was obtained from the arithmetic mean of the five players per team. These time series data, were then subjected to relative phase analysis using Hilbert transform (Palut and Zanone, 2005; Rosenblum *et al.*, 2004). The relative phase quantifies the position relations between two sinusoidal signals by measuring the phase differences between signals in their respective cycles. Thus, in-phase (0°) represents signals at the same point in their respective cycles, and anti-phase (180°) denotes signals that are a half-phase displaced from each other. Other phase relations between in-phase and anti-phase likewise expressed with values between 0° and 180° (or between 180° and 360°).

The coefficient of reliability produced data for the attackers *(R=.97)*, defenders *(R=.96)* and ball *(R=.99)* demonstrating good reliability between measurements.

## 3. RESULTS

The coordination dynamics between players and ball and between attackers and defenders revealed higher attractions to lateral than to longitudinal directions in the same phase relations. The relative phases between defenders and ball, summarized in an exemplar trial for lateral direction, reports a pronounced attractor of -30° as represented by relative phase results over time and frequency histogram (41.0%). The nature of this relation means that, understandably, the ball leads the defending player (see upper panels of Figure 1).

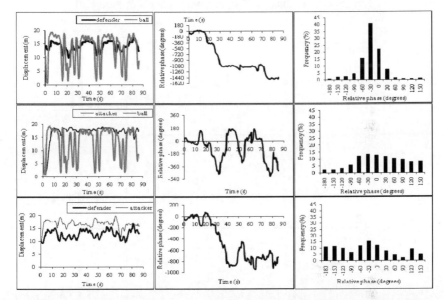

**Figure 1** Exemplar trial of players and ball displacements and between players with correspondent relative phase results: Upper panels–Defender-ball pair displacements and relative phase results; 2nd panels–Attacker-ball pair displacements and relative phase results; 3rd panels–Defender-attacker displacements and relative phase results.

Similar to the results for the defenders and ball, the relative phase of the exemplar trial for the attackers and ball in the lateral direction demonstrated attraction to -30° (14.6%), although the strength of the attraction is much weaker than for the defenders and ball. The results for the relative phase over time highlighted the low attraction to a specific mode of relation (see middle panels of Figure 1). The relative phase exemplar trial data for the defenders and attackers also demonstrated weak attractions towards -30° for the lateral (14.7%) displacements (see lower panels of Figure 1).

The coordination dynamics between teams and ball and between attacking and defending team revealed higher attractions to lateral directions than longitudinal directions to the same phase relations. The phase relations between the geometric centre of the defending team and ball, summarized in an exemplar trial for lateral direction, demonstrated -30° attractions in lateral direction as represented by relative phase result over time and frequency histogram (56.7%) (see upper panels of Figure 2). As with the results for the defending team and ball, the attacking team and ball yielded -30° phase relation in the lateral direction. Once more, the attacking team revealed weaker attraction in lateral direction (34.4%) as compared with the defending team (see middle panels of Figure 2). Similar findings were reported for the coordination patterns between the two teams with -30° phase produced in the lateral direction, with similar pattern of phase transitions over time and frequency results (25.7%) (see lower panels of Figure 2).

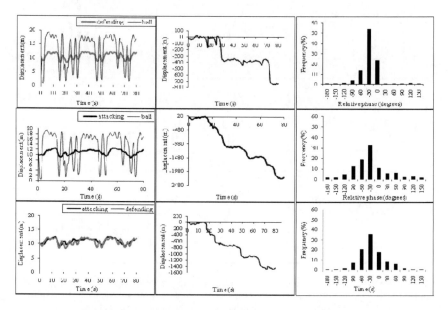

**Figure 2** Exemplar trial of teams and ball displacements and teams with correspondent relative phase results: Upper panels – Defending team and ball displacements and relative phase results; 2nd panels–Attacking team and ball displacements and relative phase results; 3rd panels–defending-attacking team displacements and relative phase results.

## 4. DISCUSSION

The nature of team sports means that the ball is an integral component of futsal game behaviour, and phase attractions observed between the players and ball, and between the teams and ball, confirm ball dynamics as an important constraint on game behaviour. This investigation has revealed higher dynamical linkages between players and ball, and teams and ball, than between players or teams, from which we deduce that attackers and defenders and their respective teams integrate ball trajectory information to coordinate actions to achieve their aims.

Varying phase attractions with the ball were observed for the players and teams, with the defenders revealing considerably stronger phase attractions for both players and teams. These different results are attributed to the contrasting aims of the two teams, namely that of preventing and scoring goals, and the different strategies used as a means of achieving these separate objectives. Thus, reduced variability and stronger attractions to in-phase for the defending players and team, and, conversely, increased variability and weaker phase attractions for the attacking players and team are explained by the different and competing aims of the two teams (Travassos *et al.*, 2011). Specifically, the attackers try to disrupt the defensive structure by exploring the various dynamical relations whereas the defenders couple themselves with the ball and teammates so as to maintain in-phase positional relations, with the ball, with each other, and with the goal area being defended (Travassos *et al.*, 2011). This plasticity of game behaviour, from the individual to the collective, is important as it allows for game objectives to be reached in functional ways (McGarry *et al.*, 2002).

The results also demonstrated that the player relations contain more variability than the team relations, with the latter exhibiting strong attraction towards in-phase in both lateral and longitudinal directions, particularly for the defending team. Accordingly, the emergence of team stability in relations was due to variability of players relations (Travassos *et al.*, 2011). From a behavioural perspective, increased variability observed for the playing dyads as compared to the team dyads, and particularly for the attacking players, may be the result of players continually engaging with their surrounding information as to produce functional adaptive behaviours at the team scale, a feature noted elsewhere for other biological systems (Kelso and Engstrøm, 2006).

The game behaviours in team sports emerges by players acting under constraints such as game rules, game strategies, changing objectives, and so on (Araújo *et al.*, 2006). In this study, contrasting results were observed to those reported previously for basketball (Bourbousson *et al.*, 2010) and small-sided football games (Frencken and Lemmink, 2008) which reported stronger in-phase attractions between dyads and teams in the longitudinal direction as opposed to the lateral direction. These differences can be attributed to the different strategies used by the defending teams. For basketball and football, the teams comprised of 5-v-5 and 4-v-4, respectively, with individual defending strategies used by both teams in both investigations, whereas in this study we investigated 5-v-4+GK futsal game practice with the defending team using zone defence. Further investigation is required in order to understand how changes in defensive or attacking strategies constrain game behaviour.

## 5. CONCLUSIONS

In summary, individual and team coordinated behaviours are the result of information exchanges between dyads with the ball dynamics serving as an important constraint. Players and teams are more constrained by ball kinematics than by the kinematic behaviours of their opponents. Future work on analysis of team sports such as futsal should consider the ball dynamics as an important constraint that allows better understanding of the emergent patterns of game coordination.

## References

Araújo, D. *et al.*, 2006, The ecological dynamics of decision making in sport. *Psych Sport Exerc*, **7**, 653–676.

Bourbousson, J. *et al.*, 2010, Space-time coordination patterns in basketball: Investigating the interaction between the two teams. *J Sport Sci*, **28**, 349–358.

Davids, K. *et al.*, 2008, *Dynamics of Skill Acquisition: A Constraints-led Approach*. Champaign IL: Human Kinetics.

Duarte, R. *et al.*, 2010, Capturing complex human behaviors in representative sports contexts with a single camera. *Medicina*, **46**, 408–414.

Fernandes, O. *et al.*, 2010, Validation of the tool for applied and contextual time-series observation. *Int J Sport Psychol*, **41**, 63–64.

Frencken, W. and Lemmink, K., 2008, Team kinematics of small-sided soccer games: a systematic approach. In *Science and Football VI*, London: Routledge, pp. 61–166.

Kelso, J.A.S. and Engstrøm, D.A., 2006, *The Complementary Nature*. Cambridge, MA: MIT Press.

McGarry, T., 2009, Applied and theoretical perspectives of performance analysis in sport: Scientific issues and challenges. *Int J Perf Analys Sport*, **9**, 128–140.

McGarry, T. *et al.*, 2002, Sport competition as a dynamical self-organizing system. *J Sports Sci*, **20**, 771–781.

Palut, Y. and Zanone, P.G., 2005, A dynamical analysis of tennis: Concepts and data. *J Sports Sci*, **23**, 1021–1032.

Passos, P., *et al.*, 2008, Information-governing dynamics of attacker-defender interactions in youth rugby union. *J Sports Sci*, **26**, 1421–1429.

Rosenblum, M. *et al.*, 2004, Synchronization approach to analysis of biological systems. *Fluctuation and Noise Lett*, **4**, L53–L62.

Travassos, B. *et al.*, 2011, Interpersonal coordination and ball dynamics in futsal (indoor football). *Human Mov Sci*, **30**, 1245–1259.

Travassos, B. *et al.*, (in press), Spatiotemporal coordination patterns in futsal are guided by informational game constraints. *Human Mov Sci*.

Winter, D., 2005, *Biomechanics and Motor Control of Human Movement* (3rd ed.). New York: John Wiley & Sons.

# CHAPTER TWENTY-SEVEN

# Score-line effect on work-rate in English Premier League soccer

P. Clark and P. O'Donoghue

Centre for Performance Analysis, Cardiff School of Sport,
University of Wales Institute Cardiff, Wales, UK

## 1. INTRODUCTION

In soccer, score-line has been shown to influence both tactical (Bloomfield *et al.*, 2004a; Jones *et al.*, 2004; Lago and Martin, 2007) and technical aspects of play (Taylor *et al.*, 2008). Score-line has also been found to influence work-rate in soccer (O'Donoghue and Tenga, 2001; McStravick and O'Donoghue, 2001; Shaw and O'Donoghue, 2004; Bloomfield *et al.*, 2004b). Previous studies have used varied time-motion analysis techniques to measure score-line effects in soccer that do not incorporate for different factors influencing the outcome, Redwood-Brown *et al.* (2009) used an automatic player tracking system that doesn't distinguish between forward, backward and sideways movements. Other studies have used data from over a decade ago (O'Donoghue and Tenga, 2001), used a semi-professional cohort (McStravick and O'Donoghue, 2001; Shaw and O'Donoghue, 2001) and excluded defenders in their analysis (Bloomfield *et al.*, 2004). Over the past decade, there have been rule changes in soccer relating to defending throw-ins and goalkeeper possession of the ball and the definition of offside. There have also been developments in player preparation with technology assisting match analysis and feedback. Clearly there is a need for up-to-date research on elite soccer players to determine the influence of score-line on elite soccer play. The purpose of the current investigation was to investigate the influence of score-line on work rate profiles in elite soccer players during the 2009–2010 season.

## 2. METHODS

### 2.1. Participants and data collection

A sample of 20 outfield English FA Premier League players was used in the current investigation. Each of these players were observed during an English FA Premier League, English FA Cup or UEFA Champions League match during the 2009–10 season. The matches used from the FA Cup were restricted to matches between English FA Premier League teams only. Players were classified into 5 positional groups with 4 players representing each group. The positional groups were central defenders, wide defenders, central midfielders, wide midfielders and forwards. The players were observed live during games at the stadium where the match was played. Permission to use a digital dictation machine was granted by the stadium management in order to comply with the terms and conditions of ticket use and it was agreed that no transmission of the match would take place and player names wouldn't be identified. One player was recorded for each match attended by the primary author. The author verbally coded player movement, recording this information onto a Sony ICD-P630F digital voice recorder. The recording was played back and simultaneously manually entered into the CAPTAIN (Computerised All Purpose Time-motion Analysis Integrated) time-motion analysis system.

The times at which goals were scored were used to determine the percentage of time players spent performing high intensity activity (%HI) when their team was level, ahead and behind. Data were only included for analysis when the score-line was constant for at least 15 minutes (Redwood-Brown *et al.*, 2009). There were only two players whose team was level, ahead and behind for at least 15 minutes during the matches observed. Therefore, two separate analyses were done; players whose teams were level and ahead during the game (LA group) and players whose teams were level and behind during the game (LB group). The LA group consisted of 12 players and the LB groups consisted of 7 players.

### 2.2. Time-motion analysis

The CAPTAIN system is a computerised time-motion analysis system that can be tailored for use with any movement classification scheme of up to 9 movement classes (O'Donoghue, 1998). The current study used a classification scheme of the following 7 movements defined by Huey *et al.* (2001):

- *Standing*, any time the subject spends stationary, this includes standing, lying or sitting down and is not in possession of the football.
- *Walking*, walking in a forward direction and not in possession of the football.
- *Backing*, low intensity backwards and sideward motion and not in possession of the football.
- *Jogging*, low intensity running in a forward direction, without possession of the football.
- *Running*, high intensity running with significant effort and not in possession of the football.
- *Shuffling*, high intensity backwards, sideways and on the spot movement requiring significant effort.
- *Football*, any time the subject has possession of the football during the match (including stoppage time).

Of these movements, running, shuffling and football were classified as high intensity activity. The CAPTAIN system represented each of these movements by a different function key on the computer's keyboard, with a keyboard overlay used to assist data entry. The system recorded a chronological timed sequence of movements for each player that was entered by the author. The system has been enhanced to provide outputs relating to the duration of high intensity activity periods and the low intensity recoveries that follow them. This was done by concatenating adjacent periods of high intensity movements (and low intensity movements) into single bursts (and recoveries). The high intensity activity periods may be composed of consecutively performed instances of different types of high intensity activity or they may be single activity instances. Similarly, recovery periods may be composed of multiple consecutively performed instances of different low intensity movement types.

## 2.3. Reliability of data collection

The authors independently observed and verbally coded a 97 minute video that followed an elite striker during an English FA Premier League soccer game. The video followed the player for the entire match irrespective of whether the player was involved in on-the-ball action or not. Each observer then played back the recording of the verbal coded movement and manually entered the data into the CAPTAIN system. The detailed results of this reliability study are described by Clark (2010), showing a good strength of inter-operator agreement ($\kappa = 0.885$).

## 2.4. Statistical analysis

A Shapiro-Wilks test found that the percentage of time spent performing high intensity activity was not normally distributed, meaning that the data was nonparametric. Therefore, Wilcoxon signed ranks tests were used to compare the %HI between score-line states.

## 3. RESULTS

The 12 players whose teams were level and ahead had similar %HI when level and ahead ($9.4 \pm 2.5\%$ vs. $8.8 \pm 2.5\%$, $p > 0.05$). The second group of 7 players had %HI of $8.3 \pm 1.9\%$ when level which was significantly ($p < 0.01$) greater than when behind ($8.3 \pm 1.9\%$ vs. $7.1 \pm 1.8\%$). Figure 1 shows that the players performed more HI activity when level than when ahead or behind.

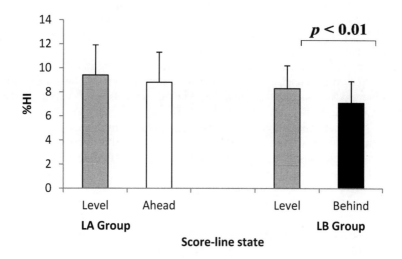

**Figure 1** Percentage of time spent performing high intensity activity in different score-line states.

## 4. DISCUSSION

The differences between score-line states can be discussed in relation to the variability in % time spent performing HI activity within performances. This was calculated from six 15-minute periods and ranged from 1.01% to 2.58% for the 20 players. The difference between % time spent performing HI in the level and behind score-line states agrees with previous research (O'Donoghue and Tenga, 2001). However, the 0.6% difference for HI activity between level and ahead score-line states was lower than the lowest within-performance standard deviation. Furthermore, the 1.2% difference for HI activity between level and behind score-line states was only greater than 3 of the 20 within-performance standard deviations.

When discussing score-line effects, it is worth considering that matches typically start level, with ahead and behind score-lines being experienced later. Previous research has reported that players perform a greater volume of HI activity in the first half than the second half of matches, with the score being more likely to be level in the first half than the second half (Redwood-Brown *et al.*, 2009). Therefore, the significant score-line effect found in the current investigation may be coincidental. Adjusting the % time spent performing HI activity to correct for the normal fatigue patterns during 0-0 draws is possible (Redwood-Brown *et al.*, 2009). However, this requires a great volume of data that is only feasible where semi-automatic player tracking systems are available.

O'Donoghue and Tenga (2001) produced a speculative model for the mechanisms behind score-line effects. The authors referred to sports psychology research in the areas of efficacy expectation (Bandura, 1977) and causal attribution (McAuley, 1992). They proposed a pathway from a goal being scored or conceded to motivation of effort that included score-line state, causal attribution and perceived locus of control. The argument was that when leading or trailing, players may attribute the score-line state to factors outside their own control. This can lead to reduced effort and a reduction in observable movement for players who are leading and trailing (Feltz, 1992). This speculative model can be criticised on a number of grounds. Firstly, there is little evidence to support such a mechanism, with the elements of the model between the score-line state and observable movement being left as 'black boxes'. Only McStravick and O'Donoghue (2001) have gathered additional data to complement the time motion data within a score-line study. The second criticism is that in the seven matches where there was no more than a single goal between the two teams at any time, the score-line can change in an instant through a goal being scored. In these matches, the outcome of the match may have been considered within the control of the players until the end of the match. This suggests that the mechanisms proposed by O'Donoghue and Tenga (2001) were not solely responsible for a reduction in observed work-rate when players were ahead or level.

The third area of criticism of O'Donoghue and Tenga's (2001) model is that it can be interpreted as placing too much emphasis on the first goal of a match. According to the model, when the first goal is scored, the scoring team and the conceding team will lose motivation as the outcome of the match becomes more obvious and outside the players' personal control. The final criticism is that the model is based on the assumptions of the normative paradigm assuming such a thing as 'the average elite soccer player'. Different players and different teams may be influenced by score-line states in completely different ways.

The current investigation has found that differences in % time spent performing HI activity between score-line states were no greater than normal within-match variability in soccer performance. Further research is needed to explore score-line effect on work-rate controlling for stoppage time. O'Donoghue and Parker (2002) found that the ball was in play for 55 minutes of 90 minute soccer matches. The current investigation has limitations due to the low number of players included, differing group sizes being used and limited reliability of human classification of player movement during live observation. Furthermore, stoppage time within matches was not controlled for and may have differed between score-line states for some players. As player tracking technology improves there will be further opportunities to exploit such systems in the investigation of player work-rate in general and score-line effect in particular.

## References

Bandura, A., 1977, Self-efficacy: Toward a unifying theory of behavioural change. *Psychology Review*, **84**, 191–215.

Bloomfield, J. *et al.*, 2004a, Effects of score-line on match performance in FA Premier League Soccer. *J Sports Sci*, **23**, 192–193.

Bloomfield, J. *et al.*, 2004b, Effects of score-line on work-rate in midfield and forward players in FA Premier League Soccer, *J Sports Sci*, **23**, 191–192.

Clark, P., 2010, Intermittent high intensity activity in English FA Premier League soccer. *Int J Perf Analysis Sport*, **10**, 139–151.

Feltz, D.L., 1992, Understanding motivation in sport: A self-efficacy perspective. In *Motivation in Sport and Exercise*, Champaign, IL: Human Kinetics Publishers, pp. 93–106.

Huey, A. *et al.*, 2001, From time-motion analysis specific intermittent high intensity training. In *Pass.com (Performance Analysis, Sports Science and Computers)*, Cardiff: CPA UWIC Press, pp. 29–34.

Jones, P.D. *et al.*, 2004, Possession as a performance indicator in soccer. *Int J Perf Analysis Sport*, **4**, 98–102.

Lago, C. and Martin, C., 2007, Determinants of possession of the ball in soccer. *J Sports Sci*, **25**, 969–974.

McAuley, E., 1992, Self-referent thought in sport and physical activity. In *Advances in Sport Psychology*, Champaign, IL: Human Kinetics Publishers, pp. 101–118.

McStravick, L. and O'Donoghue, P.G., 2001, The effect of score-line on performance: A time-motion and sports psychology investigation in Irish League soccer, *Exercise and Sports Science Association of Ireland Annual Conference*, Carlow, 27th April 2001.

O'Donoghue, P., 1998, The CAPTAIN (Computerised All-Purpose Time-motion Analysis INtegrated). In *Notational Analysis of Sport IV*, Porto: University of Porto, pp. 213–219.

O'Donoghue, P.G. and Parker, D., 2002, Time-motion analysis of FA Premier League soccer competition, *J Sports Sci*, **20**, 26.

O'Donoghue, P.G. and Tenga. A., 2001, The effect of score-line on work rate in elite soccer. *J Sports Sci*, **19**, 25–26.

Redwood-Brown, A. *et al.*, 2009, The interaction effect of positional role and score-line on work-rate in FA Premier League soccer, 3rd ISPAS International Workshop, Lincoln, UK, 6–7 April.

Shaw, J. and O'Donoghue, P.G., 2004, The effect of score-line on work rate in amateur soccer. In *Performance Analysis of Sport 6*, Cardiff: CPA UWIC Press, pp. 84–91.

Taylor, J.B. *et al.*, 2008, The influence of match location, quality of opposition, and match status on technical performance in professional association football. *J Sports Sci*, **26**, 885–895.

# CHAPTER TWENTY-EIGHT

# Addressing opposition quality in rugby league performance

A. Cullinane and P. O'Donoghue

Centre for Performance Analysis, Cardiff School of Sport,
University of Wales Institute Cardiff, Wales, UK

## 1. INTRODUCTION

In a review of research across the football codes, Reilly and Gilbourne (2003) drew attention to a dearth of literature in Rugby Football League. Soccer and rugby union still continue to dominate performance analysis research in the football codes with the exception of work from Eaves and Broad (2007), Eaves and Evers (2007) and Eaves et al. (2008). The current research stems from performance analysis support for a rugby league side and the desire for profiles of performances that could be evaluated taking into account opposition quality.

There have been three main profiling techniques developed in performance analysis; one using quantiles (O'Donoghue, 2005), one using 95% confidence interval for medians (James et al., 2005), and a third technique using separate norms for matches against different strengths of opponents (O'Donoghue et al., 2008). The techniques of O'Donoghue (2005) and James et al. (2005) both represent typical performance and the spread of performances about this typical performance. It is important to represent the spread of performances for a team or individual as sports performance indicators are not stable characteristics of performers. There are many sources of variation in sports performance with opposition effect being the largest source of variability (McGarry and Franks, 1994). The techniques of O'Donoghue (2005) and James et al. (2005) are suitable for profiles of performers using data from a representative series of matches. However, they are not suitable for the interpretation of individual performers because performance indicator values influenced by strong opponents will simply be confirmed as below average. Therefore, O'Donoghue et al. (2008) proposed classifying teams into groupings based on league position or World ranking so that different norms could be used to interpret performance in matches against opponents of different strengths However, a criticism of O'Donoghue et al.'s (2008) technique is that teams within broad groups (for example, top half of the league and bottom half of the league) are assumed to be of a similar quality. In many sports, there is a smoother increase in team quality as we go from the bottom of the league to the top. Therefore, the interpretation of performance would benefit from a finer grain approach to representing opposition quality.

The purpose of the current investigation was to develop a profiling technique where regression is used to determine expected performance indicator values for matches against opponents of given qualities. The technique would be applied to rugby league data and have applications in evaluating individual matches, producing profiles for teams and analysing trends in performance.

## 2. THE REGRESSION BASED APPROACH TO PROFILING

The approach to interpreting performance indicators uses the following 6 steps:

1. Determine a measure of quality for a performer; this could be World ranking, best time/distance or points within a league table, for example.
2. Determine whether there is a relationship between performance indicators and relative quality of the performers involved in matches. Relative quality is the difference in the quality measure between the performers involved in a match. The remaining steps only apply to those performance indicators related to relative quality.
3. Determine an equation for any relationship. This will give an expected value for a performance indicator in a match between the given performers.
4. Determine the distribution of the residual values used to create the model for the expected performance indicator value. The residuals represent how much better or worse a performer did than expected given the quality of opponent.
5. To interpret a given performance, compare each performance indicator value with the expected value given the relative quality between the performer and the opponent. The difference between observed and expected value can be assessed using the known distribution of residuals for the performance indicator to give a percentage score. For example, if residuals are normally distributed, the z-score for the residual for the given match is mapped onto a probability. Multiplying this probability by 100% gives a percentage of similar performances that have been exceeded by the performer given the quality of opposition.
6. There will be a percentage score for each performance the approach can be applied to. These performance indicators and their corresponding percentage scores are included within a performance profile for the match.

## 3. METHODS

A computerised match analysis system was developed for a rugby league squad using Sportscode Elite version 8 (Sportstec, Warriewood, Australia). The system produced a set of 57 performance indicators. An intra-operator reliability study revealed a very good strength of agreement between independent observations for all variables ($k > 0.8$). Twenty matches played by the rugby league squad during the 2010 season were analysed. The current paper focuses on five performance indicators: possession time, clean breaks, attacking errors, completed set from own 40m (Exit Set) and tries. All of these except tries are defined in Table 1.

**Table 1** Operational definitions.

| Term | Operational Definition |
|------|------------------------|
| *Possession* | When a team has control of the ball in an attacking or defensive situation. |
| *Tackle Set* | From each possession a team has 6 tackles within a tackle set to attempt to score. |
| *Completed Set* | Any occasion the team has ended a tackle set by choosing to kick the ball away on their own terms (on or before the 6th tackle). Also it is deemed a completed set if a try is scored or a penalty is awarded at any point during the 'tackle set'. |
| *Completed Set Own 40m (Exit Set)* | A completed set that begins in the team's own 40m zone. |
| *Attacking Error* | Any error while in possession of the ball; this can include a knock on, intercepted pass or a kicking error (i.e., out on the full). |
| *Clean Break* | When a player breaks through the defensive line. |

Performance indicators were determined by the system implemented in Sportscode and transferred into a Microsoft Excel (Microsoft Inc., Redmond, Washington) to apply the profiling technique described in section 2. The indicator of team quality used was league points accumulated at the end of the season. The relative quality between two teams within a match was, therefore, the difference between their league table points.

The absolute correlations for possession time (r=.503), clean breaks (r=.517), attacking errors (r=.521), completed set within own 40m (r=.488) and tries (r=.661) were high enough for a regression model to be produced for each in terms of relative quality (RQ). In each case an equation of the form $PI_{Exp} = a + b \times RQ$ was produced for the expected value of the performance indicator. The residual values for a performance indicator had a mean of 0.0 and a standard deviation, $SD_{Res}$, that could be used to produce a z-score for an observed value of a performance indicator, $PI_{Obs}$ ($z = (PI_{Obs} - PI_{Exp}) / SD_{Res}$). The percentage evaluation score, %ES was calculated using the probability distribution of the standard normal distribution; %ES = 100 x NORMDIST(z).

## 4. RESULTS

Figure 1 shows the relationship between possession time, PT, and relative quality, RQ. The regression line represents the expected value given the relative quality between the two teams within a match. Any points above the line are where a team had more possession than expected given the quality of opposition and any points below the line are where a team had less possession than expected given the quality of opposition.

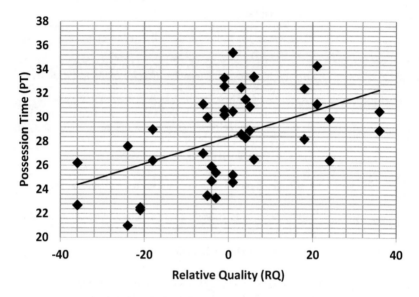

**Figure 1** Relationship between relative quality and possession time.

## 5. USES OF THE PERCENTAGE EVALUATION SCORE (%ES)

The percentage evaluation score can be used to evaluate the performances of a team and their opponents in a single match (Table 2). The same actual value for a given performance indicator does not always map onto the same evaluation score. This is because the technique takes into account the quality of the opposition. This information could be provided as a table (like Table 2) or in graphical form.

A second use of the %ES is to characterise a team's typical performance and consistency of performance over a series of matches. This is a profiling technique that represents performance as a series of relevant variables. Figure 2 shows an example of a profile for the team who participated in the current study. This profile combines the strengths of the methods of O'Donoghue (2005) and James *et al.* (2005), while also addressing the quality of opposition during performance evaluation. In the case of the team participating in the current investigation, their strongest area was clean breaks, while possession time was consistently low. Completed sets from there own 40m were the most consistent area of performance and clean breaks were the most inconsistent area. The technique can also be used to plot a single performance indicator over a series of matches giving a performance trend, which addresses opposition quality.

**Table 2** Summary of PI values and corresponding %ES scores for a match.

|                      | Team         |      | Opponents    |      |
| -------------------- | ------------ | ---- | ------------ | ---- |
|                      | Actual value | %ES  | Actual value | %ES  |
| Possession Time      | 30.5         | 74.6 | 32.6         | 92.0 |
| Clean Break          | 6            | 82.8 | 2            | 25.8 |
| Try                  | 3            | 20.8 | 3            | 23.9 |
| Comp Sets Own 40m    | 21           | 68.0 | 18           | 32.5 |
| Attacking Errors     | 7            | 63.3 | 10           | 8.2  |

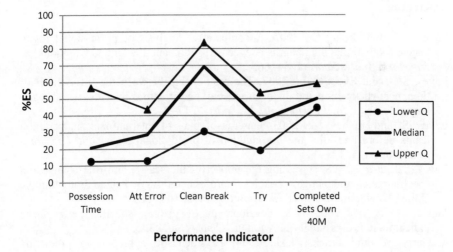

**Figure 2** A team profile over the 2009–10 season.

## 6. DISCUSSION AND CONCLUSIONS

The relationships between relative quality and performance indicators in the current investigation were linear with residual values being normally distributed. However, the approach described here is not restricted to such relationships and can be applied to curvilinear relationships between relative quality and performance indicators. Where residuals are not normally distributed, it is necessary to transform them so as they are approximately normal to permit a valid %ES to be determined. A further issue is that the distribution of residual values maybe heteroscedastistic, with greater variance for higher values of relative quality. If this is the case then a function needs to be devised for the standard deviation of the residuals in terms of relative quality. It is important to recognise that there are some performance indicators that are unrelated to opposition quality, as different tactical styles of play may exist throughout the rankings of rugby league teams. The approach described here should be combined with existing methods of analysing those performance indicators where there is no relationship with relative quality. The technique can be applied in a coaching context allowing performance indicators to be evaluated in real-terms addressing opposition quality.

The proposed technique, which considers opposition strength, has clear advantages over previous profiling methods devised by O'Donoghue (2005) and James *et al.* (2005). Coupled with this, the recognition of a smoother transition between opposition quality, when considering a league/ranking structure (compared to that assumed by O'Donoghue *et al.,* 2008) allowed for a more effective interpretation of performances.

## References

Eaves, S.J. and Broad, G., 2007, A comparative analysis of professional rugby league football playing patterns between Australia and the United Kingdom. *Int J Perform Analys Sport*, **7**, 54–66.

Eaves, S. J. and Evers, A.L., 2007, The relationship between the 'play the ball' time, post-ruck action and the occurrence of perturbations in professional rugby league football. *Int J Perform Analys Sport*, **7**, 17–24.

Eaves, S. and Hughes, M., 2003, Patterns of play of international rugby union teams before and after the introduction of professional status. *Int J Perform Analys Sport*, **3**, 103–111.

Eaves, S.J. *et al.*, 2008, Assessing the impact of the season and rule changes on specific match and tactical variables in professional rugby league football in the United Kingdom. *Int J Perform Analys Sport*, **8**, 104–118.

James, N. *et al.*, 2005, The development of position-specific performance indicators in professional rugby union. *J Sports Sci*, **23**, 63–72.

McGarry, T. and Franks, I.M., 1994, A stochastic approach to predicting competition squash match-play. *J Sports Sci*, **12**, 573–584.

O'Donoghue, P., 2005, Normative profiles of sports performance. *Int J Perform Analys Sport*, **5**, 104–119.

O'Donoghue, P. *et al.*, 2008, Performance norms for British National Super League netball. *Int J Sports Sci Coaching*, **3**, 501–511.

Reilly, T. and Gilbourne, D., 2003, Science and football: A review of applied research in the football codes. *J Sports Sci*, **21**, 693–705.

# CHAPTER TWENTY-NINE

# A method for game analysis based on dominant region

T. Taki and J. Hasegawa

School of Life System Science and Technology, Chukyo University, Japan

## 1. INTRODUCTION

In any football game, space management by players is one of the most important factors to exercise control over the game. In game analysis, the amount of player space and its location, in addition to its changing characteristics throughout the game are essential information. However, there are few methods to obtain such data regarding player space quantitatively and visually. Therefore, an automated system for analysing and quantifying this space from video sequences has been identified as necessary.

In this paper, we describe novel methods for extracting quantitative information about this space from video sequences and for analysing a game utilising the extracted results. Those methods are based on the concept of 'dominant region' (Taki and Hasegawa, 2000) and a new measure called 'time occupancy rate'. Also, the results of an analysis of an actual game using these methods are presented, and the effectiveness of our system is demonstrated.

## 2. DOMINANT REGION

The immediate region around any given player can be considered a kind of sphere of potential influence of that player. Generally, given a set of points in a space, the spatial territory of each point can be expressed by the Voronoi region (Okabe *et al.*, 1992). In actual games, the player's sphere of influence is changed according to the direction and speed of their movements. This change can be observed through frame by frame video analysis. Therefore, the sphere of influence is formulated by replacing the distance function of the Voronoi region with a time function. We call this the 'dominant region'. The dominant region of a player is defined as a region where the player can arrive earlier than any other players, on condition that the player moves at their maximal speed. Also, the physical ability of each player can be reflected by the dominant regions. Figure 1 shows an example of the changes of dominant regions in a case where a player receives the ball behind an opponent player with a checking run. In the Figures 1(a) to 1(f), the background shows the dominant region of each player, and each dominant region is distinguished by different colours. We can easily observe that player A will be able to receive the ball, because the space behind player B is becoming the dominant region of player A.

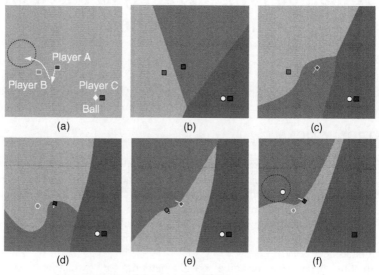

(a) movements of players and a ball
(b) initial position
(c) player A moves to the lower-left (checking run)
(d) player B also moves to the same direction
(e) player A turns in direction and moves behind player B
(f) player A receives the ball

**Figure 1** Transition of the player's positions and their dominant regions.

## 3. METHODS

Initially, player's positions and velocities are estimated from a video sequence. Subsequently, the dominant region for each player or each team is computed frame by frame. We regard every dominant region with a size larger than a given threshold as a 'space'. Furthermore, we compute a 'time occupancy rate' for representing a superiority or inferiority ranking of each player or each team. The dominant regions show the superiority level for a certain frame, while the time occupancy rate image can be regarded as a map of superiority for a specified time period of a game. The time occupancy rate is calculated from the ratio of the dominant regions for each point of the pitch from a sequence of dominant regions. For example, if a team dominates a certain place for a total of six minutes against a specified ten minutes in a game, the place becomes 60% occupation of the team.

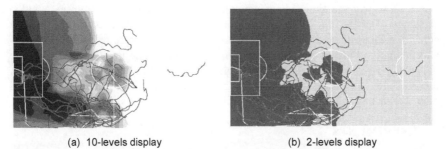

(a) 10-levels display     (b) 2-levels display

**Figure 2** An example of time occupancy rate image.

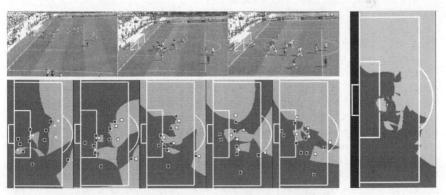

**Figure 3** Time variation of the team dominant regions and the time occupancy rate in the case of scoring a goal from a throw in.

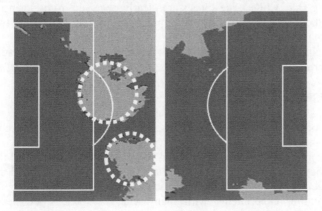

**Figure 4** Comparison between the time occupancy rate images for 45 minutes.

Figure 2 shows the time occupancy rate of each team obtained from a video sequence of about 22s. In this scene, the right end team attacked toward the left side from kick-off, and then finally scored a goal. The trajectories of all players and the ball are also displayed on the image. The left side image shows the time occupancy rate by 10-levels, and the right side image shows it by 2-levels. From these images, we can easily determine the areas on the pitch where an individual player or team has been superior or inferior in comparison to the opposition.

## 4. EXPERIMENTS

Using the proposed method, we endeavoured to extract the superior or inferior regions for each team from video sequences in 6 games including the 2006 FIFA World Cup, the English Premier League and the Japan Professional Football League. In these cases, the positions of each player and a ball are manually inputted at 30Hz from recorded media.

In Figure 3, we show an example of the video sequence in the upper left, the changes of team dominant regions in the lower left, and the time occupancy rate image represented by 2-levels in the right, respectively. In this scene, the attacking team threw in a ball from the left side to the front of the goal, attacked the dropped ball and finally scored a goal. We found that the defending team allowed a shooting space around the penalty spot in spite of numerical superiority from these images. Furthermore, we generated the time occupancy rate image for 45 minutes. From this image two very interesting spaces were obtained and visualised. Those results are shown by circles in the left side of Figure 4. In the figure, the dark colour area means the region having more than 50% of the time occupancy rate, with the left and right figures showing the losing and winning sides, respectively. From this result, we could observe that there is little space around the penalty area of the winning side, while large spaces are clearly observed in the losing side. In fact, both of these spaces were the starting point of attacking moves and two goals were made from them.

In the experiments using other video sequences, some similar results were obtained. Therefore, the effectiveness of the time occupancy rate was confirmed.

## 5. CONCLUSION

A novel method for game analysis based on a space using the dominant region was proposed. In the experiments with several video sequences, it was shown that the superiority or inferiority of each team could be quantified and visualised using the time occupancy rate image. The basic ideas and methods described here are applicable to other football competitions such as rugby, American football and so on. In the future, experiments with many video sequences are needed for evaluating the proposed system.

At present we only have some limited data sets. However, if many full data sets become available, it may be possible to make a comparison not only between both teams in a certain game, but also between two games, or to extract the characteristics of extended team tactics.

## References

Okabe, A. *et al.*, 1992, *Spatial Tessellations Concepts and Applications of Voronoi Diagrams*. New York: John Wiley & Sons.

Taki, T. and Hasegawa, J., 2000, Group motion analysis in team sports. In *Proceedings of the 4th Asian Conference on Computer Vision (ACCV2000)*, pp. 693–698.

# CHAPTER THIRTY

# Do attacking game patterns differ between first and second halves of soccer matches in the 2010 FIFA World Cup?

D. Barreira[1,2], J. Garganta[1,2], T. Pinto[1], J. Valente[1] and T. Anguera[3]

[1]Centre of Research, Education, Innovation and Intervention in Sport, Portugal
[2]Faculty of Sport, University of Porto, Portugal
[3]Faculty of Psychology, University of Barcelona, Spain

## 1. INTRODUCTION

Soccer is a 'goals game' (Hughes and Bartlett, 2002). In World Cups and European Championships—competitions that showcase the best players, coaches, and strategies, country-specific cultures, and the utmost prestige of the victory—goal patterns have been detected by quantitative (Hughes and Franks, 2005) and qualitative (Barreira et al., 2011) analysis methods. World Cup statistics point out that the average number of goals scored per game has been decreasing, with an average reduction of 1.66 goals per game, from Uruguay 1930 to Germany 2006. Because the number of goals per game is too small and the identification of statistical differences remains difficult, most studies consider shots and time of ball possession as key performance indicators (Hughes and Bartlett, 2002). The observation of game patterns provide relevant information about how the teams manage the different phases and moments of the game (Garganta, 2009). Game patterns vary according to multiple variables including match status (Barreira et al., 2011), type of competition, time gap between tournaments (Castellano et al., 2009), the country's soccer culture, and elapsed playing time. However, there is a lack of research concerning the player's behaviour in each half of the match. In the current study differences in attacking play patterns between the two halves of World Cup (WC) 2010 matches were reported.

## 2. METHODS

Two teams were followed continuously in each match. A follow-up, nomothetic and multidimensional mixed design (lag-log) was carried out (for further details, see Blanco et al., 2003). Seven WC 2010 play-off matches (from quarter-final to final phase) were observed and reported the respective data. A total of 14 observations were performed (956 offensive sequences) with an average of 137 attacks per game. Matches were observed and analysed in the regular time (i.e., 90mins, excluding extra time). The offensive sequences in which players left the camera's recording field and those during which the team was playing with ten elements or less, were excluded. Offensive sequences comprised 485 attacks, 5389 multi-events, and 20,683 events (first half); and 471 attacks, 5085 multi-events, and 19,734 events (second half). Sequential order was used to describe the matches' occurrences evolution.

Observational instrument guidelines have been used elsewhere (Barreira *et al.*, 2011; Barreira *et al.*, 2010) and follow the Organization Model of the Soccer Game proposed by Barreira *et al.* (2011). This model encompasses the offensive and defensive phases of the game, including the transitions, and afford two types of transition: interphase, when an indirect ball recovery is observed—game interruption by infraction or by the sending of the ball out of the field, and state, when the ball recovery is direct—the dynamic of the game is preserved, with no interruptions, and a player performs at least three consecutive touches of the ball, a positive pass, or shoots to the opponent's goal (Garganta, 1997) or the goalkeeper controls the ball (Castellano, 2000).

The instrument includes 80 categories concerning seven criteria: a) Start of the offensive phase (BR); b) Development of defence/attack transition state (DT); c) Progress of ball possession (DP); d) Finishing of the offensive phase (F); e) Patterns of field space position (adapted from Garganta, 1997); f) Centre of the game/ball position; and g) Spatial patterns of interaction between teams, including the position of the players holding the ball and relative to the opponents (adapted from Castellano, 2000). The first four criteria correspond to game behaviours; the fifth, is a structural criterion, dividing the field into 12 zones (adapted from Garganta, 1997); the sixth and seventh, embody the interactional contexts. Structural and interactional criteria comply with the conditions of exhaustiveness and mutual exclusivity.

Inter-observer reliability was determined by calculating Cohen's Kappa during the first half of the WC 2010 final match (Netherlands versus Spain). Values of $0.88 < k < 0.98$ were found using the SDIS-GSEQ software (v4.2.0, Bakeman and Quera, 1995). These values ensure the highest data quality, in accordance with the $k \geq 0.75$ suggested by Bakeman and Gottman (1997). SoccerEye software (Barreira *et al.*, 2010) reduces both time spent in the registration process and errors when compared with the hand-notation system. The observer categorizes match status, competition phase and match time. SoccerEye is congruent to the SDIS-GSEQ software language (Bakeman and Quera, 1995).

Data were submitted to inferential and sequential analyses. Inferential statistics—Mann-Whitney and Wilcoxon tests—was used to calculate the average occurrence of behaviour types of finishing the attack (criterion 4), in each half of the WC 2010 play-off matches. Sequential analysis provides the probability to find significant associations (positive and negative) between different events in a match. The strength of the relations between the behaviours and their sequence is determined based on the Z value (for details, see Quera and Bakeman, 2000). Attacking sequences were analysed using the SDIS-GSEQ, version 4.2.0. The conventional rules used by Sackett (1979) to determine the max-lag of behaviour patterns were not followed.

## 3. RESULTS AND DISCUSSION

The average of goals per match in WC 2010 was 2.27 which confirms the decreased number of goals scored in WC 2006, reported by Castellano *et al.* (2009). In our study, the number of goals observed in the second half (n=11, 0.4±0.5) doubled that observed in the first half (n=5, 0.8±1.0). These values do not agree with the WC overall statistics because they refer to matches taking place from the quarter-final to the final phase only. Additionally, the teams performed a higher number of attacks during the first half, compared with the second half (485 vs. 471, respectively), yet not significantly so (Table 1). On the other hand, in EURO 2008, the occurrence, on average, of unsuccessful attacking behaviours between the two halves was significantly different (Table 1). So, the loss of ball possession by the intervention of the opponent goalkeeper—Fgk—was significantly lower (p=0.009) in the second half but the opposite occurred in the first half regarding ball recovery by the opponent's violation of the laws of the game—Fi (p=0.048). When comparing each half of both competitions, the average of unsuccessful attacks was significantly different. The loss of ball possession through error by the ball carrier or the defender intervention—Fed, and by throwing the ball out of the pitch—Fo—were significantly higher in WC 2010, whereas the ball loss by the intervention of the opponent goalkeeper was significantly lower than in EURO 2008. Overall, match behaviours during the WC 2010 were similar between the two halves of each match (p>0.05).

Retrospective sequential analysis provides a mirror image to find how the behaviours preceding the criterion behaviour maintain a stable relationship with the others and, consequently, also with the actions preceding the final event. Five negative lags that preceded the end of the attack were considered to show whether the association between the behaviours is statistically significant or non-significant (Anguera *et al.*, 2003). To determine the associations with 95% of certainty, $z \geq 1.96$ and $p \leq 0.05$ were considered. Table 2 summarizes the behavioural patterns concerning the attack performance. Shots on target occurred predominantly in the defence/attack transition, contrary to EURO 2008 (Barreira *et al.*, 2010). In the first half, positive short passes were performed in mid-area of the observed team into the opponent's backward area, and a shot on target was performed in the left offensive zone. In the second half, after ball recovery by tackle ($z=3.55$) in defensive (2: $z=2.07$) or mid-defensive zones (6: $z=2.07$), a long pass during the defence/attack transition was performed ($z=2.00$). Therefore, the ball was received and controlled with no constraints ($z=2.52$), and shot from the right mid-offensive zone ($z=2.00$). Nevertheless, in the first half, shots on target occurred mostly from the opposite lateral offensive zone (10: $z=2.63$). While in WC 2010 the lateral wings were the most used to perform shots on target, in EURO 2008, the central offensive zone, in contexts of attacker(s) against goalkeeper ($z=6.67$), was the most frequent (Barreira *et al.*, 2011). Shots stopped by the opponent with no continuation of ball possession occurred predominantly during the progress of ball possession, probably because the opponent team was defensively organized. In the second half, shots were performed from between the mid area of the observed and the opponent teams ($z=1.97$) with no constraints ($z=2.30$). Goals scored in the first half showed a higher probability to be preceded by a positive long pass followed by ball carriage ($z=1.98$) or dribble ($z=1.98$), carrying the centre of the game from lateral mid-offensive (7: $z=2.42$) to lateral offensive zones and ultimately leading to situations of 1×goalkeeper ($z=1.96$). In the second half, negative short passes on zone 10 led to positive crossing in the same zone with no constraints. Then, crosses or assistances ($z=2.44$) were held from lateral offensive zones and goals were scored in the same spatial pattern of the team's interaction ($z=3.30$), as observed in the first half. Similar goal patterns were found in EURO 2008 play-off matches (*idem*, 2011). All in all, despite lack of quantitative statistical significant differences in finishing of attacking behaviours, the sequential facet showed that successful attacking patterns differ significantly from first to second halves in WC 2010 matches.

**Table 1** Comparison between first and second halves of WC 2010 play-off matches according to the types of finishing the attack; and between EURO 2008[1] and WC 2010 play-off matches regarding first and second halves and the types of finishing the attack. Values are mean±SD.

| | | EURO 2008[1] | | | WORLD CUP 2010 | | |
|---|---|---|---|---|---|---|---|
| | | 1st half | 2nd half | p | 1st half | 2nd half | p |
| Successful attack | Fws | 2.4±1.8 | 3.8±2.5* | 0.006 | 2.3±1.5 | 2.7±1.9 | 0.420 |
| | Fst | 1.2±1.3 | 1.5±1.3 | 0.510 | 0.9±0.9 | 1.1±1.1 | 0.470 |
| | Fso | 0.4±0.7 | 0.3±0.6 | 0.589 | 0.2±0.4 | 0.5±0.8 | 0.271 |
| | Fgl | 0.4±0.7 | 0.8±0.9 | 0.157 | 0.4±0.5 | 0.8±1.0 | 0.107 |
| Unsuccessful attack | Fed | 17.0±4.3 | 17.7±4.3 | 0.593 | 23.2±5.4[#] | 21.5±5.2 | 0.194 |
| | Fgk | 2.7±1.8 | 1.4±1.4* | 0.009 | 1.1±1.7[#] | 1.1±1.6 | 0.957 |
| | Fo | 1.8±1.9 | 2.0±2.7 | 0.671 | 3.9±2.7[#] | 3.7±3.6 | 0.858 |
| | Fi | 1.8±1.2 | 2.9±2.3* | 0.048 | 2.6±1.3 | 2.3±1.8 | 0.386 |

Fws: Wide shot; Fst: Shot on target; Fso: Shot stopped by the opponent with no continuation of ball possession; Fgl: goal scored. *Significantly different from first half in the same competition, $p \leq 0.05$, using Wilcoxon test [#]Significantly different from the same half in EURO 2008, $p \leq 0.05$, using Mann–Whitney test[1] Data from Barreira *et al.* (2011)

## 4. CONCLUSIONS

Although the attacking behaviours during WC 2010 proved to be quantitatively similar in both halves of the matches, sequential analysis showed differences in successful attacking patterns, including goal scoring patterns. These findings suggests that it seems relevant to consider the sequential facet of the performance when analyzing the attacking tactical behaviour in soccer.

**Table 2** Obtained adjusted residuals (z), to a p-value<0.05 according a retrospective perspective, World Cup 2010.

| Lag -5 | Lag -4 | Lag -3 | Lag -2 | Lag -1 | Lag 0 | |
|---|---|---|---|---|---|---|
| 12 (2.00) EB (2.32) | Pr (1.96) | — | — | DPpcr (2.06) 12 (2.61) | ---- | Fws 1$^{st}$hf |
| 8 (2.03) | — | — | — | — | — | Fws 2$^{nd}$hf |
| DTnlp (2.05) / DTbc (2.02) 5 (2.41) | DTpsp (2.02) / DPd (1.97) | MB (1.99) | — | — | 10 (2.63) | Fst 1$^{st}$hf |
| BRt (3.55) / DPe (2.02) 2 (2.07) / 6 (2.07) Pa (2.08) / BF (2.95) | DTplp (2.00) 6 (2.00) | DTrb (2.75) | DTpsp (3.40) | DTbc (2.21) NPa (2.52) | 9 (2.00) | Fst 2$^{nd}$hf |
| DPi (3.83) | DTplp (3.91) / DPti (2.61) | DTbc (2.06) / DPncr (2.06) | DPi (4.00) 11 (2.71) | DPbc (3.26) | — | Fso 1$^{st}$hf |
| BRt (2.90) / BRgk (2.90) / DPnlp (2.90) | 2 (3.00) / 7 (3.02) NPa (3.00) BF (3.00) | DPpcr (3.02) 7 (2,50) | DPr (2.75) 1 (3.02) NPa (2.26) | — | NPr (2.30) MM (1.97) | Fso 2$^{nd}$hf |
| BRi (2.90) NPr (3.49) BF (3.06) | DPrb (3.29) 5 (1.96) / 6 (2.96) NPe (2.16) | DPplp (3.03) | NPe (2.05) | DTrb (1.98)/ DPplp (3.10)/DPd (1.98) 7 (2.42) | 7 (1.98) FE (1.96) | Fgl 1$^{st}$hf |
| DPd (2.36) 10 (1.98) / EB (2.11) | DPrb (2.31) | DTnlp (2.33) NPr (2.74) | DPnsp (2.33) 10 (2.54) | DPpcr (2.44) NPe (2.35) / FE (2.48) | FE (3.30) | Fgl 2$^{nd}$hf |

BRi: Ball recovery (BR) by the interception; BRt: BR by tackle; BRgk: BR by the intervention of the goalkeeper in defensive phase; BRt: BR by a defensive behaviour followed by transmission; DTnlp: Development of defence/attack transition state (DT) by negative long passing; DTbc: DT by ball control; DTpsp: DT by positive short passing; DTplp: DT by positive long passing; DTrb: DT by running with the ball; DTbc: DT by ball control; DPpcr: Progress of ball possession (DP) by positive crossing; DPd: DP by dribbling (1x1); DPc: DP by corner kick; DPpsp: DP by positive short passing; DPi: DP by violation to the laws of the game; DPnsp: DP by negative short passing; DPti: DP by throw-in; DPncr: DP by negative crossing; DPrb: DP by running with the ball; DPbc: DP by ball control; DPs: DP by shooting; DPplp: DP by positive long passing; DPnlp: DP by negative long passing; 1: left defensive zone; 2: central defensive zone; 5: central mid-defensive zone; 6: right mid-defensive zone; 7: left mid-offensive zone; 8: central mid-offensive zone; 9: right mid-offensive zone; 10: left offensive zone; 11: central offensive zone; 12: right offensive zone; NPa: Absolute numerical superiority; NPr: Relative numerical superiority; NPe: No pressure in numerical equality; Pr: Relative numerical inferiority; Pa: Absolute numerical inferiority; BF: Ball is located (BL) between the backward area of the observed team and the opponent forward area; EB: BL between the exterior area of the observed team and the opponent backward area; EF: BL between the empty area of the observed team and the opponent forward area; MB: BL between the mid area of the observed team and the opponent backward area; FE: BL between the forward area of the observed team and the opponent empty area; MM: BL between the mid area of the observed and the opponent teams.

# References

Anguera, M.T. *et al.*, 2003, Evaluating links intensity in social networks in a school context through observational designs. In *Culture, Environmental Action Sustainability*, Göttingen: H & H, pp. 286–298.

Bakeman, R. *et al.*, 1997, *Observing Interaction: An Introduction to Sequential Analysis* (2nd ed.). Cambridge, UK: University Press.

Bakeman, R. *et al.*, 1995, *Analyzing Interaction: Sequential Analysis with SDIS and GSEQ.* Cambridge, UK: Cambridge University Press.

Barreira, D. *et al.*, 2010, Attacking game-patterns in soccer. A sequential analysis of European Championship 2008. Paper presented at the IV European Congress of Methodology: EAM-SMABS 2010, Potsdam, Germany.

Barreira, D. *et al.*, 2011, In search of nexus between attacking game-patterns, momentaneous score and type of ball recovery in European Soccer Championship 2008. In M. Hughes *et al.*, *Research Methods and Performance Analysis*, Szombathely, Hungary, pp. 226–237.

Blanco, A. *et al.*, 2003, Data analysis techniques in observational designs applied to the environment-behaviour relation. *Med Amb Comp Hum*, **4**, 111–126.

Castellano, J., 2000, *Observación y análisis de la acción de juego en el fútbol.* (Tesis Doctoral), Universidad del País Vasco.

Castellano, J. *et al.*, 2009, Has soccer changed in the last three World Cups? In *Science and Football VI*, London: Routledge, pp. 167–170.

Garganta, J., 1997, *Modelação táctica do jogo de Futebol. Estudo da organização da fase ofensiva em equipas de alto rendimento [Tactical modelling of Soccer game].* (Dissertação de Doutoramento), FCDEF-UP, Porto.

Garganta, J., 2009, Trends of tactical performance analysis in team sports: Bridging the gap between research, training and competition. *Revista Portuguesa de Ciências do Desporto*, **9**, 81–89.

Hughes, M. *et al.*, 2002, The use of performance indicators in performance analysis. *J Sports Sci*, **20**, 739–754.

Hughes, M. and Franks, I., 2005, Analysis of passing sequences, shots and goals in soccer. *J Sports Sci*, **23**, 509–514.

Quera, V. and Bakeman, R., 2000, GSEQ for Windows: New software for the sequential analysis of behavioral data, with an interface to the observer, *3rd Int Conf Methods and Techniques in Behavioral Research.* Nijmegen, Netherlands.

Sackett, G.P., 1979, The lag sequential analysis of contingency and cyclicity in behavioural interaction research. In *Handbook of Infant Development*, New York: Wiley, pp. 623–649.

# CHAPTER THIRTY-ONE

# The relationship between (GPS) match activity profile and performance in the AFL

J. Heasman[1], B. Dawson[1,2], G. Stewart[2] and B. Lay[1]

[1]School of Sports Science, Exercise and Health, University of Western Australia, Perth, Australia, [2]West Coast Eagles Football Club, Australia

## 1. INTRODUCTION

Many studies that have used Global Positioning System (GPS) technology have investigated its validity and reliability for use in team sports. These studies (Coutts and Duffield, 2010; Petersen *et al.*, 2009) suggest distance based measures should predominantly be used to monitor individual player workloads and intensities and that high speed running variables should be based on broad (rather than narrow) speed zone categories. Further, quantifying acceleration with current GPS technology was not supported, as the noted errors were high. No study has yet tracked individual player movement-pattern profiles within a single Australian Football League (AFL) team in relation to performance over the course of multiple seasons. This study aimed to identify the most relevant GPS match activity variables to individual performance. By better understanding the relationship between GPS derived match activity profiles and player performance, sports science staff may be able to streamline GPS use and provide more meaningful information for coaches and players.

## 2. METHODS

Due to variations in the number of GPS units available, and restrictions on the number of players able to wear GPS, the methodology varied slightly over the course of the study period. Between 10 and 22 players from one AFL team wore GPS in each game of the 2009 and 2010 AFL seasons. Each player was allocated to one of two positional zones (free-roaming or stationary) to allow for inter-positional and intra-positional comparisons.

To rate performance, possessions gained per minute of game time were recorded and objective player impact scores were produced by using a formula, previously developed and validated for use in Australian football (Heasman *et al.*, 2008), into Champion Integrated Software (CIS). The CIS is a commercial statistical analysis program which provides sophisticated player and team data on

AFL games. Individual player impact scores were produced within CIS by multiplying the frequency of selected game actions by allocated positive and negative numerical values. Derived scores were produced by dividing the total impact scores of players by the number of minutes they played.

Participants were fitted with 5-Hz SPI-Pro GPS units by sports science staff just prior to game commencement, being positioned on the upper back, above legal tackling height in Australian football using a sports-specific protective harness. GPS data in the breaks between quarters and interchange periods was omitted from analysis. After game completion, data was downloaded to a customised computer GPS analysis program (GPSports Systems TEAM AMS), which allows player match activity profiles to be analysed. Over the course of the study different variables were of interest to the AFL club involved. Therefore, there were some variations in the variables analysed. Table 1 below presents the variables that were tracked each year.

**Table 1** GPS variables analysed in the 2009 & 2010 AFL seasons.

| Year | GPS Variables |
|------|---------------|
| 2009 | Distance, distance/minute, distance/minute > 60% max speed, distance/minute > 75% max speed, distance/minute > 25 km/h. |
| 2010 | Distance, distance/minute, distance/minute > 15 km/h, distance/minute > 20 km/h, distance/minute > 75% max speed. |

Pearson correlation coefficients were calculated between GPS variables and number of possessions and derived impact points per minute of game time. Intra-positional correlations between GPS and performance variables were also calculated. A stepwise multiple regression equation was used to assess the combination of match activity variables which best predicted possessions gained per minute and derived impact points gained per minute of game time.

## 3. RESULTS

As presented in Table 2, across both 2009 ($r = 0.41$, $p < 0.01$) and 2010 ($r = 0.45$, $p < 0.01$), overall distance covered per minute of game time had the highest correlation with possessions gained per minute. Additionally, in 2010, overall distance covered per minute had a small, but significant positive correlation ($r = 0.18$, $p < 0.01$) with derived impact points per minute. Distance covered per minute above 15 km/h also had a significant positive correlation with possessions per minute ($r = 0.39$, $p < 0.01$) and derived impact points per minute ($r = 0.11$, $p < 0.05$). Distance covered per minute above 20 km/h had a weak relationship ($r = 0.11$, $p < 0.05$) with possessions per minute. Distance covered per minute above 75% of individual maximum speed had a significant negative correlation with possessions per minute in 2009 ($r = -0.16$, $p < 0.01$) and derived impact points per minute in both 2009 (r = -0.22, p < 0.01) and 2010 (r = -0.12, p < 0.05). In 2009, distance covered per minute above 25 km/h had a significant negative correlation with both possessions per minute (r = -0.13, p < 0.05) and derived impact points per minute (r = -0.26, p < 0.01).

Overall distance covered per minute had the highest positive correlation with possessions per minute in the free roaming positional group for 2009 (r = 0.31, p < 0.01) and 2010 (r = 0.27, p < 0.01) (see Table 3). Distance covered per minute above 15 km/h also had a significant positive correlation with possessions per minute in 2010 for the free roaming group (r= 0.24, p < 0.01). Distance per minute also had the highest correlation with possessions per minute in the stationary positional category for 2009 (r = 0.37, p < 0.01) and 2010 (r = 0.33, p < 0.01) (see Table 3). Across both years, there were higher correlations between the GPS variables and possessions gained per minute compared to the correlations between the GPS variables and derived impact points per minute. The only significant correlation between any GPS variables and derived impact points per minute for either of the positional categories was for free roaming (DI points/min 2010 and distance/min >15 km/h, r = -0.18, p <0.01).

As shown in Table 4, distance per minute rates accounted for 16% of the variation in possessions per minute for 2009 and 19% of the variation in 2010. Collectively, the GPS variables analysed explained 21% of the variation in possessions per minute in 2009 and 23% in 2010. Conversely, only 10% of the variation in derived impact was accounted for by variations in the GPS data.

**Table 2** Correlations with possessions per minute (Poss/Min) and derived impact (DI) points per minute.

| GPS Variable | Poss/Min 2009 (n= 279) | Poss/Min 2010 (n= 279) | DI points/min 2009 (n= 348) | DI points/min 2010 (n= 348) |
|---|---|---|---|---|
| Distance covered per min | 0.41 ** | 0.45** | 0.03 | 0.18** |
| Distance/min > 75% max speed | -0.16** | -0.09 | -0.22** | -0.12* |
| Distance/min > 15 km/h | - | 0.39** | - | 0.11* |
| Distance/min > 20 km/h | - | 0.11* | - | -0.08 |
| Distance/min > 25 km/h | -0.13* | - | -0.26** | - |

*\*\* significant at p < 0.01 level, \* significant at p < 0.05 level*

**Table 3** Correlations with possessions per minute (Poss/Min) and derived impact (DI) points per minute (free-roaming players & stationary position players).

| GPS Variable | Poss/Min *2009* | Poss/Min *2010* | DI points per min *2009* | DI points per min *2010* |
|---|---|---|---|---|
| Distance covered per min (free roaming) | 0.31** | 0.27** | -0.02 | 0.004 |
| Distance/min > 15 km/h | - | 0.24** | - | -0.18** |
| Distance covered per min (stationary) | 0.37** | 0.33** | -0.11 | 0.12 |

*\*\* significant at $p < 0.01$ level, \* significant at $p < 0.05$ level*

**Table 4** Multiple regression equations for match activity variables and performance indicators.

| 2009 Model | *2009* Poss/Min $R^2$ | *2009* DI/Min $R^2$ | 2010 Model | *2010* Poss/Min $R^2$ | *2010* DI/Min $R^2$ |
|---|---|---|---|---|---|
| 1: Dist/min | 0.16* | -0.03 | 1: Dist/min | 0.19* | 0.03 |
| 2: Dist/min<br><br>Dist/min > 60% max speed<br><br>Dist/min > 75% max speed<br><br>Dist/min > 25 km/hour | 0.21* | 0.06 | 2: Dist/min<br><br>Dist/min > 15 km/hour<br><br>Dist/min > 20 km/hour<br><br>Dist/min > 75% max speed | 0.23* | 0.06 |

*\*significant at $p < 0.05$ level*

## 4. DISCUSSION

There have been a limited number of studies relating individual performance to match activity profiles in Australian football. Wisbey and Montgomery (2006) and Wisbey *et al.* (2009) found moderate correlations between a GPS 'exertion index' and the number of possessions gained in AFL games. However, these studies collated GPS data from several different types of GPS units, from different manufacturers and with different sampling rates (1-Hz and 5-Hz). Previous studies have found significant differences in data between GPS unit types (Petersen *et al.*, 2009). Therefore, the primary aim of this study was to investigate the relationship between match activity profiles and individual Australian football performance measures, within one AFL team, using equivalent GPS technology.

Across both 2009 and 2010, the overall distance covered per minute had the highest correlation (between 0.40-0.45) with both possessions gained per minute and derived impact points per minute. Therefore, the higher a player's distance per minute, then the more times they are likely to gain possession of the ball, thus providing more opportunities to impact the game. Distance per minute also had the highest correlation with possession rate in both the free roaming and stationary positional categories. The implications of these findings suggest that, of the match activity variables measured, ability to cover an overall large amount of ground per minute is of greatest importance (irrespective of player position). Additionally, distance covered per minute above 15 km/h had a moderate relationship with possession rate, particularly in the free roaming positional group. High speed running variables, particularly distance per minute above 75% of max speed and distance per minute above 25 km/h, had a weak negative relationship with both possessions per minute and derived impact points per minute. A potential reason could be that the majority of these high speed efforts take place when the opposition is in possession and the players are chasing, attempting to lay a tackle or attempting to make position. These findings, from a team performance perspective, suggest that players with a high distance per minute, (perhaps indicative of a high aerobic capacity) and the capability of a large volume of efforts between 15 to 25 km/h are likely to have a higher possession rate, particularly in the free roaming positional group.

Across both 2009 and 2010, correlations were higher between the GPS variables and possession per minute rate compared to between the GPS data and derived impact points per minute. Derived impact per minute takes into account both the effectiveness of player possessions as well as the impact of these possessions, and other actions such as tackling and blocking, on the game. Therefore, a high possession rate does not necessarily translate to a high derived impact score as players may turn the ball over consistently with their disposals (hence accruing negative derived impact scores and reducing their game totals). As players can have higher match activity profiles and accumulate a large number of disposals, yet have a low derived impact score, this may account for the lower correlations between the GPS data and derived impact data.

Whilst the match activity variables were a significant predictor of possessions, 75% of the variation in possessions gained per minute was not accounted for. Additionally, the GPS variables accounted for less than 10% of the variation in derived impact scores. Therefore, although match activity profiles are an important component of performance, the results emphasize that Australian football performance is multi-factorial. A large variety of different factors, namely skill execution, number of games played, decision-making ability, team tactics, the opposition, environmental conditions, physiological state, training workloads and injury status can all have a significant influence on performance. However, due to limitations in current GPS technology, what is unknown at this point is how the frequency of moderate and rapid accelerations, decelerations and changes of direction relate to Australian football performance. It is probable that the frequency of moderate and rapid accelerations would be important to possession rate and may increase the predictive capacity of GPS data in relation to performance.

## References

Coutts, A. and Duffield, R., 2010, Validity and reliability of GPS devices for measuring movement demands of team sports. *J Sci Med Sport*, **13**, 133–135.

Heasman, J. *et al.*, 2008, Development and validation of a player impact ranking system in Australian football. *Int J Perf Analys Sport*, **8**, 156–171.

Petersen, C. *et al.*, 2009, Validity and reliability of GPS units to monitor cricket-specific movement patterns. *Int J Sports Physiol Perf*, **4**, 381–393.

Wisbey, B. and Montgomery, P., 2006, Quantifying AFL player demands using GPS tracking: 2006 season. *AFL Research Board Report*.

Wisbey, B. *et al.*, 2009, Quantifying AFL player demands using GPS tracking: 2009 season. AFL Research Board Report.

# CHAPTER THIRTY-TWO

# Measuring effectiveness of zone-oriented defence on preventing goal scoring in professional soccer matches

A. Tenga

Department of Coaching and Psychology,
Norwegian School of Sport Sciences, Oslo, Norway

## 1. INTRODUCTION

The zone-oriented defence is based on the defensive organization that emphasizes exerting pressure on the opponent player with the ball, at the same time providing backup and cover once the team loses ball possession in open play (Worthington, 1980; Olsen *et al.*, 1994). The empirical evidence on whether these practical guidelines really work is rarely found in the literature. The aim of this case-control study is to examine the effects of the zone-oriented defensive tactics of defensive pressure, defensive backup and defensive cover, separately and combined, on the probability of conceding a goal in real matches from Norwegian elite soccer.

## 2. METHODS

Videotapes from 163 out of 182 (90%) matches played in the Norwegian professional male league during the 2004 season were used. The league involves 14 teams and follows a double round robin competition format, which means that each team played 26 matches, 13 home and 13 away. A total of 203 goals (43%) out of 476 goals were scored from open-play. A sample included 203 goals (cases) and 1688 random team possessions (control group) obtained from open-play periods in soccer matches.

To obtain random controls, we assigned each match a computer-generated random number to indicate the beginning (in minutes) of a match period from which an estimated number of 10 team possessions was eventually collected and used in a control group.

A team possession was used as the basic unit of analysis and was defined according to Pollard and Reep (1997, p. 542):

> A team possession starts when a player gains possession of the ball by any means other than from a player of the same team. The player must have enough control over the ball to be able to have a deliberate influence on its subsequent direction. The team possession may continue with a series of passes between players of the same team but ends immediately when one of the following events occurs: a) the ball goes out of play; b) the ball touches a player of the opposing team (e.g. by means of a tackle, an intercepted pass or a shot being saved). A momentary touch that does not significantly change the direction of the ball is excluded; c) an infringement of the rules takes place (e.g. a player is offside or a foul is committed).

Four categorical variables including three independent variables defensive pressure, defensive backup, and defensive cover and one dependent variable possession outcome were used. In addition, a categorical variable overall defensive score was created from the combined probability scores of these three defensive variables.

For the variable defensive pressure, a team possession was characterized as 'tight pressure' when an estimated pressing distance(s) of not more than 1.5m was observed in all ball involvements throughout the entire team possession. In contrast, a 'loose pressure' characterizes team possession when an estimated pressing distance(s) of more than 1.5 m was observed throughout the entire team possession. For the variable defensive backup, the categories 'present backup' and 'absent backup' included team possessions completely with or without a second defender, respectively, within 5 m estimated distance from the first defender in all ball involvements throughout the entire team possession. And, for the variable defensive cover, the categories 'present cover' and 'absent cover' included team possessions completely with or without third defender(s), respectively, beyond 5m behind the first defender in all ball involvements throughout the entire team possession. This means those team possessions which involved mixed categories in each of these variables were excluded from the analyses. In addition, the estimated defensive distances were supplemented by a qualitative evaluation of players' spatial-temporal positioning in each ball involvement based on players' defensive intentions in the specific match situation. Consequently, a more pragmatic at the same time meaningful analysis of zone-oriented defensive tactics was achieved.

The two categories of the variable overall defensive score characterized team possessions as playing against a balanced defence (tight pressure, present backup, and present cover) as well as playing against an imbalanced defence (loose pressure, absent backup, and absent cover) in all ball involvements throughout the entire team possession.

The variables' reliability scores from inter-observer tests showed good kappa values for defensive pressure ($\kappa=0.68$) and team possession outcome ($\kappa=0.75$) and fair values for defensive backup ($\kappa=0.24$) and defensive cover ($\kappa=0.27$) (Altman,

1991). The association between the three defensive tactics and between the independent variables and the probability of conceding a goal was tested by a chi-square analysis. The association was tested further by univariate logistic regression analyses. We used an alpha value of < 0.05.

## 3. RESULTS AND DISCUSSION

The $\chi^2$ values show only association between defensive pressure and defensive backup tactics ($\chi^2$=29.08, P<0.001) (Table 1). In specific, loose pressure with backup (38.3%) conceded goals in lower percentages of attempts than without backup (75.1%), while tight pressure without backup (24.9%) conceded goals in lower percentages of attempts than with backup (61.7%). That tight pressure was found to be more effective in preventing goals when used alone rather than in the presence of backup may be explained as the effect of tackling action typically accompanies tight pressure especially in need situations during soccer matches.

There were differences in the probability of conceding goals between categories for all defensive tactics except defensive pressure, with tight pressure (6.2%) registered non-significantly less proportion of conceded goals compared to loose pressure (7.4%) (P=0.63) (Table 2). For the variable overall defensive score, a balanced defence (0.9%) conceded fewer goals than an imbalanced defence (21.8%) (Table 2).

**Table 1** Chi-square values ($\chi^2$) and their levels of significance (P values) from Fisher's Exact Test of Association between the three zone-oriented defensive tactics: defensive pressure, defensive backup, and defensive cover.

| Variable | **Defensive pressure** Loose (Imbalanced) Tight (Balanced) | **Defensive backup** Absent (Imbalanced) Present (Balanced) | **Defensive cover** Absent (Imbalanced) Present (Balanced) |
|---|---|---|---|
| **Defensive pressure** Loose (Imbalanced) Tight (Balanced) | - | $\chi^2$=29.08, P<0.001 | $\chi^2$=2.15, P=0.20* |
| **Defensive backup** Absent (Imbalanced) Present (Balanced) | $\chi^2$=29.08, P<0.001 | - | $\chi^2$=2.79, P=0.14* |
| **Defensive cover** Absent (Imbalanced) Present (Balanced) | $\chi^2$=2.15, P=0.20* | $\chi^2$=2.79, P=0.14* | - |

*25% of cells had expected count less than five.

**Table 2** Number of goals (n=203) and controls (n=1688) plus percentages of goals conceded through the three zone-oriented defensive tactics (N=1891).

| Variable | N (%) | Goal | Control | Goal % | P* |
|---|---|---|---|---|---|
| **Defensive pressure** | | | | | 0.63 |
| Loose (Imbalanced) | 487 (69.9) | 36 | 451 | 7.4 | |
| Tight (Balanced) | 210 (30.1) | 13 | 197 | 6.2 | |
| **Defensive backup** | | | | | 0.016 |
| Absent (Imbalanced) | 1134 (95.2) | 134 | 1000 | 11.8 | |
| Present (Balanced) | 57 (4.8) | 1 | 56 | 1.8 | |
| **Defensive cover** | | | | | <0.001 |
| Absent (Imbalanced) | 15 (1.0) | 7 | 8 | 46.7 | |
| Present (Balanced) | 1442 (99.0) | 26 | 1416 | 1.8 | |
| **Overall defensive score** | | | | | <0.001 |
| Imbalanced defence | 878 (62.5) | 191 | 687 | 21.8 | |
| Balanced defence | 527 (37.5) | 5 | 522 | 0.9 | |

*Fisher's Exact Test.

**Table 3** Odds ratio (OR) for conceding a goal through the three zone-oriented defensive tactics (N=1891).

| | Univariate analysis | |
|---|---|---|
| Variable | OR (95% CI) | P |
| **Defensive pressure** | | |
| Loose (Imbalanced) | 1.21(0.63-233) | 0.57 |
| Tight (Balanced) | 1 | |
| **Defensive backup** | | |
| Absent (Imbalanced) | 7.50 (1.03-54.65) | 0.047 |
| Present (Balanced) | 1 | |
| **Defensive cover** | | |
| Absent (Imbalanced) | 47.65 (16.09-141.17) | <0.001 |
| Present (Balanced) | 1 | |
| **Overall defensive score** | | |
| Imbalanced defence | 29.03 (11.86-71.05) | <0.001 |
| Balanced defence | 1 | |

Note: The odds ratio (OR) reflects the chance of conceding a goal, compared with the reference category[a].

Similar differences were observed in the odds ratio for conceding a goal. The defensive tactics absent backup and absent cover had higher odds ratios than their respective opposite tactics present backup and present cover (Table 3). The results of variable overall defensive score show over 29 times more chances to prevent a goal by a balanced defence compared to an imbalanced defence (OR=29.03; 95% confidence interval: 11.86 to 71.05; P<0.001) (Table 3).

It should be noted that the use of variables defensive backup and defensive cover, which have only fair inter-observer reproducibility (kappa correlation coefficients of 0.24 and 0.27, respectively), represents a limitation. However, the combined variable overall defensive score was still useful. In fact, these variables' relatively poor inter-observer reproducibility mainly stems from the observational limitations experienced when evaluating positional characteristics of dynamically interacting players by using video recordings from live TV broadcasts. A more emphasis on user training for the current analysis system and the use of increasingly common positional data from automatic player tracking systems may both produce more reliable data for future research.

In sum, the results show overwhelming evidence of effectiveness in preventing goals by zone-oriented defensive tactics, namely tight pressure, present backup, and present cover. This is the case especially when the effects of these tactics are considered together rather than separately. Further, only relationship between defensive pressure and defensive backup was found. Specifically, loose pressure was more effective in preventing goals in the presence of backup rather than when employed alone, while tight pressure was more effective when employed alone rather than in the presence of backup.

## 4. CONCLUSION

The zone-oriented defensive tactics of a balanced defence, i.e. tight pressure (estimated within 1.5 m), present backup (estimated within 5 m) and cover (estimated beyond 5 m), appear to be effective in preventing goals in real matches from Norwegian elite soccer. The effects of these tactics were especially stronger when considered together rather than in isolation from each other.

### References

Altman, D. G., 1991, Some common problems in medical research. In *Practical Statistics for Medical Research*, London: Chapman & Hall, pp. 403–409.

Olsen, E. *et al.*, 1994, *Effektiv Fotball*, Norway: Gyldendal Norsk Forlag A/S.

Pollard, R. and Reep, C., 1997, Measuring the effectiveness of playing strategies at soccer. *The Statistician*, **46**, 541–550.

Worthington, E., 1980, *Teaching Soccer Skills*, 2nd ed., London: Henry Kimpton Publishers Ltd.

# CHAPTER THIRTY-THREE

# Differences between winning, drawing and losing teams in the 2010 World Cup

D. Casamichana, J. Castellano, J. Calleja-González and J. San Román

University of the Basque Country (UPV-EHU), Spain

## 1. INTRODUCTION

Match analysis is commonly used in many sports and is viewed as a vital process that enables coaches to collect objective information which can be used to provide feedback on performance (Carling *et al.,* 2005). As coaches are prone to making subjective judgments and may be unable to recall events reliably, they are increasingly turning to match analysis as a way of optimizing the training process of their players and teams (Hughes and Franks, 2004). The main aim of match analysis is to identify the strengths and weaknesses of one's own team, thereby enabling the former to be further developed and the latter to be worked upon. Similarly, a coach analysing the performance of an opposing side will use the data to identify ways of countering that team's strengths and exploiting its weaknesses (Carling *et al.,* 2008).

Performance indicators in sport can be defined as the selection and combination of variables that define some aspect of performance and which help to achieve success (Hughes and Bartlett, 2002). These indicators have been suggested as useful for coaches and analysts can compare the expected performance (Sajadi and Rahnama, 2007; Rowlinson and O'Donoghue, 2009), with other teams, or predict future performance to constitute an ideal profile that can be used to predict future behaviour in a given sporting activity (O'Donoghue, 2005). In the context of soccer the World Cup is undoubtedly the greatest prize and it provides an opportunity to examine the best teams and players in the world. After a World Cup it is usually the successful teams which set the trend in terms of training and playing style. Indeed, others will tend to imitate the tactics and play of winning teams, seeking to master those aspects of performance which are deemed to underlie their success (Hughes and Franks, 2005).

They are currently some studies that have related these aspects to the match result (winning or losing) (Hughes *et al.,* 1988) in Italy 1990 (Bishovets *et al.,* 1993; Yamanaka *et al.,* 1993), France 1998 and Korea/Japan 2002 (Lawlor *et al.,* 2003). However, although these studies examined indicators of success in soccer their results remain inconclusive due to certain limitations and/or methodological problems. For instance, some of these studies are based on small sample sizes and usually conduct a univariate analysis of the observed variable. These factors are likely to influence the results regarding a team's performance and thus may contribute to the differences found in existing studies.

The aim of the present study is to identify, by means of different multivariate analyses, the performance indicators that allow us to differentiate between winning, drawing and losing teams in the 2010 FIFA World Cup.

## 2. METHODS

The collected data from all matches (64) were provided by FIFA website (http://fifa.com/worldcup/index.html). Two categories of variables were studied: those related to attacking play and those related to defence (Table 1). Their reliability was studied by coding five randomly-chosen matches and comparing the data obtained with those from the FIFA website. The resulting values of Cohen's kappa ($K$) were between 0.93 and 0.97.

A descriptive analysis was first carried out. Secondly, the homogeneity of variances was examined by means of Levene's test and an analysis of variance (ANOVA) was then used to determine which variables revealed differences between the three categories of teams (winning, drawing and losing). Whenever a significant difference was found we applied either the post hoc Bonferroni test or, if the variances were not homogeneous, Dunnett's T3 post-hoc test. Finally, a discriminant analysis was then performed in order to identify the variables which best discriminated between winning, drawing and losing teams (Ntoumanis, 2001). This was done by calculating the structural coefficients (SC), with values >0.30 being regarded as significant (Tabachnick and Fidell, 2007). All the statistical analyses were performed using *SPSS 16.0 for Windows*, with significance being set at $p<0.05$.

## 3. RESULTS AND DISCUSSION

Table 1 shows the descriptive results derived from the match statistics for winning, drawing and losing teams. In the performance indicators of attacking play, the averages for winning teams were significantly higher than those of both drawing and losing teams for the following match statistics: *total shots, shots on target* and *red cards against team*. However, on the variables *ball possession, passes, completed passes* and *completed crosses* they were only higher than the averages of losing teams ($p<0.05$). In the performance indicators of defence, the averages of losing teams were significantly higher than those of both winning and drawing teams for the match statistics *total shots against, shots on target against team,* and *red cards* ($p<0.05$).

Table 2 presents the results of the discriminant analysis for the last soccer World Cup. The discriminant functions correctly classified 82.6% of winning, drawing and losing teams, and one of the two discriminant functions obtained was significant ($p<0.05$). In the first discriminant function the variables with the greatest discriminatory power were *shots on target* (SC = 0.51) and *shots on target against team* (SC = -0.49).

**Table 1** Descriptive results and univariate differences between winning, drawing and losing teams in 2010 FIFA World Cup.

| | Winning (n = 46) | Drawing (n = 28) | Losing (n = 46) |
|---|---|---|---|
| Variables related to attacking play | | | |
| **Total shots** | **16.0 ±5.5**[ab] | 12.1 ±5.4 | 12.7 ±4.7 |
| Shots off target | 8.9 ±3.8 | 8.1 ±4.0 | 8.8 ±3.4 |
| **Shots on target** | **7.1 ±2.7**[ab] | 3.9 ±2.2 | 3.9 ±2.0 |
| Fouls received | 16.0 ±5.8 | 15.3 ±3.5 | 13.8 ±4.5 |
| **(%) Ball possession** | **52.4 ±6.0**[b] | 49.7 ±5.3 | 47.8 ±6.0 |
| Offsides | 2.4 ±2.0 | 2.3 ±2.0 | 2.1 ±1.5 |
| Corners | 5.2 ±4.5 | 4.4 ±3.5 | 4.5 ±2.6 |
| Yellow cards against team | 1.87 ±1.13 | 2.0 ±1.1 | 1.8 ±1.4 |
| **Red cards against team** | **0.3 ±0.4**[ab] | 0.1 ±0.3 | 0.0 ±0.1 |
| **Passes** | **533.5 ±114.7**[b] | 480.8±95.8 | 473.7±94.4 |
| **Completed passes** | **391.7 ±115.3**[b] | 342.1±99.1 | 334.1 ±89.6 |
| Successful passes (%) | 72.3 ±7.1 | 69.9 ±7.5 | 69.2 ±6.9 |
| Crosses | 16.6 ±7.1 | 15.5 ±6.5 | 14.4 ±7.3 |
| **Completed crosses** | **4.7 ±3.3**[b] | 3.8 ±2.8 | 3.1 ±2.1 |
| Successful crosses (%) | 28.3 ±17.1 | 22.4 ±13.5 | 22.6 ±16.2 |
| Variables related to defence | | | |
| **Total shots against** | 12.7 ±4.7 | 12.1 ±5.4 | **15.9 ±5.4**[bc] |
| Shots off target against team | 8.8 ±3.4 | 8.1 ±4.0 | 8.9 ±3.8 |
| **Shots on target against team** | 3.9 ±2.0 | 3.9 ±2.2 | **7.1 ±2.7**[bc] |
| **Fouls committed** | 14.1 ±4.8 | **16.1 ±3.7**[c] | 16.3 ±5.9 |
| Offsides against team | 2.3 ±1.6 | 2.4 ±2.0 | 2.5 ±2.1 |
| Corners against team | 4.4 ±2.5 | 4.9 ±3.4 | 5.1 ±2.9 |
| Yellow cards | 1.8 ±1.4 | 2.1 ±1.1 | 1.9 ±1.1 |
| **Red cards** | 0.02 ±0.1 | 0.1 ±0.3 | **0.3 ±0.4**[bc] |

**Note**:   [a] Significantly different from drawing teams; [b] Significantly different from losing teams; [c] Significantly different from winning teams.

The aim of this study was to identify the performance indicators that best discriminated between winning, drawing and losing teams in the last soccer World Cup (South Africa 2010). In this context, the study is the first to have applied a multivariate analysis to performance indicators of World Cup matches. The results of the initial univariate analysis identified eleven variables that differed between winning, drawing and losing teams (Table 1), while in the subsequent multivariate analysis only two variables were found to discriminate teams in relation to their performance (Table 2). The variable with the greatest discriminatory power was *shots on target* (both *made* and *against*).

**Table 2** Standardized coefficients from the discriminant analysis of match statistics for winning, drawing and losing teams from the whole sample of matches played in 2010 FIFA World Cup.

|  | Function 1 | Function 2 |
|---|---|---|
| Total shots | 0.246 | 0.336* |
| Shots off target | 0.016 | 0.155 |
| **Shots on target** | **0.511*** | 0.490* |
| Fouls received | 0.174 | -0.078 |
| (%) Ball possession | 0.297 | 0.030 |
| Offsides | 0.048 | -0.049 |
| Corners | 0.096 | 0.111 |
| Yellow cards against team | 0.032 | -0.097 |
| Red cards against team | 0.287 | 0.155 |
| Passes | 0.221 | 0.161 |
| Completed passes | 0.214 | 0.146 |
| Successful passes (%) | 0.165 | 0.083 |
| Crosses | 0.117 | -0.011 |
| Completed crosses | 0.205 | 0.022 |
| Successful crosses (%) | 0.136 | 0.138 |
| Total shots against | -0.233 | 0.336* |
| Shots off target against team | -0.011 | 0.157 |
| **Shots on target against team** | **-0.494*** | 0.550* |
| Fouls committed | -0.171 | -0.128 |
| Offsides against team | -0.047 | -0.017 |
| Corners against team | -0.097 | -0.020 |
| Yellow cards | -0.036 | -0.184 |
| Red cards | -0.282 | 0.194 |
| Eigenvalue | 1.391 | 0.293 |
| Wilks' lambda | 0.323 | 0.773 |
| Canonical correlation | 0.763 | 0.476 |
| Chi-squared | 120.804 | 27.532 |
| Significance | 0.000 | 0.121 |
| % of variance | 82.6 | 17.4 |

*SC discriminant value $\geq$.30

Ball possession is one of the most widely-studied performance indicators (Lago and Martin, 2007), although its relationship to team performance requires further clarification. In the present study, ball possession was not a discriminating variable, but it did show differences between winning and losing teams (Table 1).

In line with the present findings, Lago *et al.* (2010) also found that the variable *shots on target* had the greatest discriminatory power as regards matches played in the Spanish league, and statistically significant differences in its value have been reported between top and middle/lower ranking teams in the same league (Lago-Ballesteros and Lago, 2010). The same variable has also been shown to be one of the best at discriminating between successful and unsuccessful teams in Italy (Rampinini *et al.,* 2009), as well as between national sides in the 2002 World Cup (Lawlor *et al.,* 2003). It would seem, therefore, that what best discriminates team performance is the number of shots on target, and not the total number of shots made. This is consistent with the findings of Szwarc (2004), who reported that winning teams made only four more shots overall than did less successful teams, but the effectiveness of their shots was three-fold greater. Similar results were found by Yamanaka *et al.* (1993) and Bishovets *et al.* (1993) for national sides competing in the 1990 World Cup in Italy, as well as by research that analysed the shot variable in World Cups (Hughes *et al.,* 1988).

As regards the variables related to defensive play, differences were found (Table 1) for *total shots against, shots on target against* and *red cards.* Similarly, a recent study by Lago-Ballesteros and Lago (2010) found no defence-related variable that differed between top, mid-table and bottom teams in the Spanish league, although it should be noted that this study did not consider shots received by the opposing team as a defence-related variable.

## 4. CONCLUSION

This study has analysed match statistics related to the attacking and defensive play of winning, drawing and losing teams in the last World Cup tournament. The results may be of use to coaches in terms of designing their training programmes, providing them with information about what attacking players need to achieve, and what needs to be avoided defensively, if a team is to increase its chances of winning. The effectiveness of attacking play (in terms of *shots on target*) and defensive play (in terms of *shots on target against team*), appear to be the performance indicators that constitute the keys to success in today's soccer.

### Acknowledgements

We gratefully acknowledge the support of the Spanish government project Innovaciones en la evaluación de contextos naturales: Aplicaciones al ámbito del deporte (Dirección General de Investigación, Ministerio de Ciencia y Tecnología) [Grant number BSO2001-3368].

### References

Bishovets, A. *et al.*, 1993, Computer analysis of the effectiveness of collective technical and tactical moves of footballers in the matches of 1988 Olympics and 1990 World Cup. In *Science and Football II*, London: E. and F.N. Spon, pp. 232–238.

Carling, C. *et al.*, 2008, The role of motion analysis in elite soccer. *Sports Med*, **38**, 839–862.

Carling, C. *et al.*, 2005, *Handbook of Soccer Match Analysis*, London: Routledge.

Hughes, M. and Bartlett, R., 2002, The use of performance indicators in performance analysis. *J Sports Sci*, **20**, 739–754.

Hughes, M. and Franks, I., 2004, *Notational Analysis of Sport Systems for Better Coaching and Performance in Sport*, London: Routledge.

Hughes, M. and Franks, I., 2005, Analysis of passing sequences, shots and goals in soccer. *J Sports Sci*, **23**, 509–514.

Hughes, M. *et al.*, 1988, Comparison of patterns of play of successful and unsuccessful teams in the 1986 World Cup for soccer. In *Science and Football*, London: E. and F.N. Spon, pp. 363–367.

Lago, C. and Martín, R., 2007, Determinants of possession of the ball in soccer. *J Sports Sci*, **25**, 969–974.

Lago-Ballesteros, J. and Lago, C., 2010, Performance in team sports: Identifying the keys to success in soccer. *J Human Kinetics*, **25**, 85–91.

Lago, C. *et al.*, 2010, Game-related statistics discriminated winning, drawing and losing teams from the Spanish soccer league. *J Sports Sci Med*, **9**, 288–293.

Lawlor, J. *et al.*, 2003, The FIFA World Cup 2002: An analysis of successful versus unsuccessful teams. *J Sports Sci*, **22**, 500–520.

Ntoumanis, N. 2001, *A Step-by-Step Guide to SPSS for Sport and Exercise Studies*, London: Routledge.

O'Donoghue, P., 2005, Normative profiles of sports performance. *Int J Perf Analys Sport*, **5**, 104–119.

Rampinini, E. *et al.*, 2009, Technical performance during soccer matches of the Italian Serie A league: effect to fatigue and competitive level. *J Sci Med Sport*, **12**, 227–233.

Rowlinson, M. and O'Donoghue, P., 2009. Performance profiles of soccer players in the 2006 UEFA Champions League and the 2006 FIFA World Cup tournaments. In *Science and Football VI*, London: Routledge, pp. 229–234.

Sajadi, N. and Rahnama, N., 2007, Analysis of goals in 2006 FIFA World Cup. *J Sports Sci Med*, **6**, 3.

Szwarc, A., 2004, Effectiveness of Brazilian and German teams and the teams defeated by them during the 17th FIFA World Cup. *Kinesiology*, **36**, 83–89.

Tabachnick, B.G. and Fidell, L.S. 2007, *Using Multivariate Statistics*, New York: Harper Collins.

Yamanaka, K. *et al.*, 1993, An analysis of playing patterns in the 1990 World Cup for association football. In *Science and Football II*. London: E. and F.N. Spon, pp. 206–214.

# CHAPTER THIRTY-FOUR

# Contextual effects on the free kick performance: a case study with a Portuguese professional soccer team

F. Corbellini[1], A. Volossovitch[1], C. Andrade[1], O. Fernandes[2] and A.P. Ferreira[1]

[1]Faculty of Human Kinetics, Technical University of Lisbon, Portugal
[2]Sport and Health Department, University of Évora, Portugal

## 1. INTRODUCTION

The free kick represents one of the most relevant events for the offensive process efficacy in high performance soccer, providing from 15 to 20 percent of the goals scored (Acar *et al.*, 2009; Alcock, 2010). Recent studies provide evidence in support of the influence of contextual variables, such as match location (Tucker *et al.*, 2005; Taylor *et al.*, 2008; Lago, 2009), match status (O'Donoghue and Tenga, 2001; Bloomfield *et al.*, 2005a; Taylor *et al.*, 2008; Lago, 2009) and opponent quality (Taylor *et al.*, 2008; Lago, 2009) on football performances. Although numerous studies have analyzed key-indicators of 'set play' in soccer (Grant *et al.*, 1999; Carling *et al.*, 2005; Taylor *et al.*, 2005; Acar *et al.*, 2009; Alcock, 2010), very few have examined the effects of contextual variables on the technical and tactical aspects of team performance, and none has evaluated the contextual influence on team performance in free kick situations.

The aim of this study was to assess the effect of match status and quality of opposition on performance and subsequent success of free kicks in matches of a Portuguese professional soccer team.

## 2. METHODS

The sample consisted of 89 free kicks, marked in the offensive field, in ten matches of the Portuguese Professional Soccer League and Portugal Cup 2009/2010 played by the observed team. The free kicks were classified as 'successful', 'unsuccessful' and 'neutral', according to the development of the play, from the free kick to the end of ball possession. To facilitate the analysis, the playing field was divided into four equal parts: the defensive zone (DZ), defensive midfielder zone (DMZ), offensive midfielder zone (OMZ), and offensive zone (OZ).

A free kick was considered 'successful' when it resulted in a shot been played by one or more attackers, and also when the possession of the ball ended with a direct shot made from the OZ (regardless of whether the team scored or not). A free kick was considered 'unsuccessful' when the defense cleared the ball immediately after the free kick, or when the direct shot was made from the OMZ. Finally, a free kick was considered 'neutral' when the ball carrier made the short pass to the nearest teammate. The observation system developed for this study included seven categories and 37 performance indicators (Table 1).

**Table 1** Categories and performance indicators analyzed in the study.

| Categories | Performance Indicators |
|---|---|
| Time periods | 0'–15', 16'–30', 31'–45'<br>46'–60', 61'–75', 76'–90' |
| Zone of the free kick | Right offensive midfielder zone (ROMZ)<br>Central offensive midfielder zone (COMZ)<br>Left offensive midfielder zone (LOMZ)<br>Right offensive zone (ROZ)<br>Central offensive zone (COZ)<br>Left offensive zone (LOZ) |
| Style of shot | Inswing, outswing, straight |
| Number of attackers | Less than six, six or more |
| Number of defenders | Less than eight, eight or more |
| Area of the first contact with the ball after free kick shot | 1, 2, 3, 4, 5, 6, 7, 8 |
| Final action of free kick sequence | Goal;<br>Goalkeeper defense after a direct free kick shot;<br>Direct shot to the post;<br>Defenders clear the ball;<br>Foul by attackers;<br>Shot to the penalty area where the ball goes through all the players and nobody touches it;<br>Shot out from goal;<br>Goal after one or more players touched the ball after the free kick;<br>Goalkeeper saves after one or more players touched the ball;<br>Final shot out after one or more attackers touched the ball. |

Expert coaches' opinions have been used to validate the observation system. The data reliability was defined as the degree of agreement between two different observations of the same event, using the same registration instrument (Hill and Hill, 2002). Intra-observer reliability was assessed to validate the single-observer analysis. Free kicks from two matches from the sample have been analyzed twice with 15 days interval. After this procedure, the number of agreements and disagreements has been compared, using the Bellack formula (Van der Mars, 1989). The rates of reliability for all variables were above 90%.

The players' actions have been registered using software Match Vision Studio (Perea *et al.*, 2006). The images have been reordered *in situ* in the stadium, when the observed team played as the host. The collection of images was authorized by the Portuguese Professional Football League and the observed team's club directors.

All performance indicators observed during free kick situations have been analyzed as a function of two contextual variables – match status and quality of opposition. The Cluster analysis has been applied to categorize the matches in two groups as a function of opponent quality based on the teams' ranking before the match. Descriptive statistics and hierarchical log-linear models have been used for analysis of the relationship between performance and contextual variables.

## 3. RESULTS

The results of the log-linear model revealed the significant relationship between the match status and: 1) time of free kick occurrence ($p < 0.001$), 2) field zones where free kicks were marked ($p < 0.035$), and 3) success of free kicks ($p < 0.005$). When the match was drawn, free kicks mostly occurred during the first half of matches. However, when the observed team was losing, significantly more free kicks were taken during the last periods of matches (Figure 1). More than 40% of free kicks were taken during the last 15 minutes (76'–90' period).

The analysis of the field zones where the free kicks were taken showed that the team took more free kicks from the OMZ when drawing or winning. When the team was losing, over 40% of fouls were made in the OCZ, followed by the COMZ. No significant relationship was observed between match status and other performance indicators. However, the free kick success rate was significantly related to the match status and showed a significant link between the number of attackers that participated in free kick sequences, the number of defenders and the final action of free kick sequences.

The quality of opposition did not show any direct effect on any performance indicator, but the log-linear model estimated for quality of opposition and performance indicators revealed that success of a final shot in a free kick sequence was dependent on the zone of the free kick, the style of the shot, the number of attackers that participated in the free kick, the number of defenders and the final action of the free kick sequence.

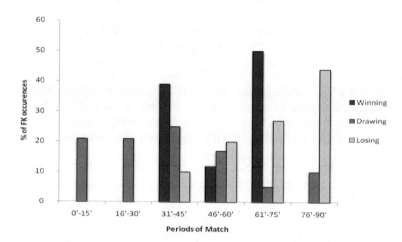

**Figure 1** Percentage of free kick occurrences as a function of match status.

## 4. DISCUSSION AND CONCLUSION

Results suggest that team performance varies as a function of the match status and time period of the match. When behind, the team suffered more fouls in the final periods of the match, which might indicate the team's attempt to 'control' the game, playing more offensively. In line with Bloomfield *et al.* (2005b), Jones *et al.* (2004), Lago and Martin (2007) and Lago (2009), the findings of the present study support the notion that team strategies in soccer are influenced by score-line; however, it has also been shown that this influence altered in different game periods.

The change of team strategy, in consequence of the current result, was revealed by the field zone where the free kicks were taken. When ahead or drawing, the team concentrated its play in the OMZ, where it suffered the highest number of fouls. However, when behind, the team performed more than 40% of free kicks in the OCZ, followed by the COMZ. These results suggest that, in score disadvantage, the team probably used more offensive strategies, trying to explore the central field zones more.

The results of the log-linear model did not demonstrate any significant interaction between performance indicators and quality of opposition. This fact might be explained by the low ranking of the observed team, lacking the sensitivity of the opposition quality variable, which classified opponents as stronger and less strong. Another explanation might be the absence of well-defined strategies for free kick situations, when the team played against different opponents. It should be noted that similar results were reported by Ensum *et al.* (2002), who had not observed any significant variety of 'set plays' such as corners, free kicks, and throw-ins as a function of any of the situation variables. Similarly, in the study of Taylor *et al.* (2008), the quality of opposition had not shown any significant effects on the behavior incidence, excluding aerial challenges, dribbles, and passes.

Analyzing the free kick as a specific soccer game situation, and considering the pitch surface where free kicks were executed, the results of this study provide a new insight into strategic and tactical changes in a team's play in different competitive contexts, as Ensum *et al.* (2002) and Hughes and Franks (2004) have suggested.

The findings of this study have some practical implications. For example, it could be suggested that a coach design free kick drills taking into consideration the different field zones; given the variability of where the team suffered the fouls. Taking into account that the central zones of the penalty area were most frequently used in the successful free kicks, it is necessary to prepare the players to explore these areas more while practicing free kick situations. Attending to the high level of free kick success observed not only in the COZ, but also in the ROZ and LOZ, these field areas might be used as alternatives to beat the opposition defense and finish the ball possession successfully.

In conclusion, our results emphasize the importance of accounting for quality of opposition and match status during the assessment of soccer-specific game situations for the free kick (Carling *et al.*, 2005; Taylor *et al.*, 2008; Lago, 2009).

# References

Acar, M.F. *et al.*, 2009, Analysis of goals scored in the 2006 World Cup. In *Science and Football VI*, London: Routledge, pp. 235–242.

Alcock, A., 2010, Analysis of direct free kicks in the women's football World Cup 2007. *Eur J Sport Sci*, **10**, 279–284.

Bloomfield, J. *et al.*, 2005a, Effects of score-line on intensity of play in midfield and forward players in the FA Premier League. *J Sports Sci*, **23**, 191–192.

Bloomfield, J. *et al.*, 2005b, Effects of score-line on team strategies in FA Premier League Soccer. *J Sports Sci*, **23**, 192–193.

Carling, C. *et al.*, 2005, *Handbook of Soccer Match Analysis: A Systematic Approach to Improving Performance*, London and New York: Routledge.

Ensum, J. *et al.*, 2002, A quantitative analysis of attacking set plays. *Insight*, **4**, 68–72.

Grant, A.G. *et al.*, 1999, Analysis of goals scored in the 1998 World Cup. *J Sports Sci*, **17**, 826–827.

Hill, M.M. and Hill, A., 2002, *Investigação por questionário*, Lisboa: Silabo.

Hughes, M.D. and Franks, I.M., 2004, Notational analysis: A review of literature. In *Notational Analysis of Sports: Systems for Better Coaching and Performance in Sport*, 2nd ed., London: Routledge, pp. 99–107.

Jones, P.D. *et al.*, 2004, Possession as a performance indicator on soccer. *Int J Perf Analys Sport*, **4**, 98–102.

Lago, C., 2009, The influence of match location, quality of opposition, and match status on possession strategies in professional association football. *J Sports Sci*, **27**, 1463–1469.

Lago, C. and Martin, R., 2007, Determinants of possession of the ball on soccer. *J Sports Sci*, **25**, 969–974.

O'Donoghue, P. G. and Tenga, A., 2001, The effect of score-line on work rate in elite soccer. *J Sports Sci*, **19**, 14–30.

Perea, A.E. *et al.*, 2006, Registro de datos observacionales a partir del Match Vision Studyo v1.0. In *Socialización y deporte: revisión crítica*, Diputación Foral del Álava.

Taylor, J.B. *et al.*, 2005, Notational analysis of corner kicks in English Premier League Soccer. In *Science and Football V*, London: Routledge, pp. 225–230.

Taylor, J.B. *et al.*, 2008, The influence of match location, quality of opposition and match status on technical performance in professional association football. *J Sports Sci*, **26**, 885–895.

Tucker, W. *et al.*, 2005, Game location effects in professional soccer: A case study. *Int J Perf Analys Sport*, **5**, 23–35.

Van der Mars, H., 1989, Observer reliability: Issues and procedures, In *Analyzing Physical Education and Sport Instruction*, Champaign, IL: Human Kinetics, pp. 19–51.

# CHAPTER THIRTY-FIVE

# Analysis of Finnish young soccer players' passing and dribbling skills

T. Vänttinen

Research Institute for Olympic Sports, Jyväskylä, Finland

## 1. INTRODUCTION

The most important variables for measuring performance in soccer are physical condition, technical skills and tactical performance (Rösch et al., 2000). As player's physical fitness capacity during puberty is mainly related to player's maturity (Mendez-Villanueva et al., 2011), it has been suggested that the focus in youth soccer should be placed on ball-handling and game skills (Lindquist and Bangsbo, 1991). Most of the studies concerning the development of ball-handling skills have been carried out on youth teams in professional soccer clubs (e.g. Malina et al., 2005, Huijgen et al., 2010). However, youth soccer in Finland has been based on the 'All Stars' ideology since the year 2000. This ideology emphasizes that every child on a team has the right to participate and guarantees equal opportunities for each player regardless of their abilities. For example, the rules of All Stars administered by the FA of Finland obligates that each player must have equal playing time during the game and no league tables are allowed in the age groups under 12 years of age. Therefore, the aims of the present study were: (1) to examine changes in the rate of dribbling and passing skill development between ages 10 to 15 years in both genders; (2) to examine the differences in dribbling and passing skills between genders; and (3) to examine how young soccer players dribbling and passing skills have changed across a decade (between 2000–2010) when players training background changed from the system that emphasized competitiveness to 'All Stars' which emphasizes participation.

## 2. METHODS

The passing (Figure 1) and dribbling tests (Figure 2) were analyzed from the annually organized Finnish youth soccer skill championships held between the years of 2002 to 2010. In the championships, the players qualified from regional competitions compete in six age categories from 10 to 15y in both genders. In the passing and dribbling tests, the performance time was measured with a stopwatch and the best out of two trials (more than 3 min recovery between trials) was recorded as a score (FA of Finland, 2010). Test results were analyzed for both genders in a 6 x 9 (age group x year) analysis of variance and the gender difference was analyzed in a 2 x 6 (sex x age group) analysis of variance.

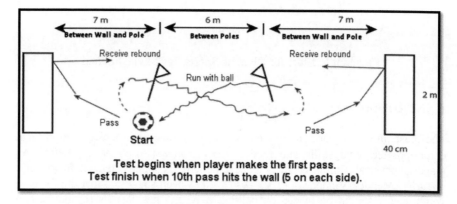

**Figure 1** Diagram of the passing test used in Finnish youth skill competitions.

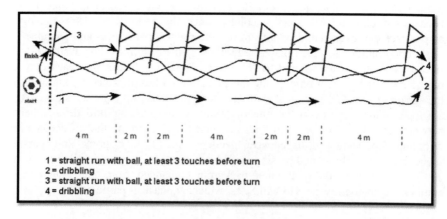

**Figure 2** Diagram of the dribbling test used in Finnish youth skill competitions.

## 3. RESULTS

The results of the passing and dribbling tests for both genders by year and by age are presented in Table 1 and 2 and Figure 3. Relative development with age for both genders is also presented in Figure 3.

In the passing test, a significant main effect for age ($F_{5,921}$=93.78, $p<0.001$) and year ($F_{8,921}$=2.74, $p<0.01$) was found in boys and for age ($F_{5,679}$=95.82, $p<0.001$), year ($F_{8,679}$=5.13, $p<0.001$) and age x year ($F_{40,679}$=1.53, $p<0.05$) in girls. Between genders, a significant main effect was found for sex ($F_{1,1696}$=617.55, $p<0.001$), age ($F_{5,1696}$=186.06, $p<0.001$) and sex x age ($F_{1,1696}$=4.47, $p<0.001$).

In the dribbling test, a significant main effect for age ($F_{5,921}$=97.27, $p<0.001$) and year ($F_{8,921}$=3.88, $p<0.001$) was found in boys and for age ($F_{5,679}$=81.30, $p<0.001$), year ($F_{8,679}$=3.62, $p<0.001$) and age x year ($F_{40,679}$=1.48, $p<0.05$) in girls. Between genders, a significant main effect was found for sex ($F_{1,1696}$=1014.55, $p<0.001$), age ($F_{5,1696}$=181.35, $p<0.001$) and sex x age ($F_{1,1696}$=8.22, $p<0.001$), age ($F_{5,1696}$=186.06, $p<0.001$) and sex x age ($F_{1,1696}$=4.47, $p<0.001$). In the dribbling test, a significant main effect for age ($F_{5,921}$=97.27, $p<0.001$) and year ($F_{8,921}$=3.88, $p<0.001$) was found in boys and for age ($F_{5,679}$=81.30, $p<0.001$), year ($F_{8,679}$=3.62, $p<0.001$) and age x year ($F_{40,679}$=1.48, $p<0.05$) in girls. Between genders, a significant main effect was found for sex ($F_{1,1696}$=1014.55, $p<0.001$), age ($F_{5,1696}$=181.35, $p<0.001$) and sex x age ($F_{1,1696}$=8.22, $p<0.001$).

**Table 1** Time (mean ± SD) in passing and dribbling tests by year for boys and girls.

|  |  | 2002 (n=142) | 2003 (n=165) | 2004 (n=187) | 2005 (n=183) | 2006 (n=204) | 2007 (n=205) | 2008 (n=196) | 2009 (n=211) | 2010 (n=215) |
|---|---|---|---|---|---|---|---|---|---|---|
| Passing (s) | Boys (n=975) | 37.6 ±5.7 | 35.6 ±6.0 | 36.4 ±3.9 | 35.8 ±3.9 | 35.5 ±3.9 | 36.9 ±4.2 | 35.8 ±4.1 | 36.8 ±4.0 | 36.5 ±6.4 |
| | Girls (n=733) | 42.6 ±5.7 | 40.2 ±6.6 | 41.1 ±5.2 | 40.4 ±6.1 | 41.0 ±5.8 | 41.2 ±6.1 | 39.1 ±5.7 | 41.7 ±5.2 | 40.6 ±5.5 |
| Dribbling (s) | Boys (n=975) | 25.4 ±1.9 | 25.4 ±1.9 | 25.2 ±1.5 | 25.4 ±1.8 | 24.9 ±1.7 | 25.4 ±1.7 | 25.1 ±1.5 | 25.8 ±1.2 | 25.4 ±1.8 |
| | Girls (n=733) | 28.7 ±2.4 | 28.2 ±2.9 | 28.2 ±2.7 | 28.0 ±2.7 | 27.9 ±2.8 | 28.1 ±2.4 | 27.4 ±2.6 | 28.8 ±1.8 | 28.3 ±2.6 |

**Table 2** Time (mean ± SD) in passing and dribbling tests by age for boys and girls.

|  |  | 10y (n=316) | 11y (n=251) | 12y (n=317) | 13y (n=377) | 14y (n=254) | 15y (n=193) |
|---|---|---|---|---|---|---|---|
| Passing (s) | Boys (n=975) | 40.2±4.5 | 36.8±3.1 | 35.9±3.2 | 35.2±4.2 | 33.7±2.4 | 33.2±2.4 |
|  | Girls (n=733) | 46.8±5.0 | 42.4±3.9 | 40.9±4.2 | 38.6±3.4 | 38.0±4.3 | 37.6±3.7 |
| Dribbling (s) | Boys (n=975) | 27.3±1.8 | 25.8±1.5 | 25.4±1.5 | 24.8±1.3 | 24.2±1.1 | 24.3±1.3 |
|  | Girls (n=733) | 31.1±2.4 | 29.0±2.2 | 28.2±2.5 | 27.1±1.9 | 26.6±1.8 | 26.8±2.1 |

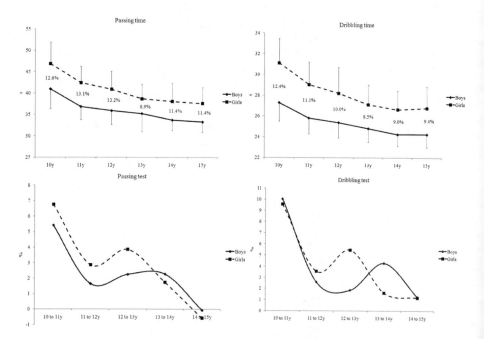

**Figure 3** Passing and dribbling time in addition with relative difference between genders (upper pics), and the relative development of passing and dribbling tests with age (lower pics).

## 4. DISCUSSION

Performance in the present passing and dribbling tests improved with age from 10 to 14y in both genders. Subsequently, no further improvement was observed in passing test time, however, an appropriate 1% improvement in dribbling test time was evident between the years of 14 to 15. The greatest relative improvement occurred between the youngest age groups (from 10 to 11 years) which suggest that the fastest development in passing and dribbling skills is likely to occur already before the age of 10 years. It also appeared that the performance time in the skill tests improved more rapidly around the peak height velocity which occurs at the age of around 12 years in girls and around 14 years in boys in Finland. The rate of improvement during this growth spurt was likely related more to development of physical abilities than actual ball-handling skills as previous research has shown that the peak development of speed and agility occurs at the same time as the growth spurt (Philippaerts *et al.*, 2006). Although, it is worth remembering that no data about the players' anthropometrics or physical performance characteristics was available in the present study. That is, no actual evidence exists about the connection between the skill tests and growth spurt and therefore the interpretations about this linkage need to be treated with caution.

Boys were around 10% faster than girls in passing and dribbling tests in all age categories. Actually, 11 year-old boys (pre-puberty) were already faster than 15 year-old girls (late puberty) in both skill tests. This indicates that boys were superior compared to girls in ball-handling skills; however, the difference cannot be explained by physical abilities in which 15y girls are known to be ahead of 10y boys (Malina, 2004). In other words, boys are performing closer to their maximal trainable potentiality than girls which suggests that girls should focus more on skill training in Finland. Although it is also important to remember that boys are usually engaged to soccer earlier than girls and around 35% more boys are playing soccer in Finland than girls in the 10–15 year-old age groups. That is, boys might be faster than girls because they have practised for a longer period of time and/or because more naturally gifted individuals exists in a bigger pool of male players.

Youth soccer in Finland has been based on the 'All Stars' ideology for more than ten years. This ideology guarantees equal opportunities for each player regardless of their abilities, which in addition to having widely acknowledged pedagogical benefits, has raised doubts about whether the system serves talented players or not. In the present study, it was found that the level of skill was not constant across the examined time period even though only the most skilful players of Finland were examined each year. However, no clear tendency for improvement nor regression could be detected in the passing or dribbling test results between 2002–2010 in either gender. In addition, as no differences were found between those players who competed in the Finnish youth soccer skill championships in the early 2000s (2002–2004) and practiced most of their time in competitive environments, and those who competed in the last years (2008–2010) and played all their career (so far) under the 'All Stars' ideology, it can be concluded that training under the 'All Stars' ideology did not affected the players' skill level. The year-to-year variation in the test results can rather be considered to arise from issues relating to test reliability, such as using hand timing and changes in environmental factors (field surface, balls and other similar variables).

To conclude, passing and dribbling test times improved uptil the age of 14 years. The rate of development increased temporarily at the same time as the growth spurt. This was likely to be related to improved physical performance abilities which are known to improve rapidly at the onset of peak height velocity (Philippaerts *et al.*, 2006). From the results of the present study, it can also be recommended that special attention should be placed on developing ball-handling skills among girl players because the difference between genders in the skill tests was greater than to be expected based on the differences in general physical characteristics (Malina, 2004). Although traditional ball-handling tests provides valuable information about young players' development, future research should focus on developing skill tests that include perceptual and decision making factors which are essential parts of skilful soccer performance and are ignored in the closed test environment.

## References

FA of Finland, 2010, The rules of youth soccer skill competitions, available from The Football Association of Finland website: http://www. palloliitto.fi/mp/ db/ file_library/x/IMG/159785/file/Taitokilpailusaannot10.pdf

Huijgen, B.C. *et al.*, 2010, Development of dribbling in talented youth soccer players aged 12–19 years: A longitudinal study. *J Sports Sci*, **28**, 689–698.

Lindquist, F. and Bangsbo, J., 1991, Do young soccer players need specific physical training? In: *Science and Football II*, London: E. & F.N. Spon, pp. 275–280.

Malina, R.M. *et al.*, 2004, Strength and motor performance. In *Growth, Maturation and Physical Activity* (2nd edition), Champaign, IL: Human Kinetics, pp. 215–233.

Mendez-Villanueva, A. *et al.*, 2011, Age-related differences in acceleration, maximum running speed, and repeated-sprint performance in young soccer players. *J Sports Sci*, **29**, 477–484.

Philippaerts, R. *et al.*, 2006, The relationship between peak height velocity and physical performance in youth soccer players. *J Sports Sci*, **24**, 221–230.

Rösch, D. *et al.*, 2000, Assessment and evaluation of football performance. *Am J Sports Med*, **28**, 29–39.

# Part IV

# Motor behaviour

# CHAPTER THIRTY-SIX

# How skilled Gaelic football players practice kicking: deliberate or not?

E. Coughlan, P. R. Ford, A. McRobert and A. M. Williams

Research Institute for Sport and Exercise Sciences,
Liverpool John Moores University, UK

## 1. INTRODUCTION

The superior performance of experts compared to their lesser skilled counterparts can be linked to the domain specific training undertaken throughout their careers (Ericsson *et al.*, 1993). This domain specific activity is known as deliberate practice and it is activity designed to advance a current aspect of an individual's performance that requires improvement, e.g. improving an identified weakness in kicking accuracy. It is characterized as being mentally and physically effortful, highly relevant to improving performance, not immediately rewarding, or inherently enjoyable (Ericsson *et al.*, 1993).

These tenets have been challenged and consequently contradicted in some studies, e.g. Hodges and Starkes (1996) and Ward *et al.* (2007) where they found that when athletes retrospectively recall their practice histories they rate these deliberate practice activities as enjoyable and rewarding. These findings may not have transpired if the data was collected during the practice session (and not retrospectively). Furthermore, the practice may not have been deliberate in nature. Practice designed to induce a lasting performance improvement requires constant attention (Auer, 1921) and also the mindfulness of both coach and athlete to know when to progress the training stimulus to match the rate of development (Guadagnoli and Lee, 2004).

When allowed to self-select their practice schedule, skilled athletes may engage in deliberate practice activity to improve their performance and rectify weaknesses, which should have the predicted deliberate practice characteristics. This is expected to counter the findings for the less skilled. The objective of this study is to test this hypothesis in a controlled environment using skilled and less-skilled Gaelic football players as they practise two different free-kick tasks.

## 2. METHODS

Forty-five adult Gaelic football players were divided equally into three groups: skilled (SK), less-skilled (LSK) and control skilled (CSK). Players completed pre-, post- and retention-tests involving two free-kick skills (out of hands, off ground – 10 trials of each) 25m from a graded set of Gaelic football posts (see Figure 1). The highest and lowest scores possible for a kick-type are 30-points and 10-points respectively. Following the pre-test and for subsequent practice sessions, participants were informed of the scores attained for both kicks. The kick-type with the lower pre-test score was deemed the weak kick and the kick-type with the higher pre-test score was deemed the strong kick. The SK and LSK groups practised the two skills over four practice sessions across four weeks, each 30 min in duration. The SK and LSK groups were required to attempt to improve their pre-test scores of both skills throughout the acquisition phase. They were free to self-select their practice schedule during practice sessions. In a novel development, the tenets of deliberate practice were examined in-situ midway through each practice session using established measures of mental effort (Rating Scale of Mental Effort – RSME, Zijlstra and van Dorn, 1985), physical effort (Rate of Perceived Exertion – RPE, Borg, 1985), motivation (Situational Motivational Scale – SIMS, Standage, *et al.*, 2003) and enjoyment (Physical Activity Enjoyment Scale – PACES, Kendzierski and DeCarlo, 1991). Concurrent verbal report data was collected to examine the cognitive thought processes occurring during practice.

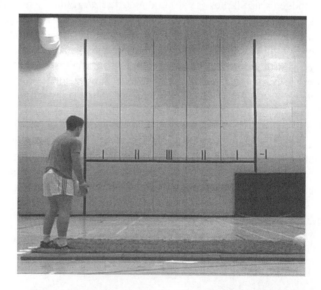

**Figure 1** Experimental set-up with graded Gaelic football posts.

A 3 (test) x 2 (kick) x 2 (group) ANOVA was used to analyze the test data. Independent samples *t*-tests were used to calculate the differences between groups for each of the tenets of deliberate practice. A 3 (statements) x 2 (group) ANOVA was used to analyze the verbal report data.

## 3. RESULTS

### Testing and acquisition data

Both the SK and the LSK groups significantly improved their overall outcome scores for kicking from pre- to post-test, whereas the CSK group did not improve their pre- to post-test scores (see Figures 2 and 3). The SK group practised the skill they were weakest on from the pre-test on 66% of the acquisition trials in comparison to 27% for the LSK group.

### Deliberate practice data

The SK group rated their practice as 31% less enjoyable (PACES), 47% more mentally effortful (RSME), 22% more challenging to motivation (SIMS), 20% more physically exertive (RPE) compared to the LSK group (see Figure 4).

### Verbal report data

In concurrence with the RSME data for mental effort the SK group recorded more verbal report statements per trial than the LSK group during acquisition (see Figure 5).

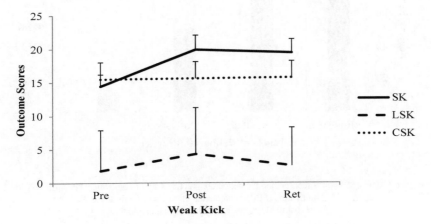

**Figure 2** Mean (SD) points scored for the weak kick of the skilled, less-skilled and control-skilled for pre-, post- and retention tests.

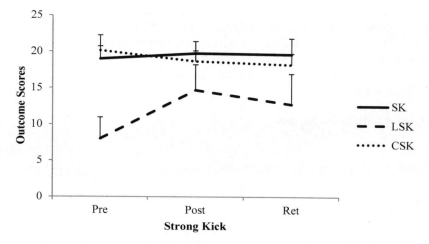

**Figure 3** Mean (SD) points scored for the strong kick of the skilled, less-skilled and control-skilled for pre-, post- and retention tests.

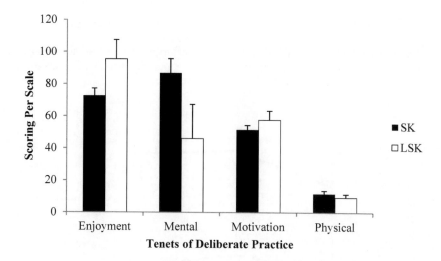

**Figure 4** Mean (SE) points recorded on the deliberate practice scales of enjoyment (PACES), physical effort (RPE), motivation (SIMS) and mental effort (RSME) for the skilled and less-skilled groups during the acquisition phase.

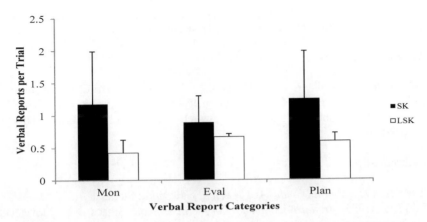

**Figure 5** Mean (SD) number of verbal report statements per trial (monitoring, evaluation, planning) for the skilled and less-skilled groups during the acquisition phase.

## 4. DISCUSSION

Participants that focused on improving the performance of an identified weakness experienced the tenets of deliberate practice as predicted by Ericsson *et al.* (1993). The novel in-situ data collection protocol accurately measured the tenets of deliberate practice of the practice session in question thereby eliminating any aggregation of previous practice experiences.

The acquisition data showed that on a greater amount of their practice trials the SK group practised their weak kick. In comparison, the LSK group practised their strong kick on the majority of their practice trials. In addition, the deliberate practise data shows how the group that chose to practice the skill that was identified as a weakness also exhibited the predicted tenets of deliberate practice i.e. the SK group. Even though the LSK group experienced significant gains in their strong kick, they did not exhibit the predicted tenets of deliberate practice, thereby assigning this practice to a more generic-type practice resulting in it being more enjoyable as the data revealed. Furthermore, the greater mental effort exhibited by the SK group compared to the LSK group is supported by the greater proportion of verbal reports the SK group dedicate to monitoring and planning during the acquisition phase.

Implications of this study will better inform athletes and coaches on how to measure the nature of the practice they engage in and prescribe respectively. This will ensure that the quality and the goals of practice are better aligned to the areas that require the most work. Future research directions may be to investigate other activities that skilled performers engage in that contribute to the gap between them and their lesser skilled counterparts e.g. reflective practice.

In conclusion, this study has shown that when a skilled group of Gaelic football players practice to improve a weakness, they experience the tenets of deliberate practice as proposed by Ericsson *et al.* (1993). Furthermore, less skilled

Gaelic football players practice in a manner that is less challenging from a physical and mental effort perspective, focusing on tasks that are more enjoyable.

## Acknowledgements

The authors would like to acknowledge the exceptional support of Ken Robinson, CEO of DCU Sport, Prof. Niall Moyna of Dublin City University, and the DCU GAA club throughout this study. This research was funded by the Gaelic Athletic Association.

## References

Auer, L., 1921, *Violin Playing As I Teach It.* New York: Stokes.

Borg, G., 1985, *An Introduction to Borg's RPE Scale.* Ithaca, NY: Movement Publications.

Ericsson, K.A. *et al.*, 1993, The role of deliberate practice in the acquisition of expert performance. *Psychological Review*, **100**, 363–406.

Guadagnoli, M.A. and Lee, T.D., 2004, Challenge point: Framework for conceptualizing the effects of various practice conditions in motor learning. *J Motor Behav*, **36**, 212–224.

Hodges, N.J. and Starkes, J.L., 1996, Wrestling with the nature of expertise: A sport-specific test of Ericsson, Krampe and Tesch-Römer's (1993) theory of 'deliberate practice'. *Int J Sport Psychol*, **27**, 400–424.

Kendzierski, D. and DeCarlo, K.J., 1991, Physical Activity Enjoyment Scale: Two validation studies. *J Sport Exerc Psychol*, **13**, 30–64.

Standage, M. *et al.*, 2003, Validity, reliability, and invariance of the situational motivation scale (SIMS) across diverse physical activity contexts. *J Sport Exerc Psychol*, **25**, 19–43.

Ward, P. *et al.*, 2007, The road to excellence: Deliberate practice and the development of expertise. *High Ability Studies*, **18**, 119–153.

Zijlstra, F. and Van Dorn, L., 1985, *The Construction of a Scale to Measure Perceived Effort.* Delft University of Technology, The Netherlands.

# CHAPTER THIRTY-SEVEN

# Factors influencing penalty kick success in elite soccer

S. White and P. O'Donoghue

Cardiff School of Sport
University of Wales Institute Cardiff, Wales, UK

## 1. INTRODUCTION

When a penalty is taken in soccer, the ball may reach the goal just 0.2s after it is kicked (Chiappori *et al.*, 2002). The reported conversion rates of penalty kicks are 63.6% (Kuhn, 1988), 76% (Morya *et al.*, 2005) and 78.9% (Jordet *et al.*, 2007). There is debate about the penalty taking strategy most likely to result in a goal. Some suggest that striking the ball low as close to the post as possible gives the best chance of a goal (McMorris and Hauxwell, 1997) while others suggest that shooting high is optimal (Bar-Eli and Azar, 2009).

Many factors can affect the success of a penalty kick including pressure and psychological stress (Jordet *et al.*, 2007; Geisler and Leith, 1997). The increased level of anxiety associated with a stressful event may lead to decreased performance (McGarry and Franks, 2000; Jordet, 2009). Penalty takers, despite being elite professional players, have been found to aim only low proportions of penalties to the areas determined the most difficult for a goalkeeper to save (Bar-Eli and Azar, 2009). A logical suggestion is that aiming towards an area where the goalkeeper has a minimal chance of making a save, such as the top corners, increases the risk of missing the goal.

Due to the importance of penalty kicks, goalkeepers strive to improve their performance in penalty kick scenarios. Goalkeeper's when facing a penalty kick dive to the left or the right in 95% of instances (Bar-Eli *et al.*, 2007). A third option which is rarely employed by goalkeepers is remaining in the middle of the goal. Goalkeepers are allowed to move along the goal line before the ball is kicked as long as they do not move forwards. Goalkeepers move in the correct direction on 69% of occasions when delaying movement compared to 30% of occasions when moving early (Morya *et al.*, 2005). These results illustrating increased performance when initiating later movement are in contrast to many other sources which state that goalkeepers need to begin their movement no later than ball contact and therefore have to make a decision on their action before the ball is kicked (McMorris *et al.*, 1993; McMorris and Hauxwell, 1997; Miller, 1998). Much of this evidence is based on analysing ball speed, reaction times and movement times from penalty kicks, with an analysis of such factors in four World Cups finding that the typical penalty kick would reach the goal in less time than the combined reaction and movement times of a goalkeeper (Miller, 1998). It can therefore be argued that anticipating kick direction and initiating early movement would appear to be the most effective tactic for goalkeepers facing penalty kicks.

It has previously been recommended that computerised notational analysis be used to obtain objective data on penalty kick strategies (Kuhn, 1988) and that research is needed to help goalkeepers decide which way to move as early as possible when facing penalty kicks (Morya *et al.*, 2005). Research on penalty kicks has investigated factors such as areas of the goal that penalty takers commonly aim for (Morya *et al.*, 2005; Bar-Eli and Azar, 2009) and the effects of factors such as footedness (McMorris and Colenso, 1996) and style of kick (Morya *et al.*, 2005*)*. The effects of time have been briefly touched on in previous literature where it has been stated that the scoring probability is greater for a penalty kick during the first 15 minutes of a game and lower for a penalty kick in the last 30 minutes (Chiappori *et al.*, 2002).

Penalty takers in professional soccer are very aware of the need to prevent their actions being predicted by an opponent (Palacios-Huerta, 2003). To avoid becoming predictable, penalty takers should randomize their actions (Bar-Eli and Azar, 2009). Very few penalty takers always kick in the same direction (Chiappori *et al.*, 2002) and choices appear to be independent of previous action or outcome (Palacios-Huerta, 2003). The aims of the current study were to investigate the following:

1. The observed use of strategies by both penalty takers and goalkeepers compared to expected uniform distributions.
2. Whether certain strategies are more successful than others.
3. Whether certain factors influence both use and success of strategies.

The scope of the present study was penalties in the top divisions in England (Premier League), Germany (Bundesliga 1), Italy (Serie A) and Spain (La Liga Primera Division) during the 2009/10 season.

## 2. METHODS

Factual data was collected from a specialist football website, www.soccernet. espn.go.com. This source was used to identify matches in which penalties were taken and collect the data for date, competition, teams, taker, score, score difference and time. This data was provided to the data collectors prior to the other fields being completed from observation of video footage of the penalty kicks. The video footage was collected using recordings of television highlight programmes and where necessary internet sites such as www.footytube.com, www.youtube .com, www.soccer360.co.uk, www.football-highlight.com. Video recordings of 286 penalties taken during soccer matches in the top professional leagues in

England, Germany, Italy and Spain in 2009–10 were analysed in the current investigation. The goal was divided into six 4ft high x 6ft wide zones as shown in Figure 1. The instances collected were used to gather data on the following variables:

- Kick direction – the zone the penalty was placed in.
- Goalkeeper's actions – the zone the goalkeeper moved to.
- Footedness – right and left footed penalty taker.
- Match time – the first and second halves of matches.
- Match score.
- The time the penalty was taken.
- Outcome – scored or not.

Chi square goodness of fit tests were used to analyse penalty taker and goalkeeper action. A series of chi square tests of independence was used to compare the 217 (75.9%) of penalties that resulted in a goal with the remaining 69 that were unsuccessful. Three independent people were used to collect the observational data. Where responses were in disagreement, the response with a majority verdict (2 out of 3 matching responses) was recorded as the result. In the events where all three data collectors reported varying observations to a given field (n=6), the penalty kicks in question were excluded from the study.

## 3. RESULTS

Penalty kicks were distributed to significantly different areas to those of an expected uniform distribution ($p < 0.001$) with 36.7% placed in the bottom-left zone and 30.1% placed in the bottom-right zone. While there were no significant differences in the outcome of penalty kicks placed in different zones ($p = 0.231$), the 86.2% scored in the upper three zones was noticeably higher than when the ball was placed in the three lower zones as shown in Figure 1.

| | | |
|---|---|---|
| 13/16 =81.3% | 11/11 =100.0% | 20/25 =80.0% |
| 76/105 =72.4% | 27/37 =73.0% | 64/86 =74.4% |

**Figure 1** Success rates of penalties placed in different zones.

There were 175 (61.2%) penalties taken in the second half which was significantly greater than the expected 50% (p < 0.001). However, the 77.7% of penalties scored in the second half was not significantly greater than the 73.0% scored in the first half (p = 0.434). None of footedness of the penalty taker (p = 0.734), goalkeeper action (p = 0.856) or score in the match (p = 0.176) had a significant influence on outcome. However, there was a significant difference in the placement of penalties by left and right footed players (p < 0.001) with left footed players placing 23.9% of kicks to the left, 10.9% in the middle and 65.2% to the right compared to 45.8% to the left, 20.4% to the middle and 33.8% to the right by right footed players.

There were 134 penalties taken by players who had taken a previous penalty with 32 (23.9%) of these being placed in the same zone as the previous penalty. Placement of the previous penalty kick was not found to significantly influence kick placement (p = 0.178). Furthermore, whether the penalty taker placed the penalty in the same zone as the previous penalty or not had no influence on the outcome (p = 0.649).

| 0<br>=0.0% | 0<br>=0.0% | 0<br>=0.0% |
|---|---|---|
| 151<br>=52.8% | 11<br>=3.9% | 124<br>=43.4% |

**Figure 2** Distribution of goalkeeper movement.

Figure 2 summarises the action of the keepers during the penalty kicks. When placement of the penalty and goalkeeper action were considered together, the 58 out of 110 (52.7%) penalties scored when the keeper moved to the correct zone was a significantly lower proportion than the 159 out of 176 (90.3%) when he did not (p < 0.001).

## 4. DISCUSSION

With 75.9% of the penalties being scored, the current investigation agrees with the findings of previous research that penalty kicks are likely to result in goals (Kuhn, 1988; Morya *et al.*, 2005; Jordet *et al.*, 2007). Goalkeepers' actions can substantially enhance their chance of preventing a goal, as shown by the significant difference in outcome when the goalkeeper moved to the correct zone. The reduction in goals scored when goalkeepers moved in the correct direction was greater than that reported in previous research (Palacios-Huerta, 2003). The most striking result of the current investigation was that there were no occasions where goalkeepers moved to the upper three zones. This would suggest that these would be successful areas for penalty takers to place penalties. The conversion percentages shown in Figure 1 confirm this and disagree with the finding of Bar-Eli and Azar (2009) that striking the ball low and close to the post is the most successful strategy. Practice is required to place penalties in these areas without the ball going over the bar. There are three explanations for goalkeepers not moving to these areas. Firstly, penalties tend to only be placed in these areas on 20.3% of penalty kicks. Secondly, the keeper has further to move to reach the top-left and top-right zones 1 and 5 meaning that a goal is more likely to be conceded even if the goalkeeper anticipates correctly. The third reason is that penalties aimed at these areas could miss the target more than penalties placed in the lower three zones.

The current investigation suggests that knowledge of placement of previous penalty kicks is of limited benefit to goalkeepers, which supports the conclusions of a previous research study (Palacios-Huerta, 2003). A pertinent and readily accessible piece of information available on penalty takers which effects kick placement is footedness. Right footed players kicking left and left footed players kicking right is deemed to be naturally easier with such kicks less likely to be saved and also less likely to be missed (Chiappori *et al.*, 2002).

The importance of a goalkeeper's actions when facing a penalty kick and the evidence to show that goalkeepers need to anticipate kick direction as opposed to reacting to kick direction (McMorris *et al.*, 1993; McMorris and Hauxwell, 1997; Miller, 1998) illustrate the importance of developing anticipation based on visual cues. If a goalkeeper can use such information to correctly anticipate a player's likely kick direction, they can move earlier and give themselves a far greater chance of being successful. Sports science support may have an important role to play in such preparation.

## References

Bar-Eli, M. and Azar, O.H., 2009, Penalty kicks in soccer: An empirical analysis of shooting strategies and goalkeepers' preferences. *Soccer and Society*, **10**, 183–191.

Bar-Eli, M. *et al.*, 2007, Action bias among elite soccer goalkeepers: The case of penalty kicks. *J Econom Psychol*, **28**, 606–621.

Chiappori, P.A. *et al.*, 2002, Testing mixed-strategy equilibria when players are heterogeneous: The case of penalty kicks in soccer. *American Economic Review*, **92**, 1138–1151.

Geisler, G.W.W. and Leith, G.M., 1997, The effects of self-esteem, self-efficacy and audience presence on soccer penalty shot performance. *J Sport Behav*, **20**, 322–337.

Hartmann, D.P., 1977, Considerations in the choice of inter-observer reliability estimates. *J Appl Behav Analysis*, **10**, 103–116.

Johnson, S.M. and Bolstad, O.D., 1973, Methodological issues in naturalistic observation: Some problems and solutions for field research. In *Behaviour Change: Methodology, Concepts, and Practice*, Champaign, Il: Human Kinetics, pp. 7–67.

Jordet, G., 2009, When superstars flop: Public status and choking under pressure in international soccer penalty shootouts. *J Appl Sport Psychol*, **21**, 125–130.

Jordet, G. *et al.*, 2007, Kicks from the penalty mark in soccer: The roles of stress, skill and fatigue for kick outcomes. *J Sports Sci*, **25**, 121–129.

Kuhn, W., 1988, Penalty kick strategies for shooters and goalkeepers. In *Science and Football*, London: E. & F.N. Spon, pp. 489–492.

McGarry, T. and Franks, I.M., 2000, On winning the penalty shoot-out in soccer. *J Sports Sci*, **18**, 401–409.

McMorris, T. and Colenso, S., 1996, Anticipation of professional goalkeepers when facing right- and left-footed penalty kicks. *Percep Motor Skill*, **82**, 931–934.

McMorris, T. *et al.*, 1993, Anticipation of soccer goalkeepers facing penalty kicks. In *Science and Football II*, London: E. & F.N. Spon, pp. 250–253.

McMorris, T. and Hauxwell, B., 1997, Improving anticipation of soccer goalkeepers using video observation. In *Science and Football III*, London: E. & F.N. Spon, pp. 290–294.

Miller, C., 1998, *He Always Puts It to the Right: A History of the Penalty Kick*, London: Orion Books.

Morya, E. *et al.*, 2005, Evolving penalty kick strategies: World Cup and club matches 2000–2002. In *Science and Football V*, London: E. & F.N. Spon, pp. 237–243.

Palacios-Huerta, I., 2003, Professionals Play Minimax. *Rev Econ Studies*, **70**, 395–415.

Tabakin, D., 2009, *Video Analysis of Soccer Penalty Kicks.* http://www.articlesbase.com/soccer-articles/video-analysis-of-soccer-penalty-kick-876350.html.

van der Mars, H., 1989, Observer reliability: Issues and procedures. In *Analyzing Physical Education and Sport Instruction, Second Edition*, Champaign, Il: Human Kinetics, pp. 53–80.

# CHAPTER THIRTY-EIGHT

# Above real time decision making in Australian football

M. Lorains, K. Ball and C. MacMahon

School of Sport and Exercise Science, Victoria University, Melbourne, Australia

## 1. INTRODUCTION

Video-based decision training in sport has been shown to improve decision accuracy in as little as six 30 minute sessions (Starkes and Lindley, 1994). One issue in the design of a video-based decision making task, is making it 'game-like'. This has led to skill acquisition research suggesting that video-based tasks do not elicit real world behaviors (Araujo *et al.*, 2006). One possibility for enhancing the 'game-like' aspects of video-based simulations involves manipulating the speed at which videos are played, to create above real time (ART) simulations. ART places the subject in an environment that functions faster than normal time and is widely used in military and aviation training (Vidulich *et al.*, 1983). Anecdotal evidence from aviation pilot training suggests that pilots felt that simulations played in ART were more real life than those simulations played in real time (Vidulich *et al.*, 1983).

In cognitive skills such as decision making, creating above-real-time demands may allow elite athletes to perform more automatically, a key characteristic of elite performance. Lorains and MacMahon (2009) employed the ART method to compare decision making accuracy on video clips played in normal and one ART speed. Results revealed that elite Australian football (AF) players performed more accurately on the ART clips compared to their lesser skilled counterparts.

This current research further explores the effect a range of video speeds, including ART, have on expert decision making performance in AF. Elite AF players were tested on a video-based decision making task, with video clips played in slow speed, normal speed and ART.

## 2. METHODS

### Participants and testing materials

Forty-five male elite AF players, currently training and/or competing in the Australian Football League (AFL, the highest level of play for the sport) completed a video-based decision simulation task.

The decision making test included 72 test clips, each played in different speeds (.75, 1.0, 1.25, 1.5, 1.75 and 2.0). The videos were sourced from aerial broadcast footage (behind the goals and side on view) from AFL matches. Each video clip was occluded at a critical decision point, in order to prompt players to decide where to kick or handball. At this point a loud beep was heard to indicate the players needed to make a response. They had a maximum of three seconds to respond, before they could no longer record a response. A second and third beep sounded to indicate they were running out of time. This was included to increase the level of time pressure they were under to make a decision.

The video clips ranged in length from two seconds to 23 seconds, depending on the speed. A range of teams were featured in the clips. Each video clip was edited within Adobe Premiere Elements version 9.0, using the time stretch feature, to change the speed of each clip. For example, if a normal speed clip was seven seconds in duration, the ART clip edited to 150% of that speed would be for a duration of four seconds.

Before editing the clips, each was viewed in full by three AFL coaches. They individually rated each video clip and assigned three points to the best decision making option, two points to the second best option and one point to the third best option. This process was used to measure decision accuracy of players. The presentation and data collection was completed through Experimental Psychological Software Testing tool E-Prime V2 Professional. This software recorded and automatically scored each response. The testing was completed on individual laptops, using a mouse click to record responses.

## Procedure

Players were seated at an individual laptop (see Figure 1) and used the computer mouse to select where on the screen they would kick/handball to if they were the player in possession of the ball. The clip played, and paused, a beep was heard and players could then respond. They had a maximum of three seconds to respond. Subsequent beeps played to indicate the three seconds were running out, and thus to induce time pressure. Responses could be anywhere on the screen, a specific player, space on the field, between the goals, or to play on (clicking on the player with the ball). Participants were instructed to make their decision as quickly as possible within the allocated three seconds.

Decision accuracy (% correct) and decision time (s) were measured. The best option was awarded three points, the second best option two points and the third best option scored one point. Any responses outside of these areas received zero points. Decision time was measured from the point that the video paused to when players clicked on the screen to respond. For analysis, speeds above 1.0 were collapsed together to make up the ART condition.

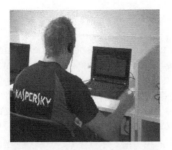

**Figure 1** Photograph of testing set up.

## 3. RESULTS

A one way repeated measures ANOVA comparing normal time and ART revealed a significant effect for accuracy [Wilks' Lambda = .56, $F(2, 43) = 16.82$, $p < .005$, partial $\eta^2 = .44$]. Post-hoc testing revealed that the athletes performed more accurately on ART clips (M = 68.53%, SD = 10.98%) compared to normal (M = 52.00%, SD = 16.91%) and slow speed clips (M = 55.94%, SD = 19.12), $p < .005$. This finding is illustrated in Figure 2. Main effects for decision time were also found [Wilks' Lambda = .86, $F(2, 43) = 3.59$, $p < .04$, partial $\eta^2 = .14$]. Decision times were significantly slower for ART clips (M = 1.43, SD = .28) and normal speed clips (M = 1.42, SD = .36) compared to slow speed clips (M = 1.33, SD = .35, $p = .03$). Decision time did not differ between normal and ART speed.

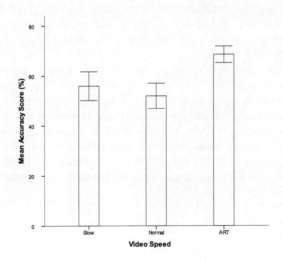

**Figure 2** Mean accuracy score across video speeds.

## 4. DISCUSSION

Decision making is a key aspect in elite sporting performance. Moreover, sport is a domain in which making decisions under immense time pressure is particularly crucial. These results lend support for previous findings (Lorains and MacMahon, 2009) which suggest that decisions made in a faster environment are more accurate due to athletes having less time to think about the action, allowing them to perform more automatically. Specifically, Johnson and Raab (2003) found that athletes performed more accurately in their decisions when they took the first option that came to mind, compared to a more deliberative process in which they generated as many options as they could. These findings were also apparent in research in AF, as discussed earlier (Lorains and MacMahon, 2009), where elite athletes performed not only significantly more accurate on ART simulations compared to their lesser skilled counterparts, but more accurately on ART clips compared to normal speeded clips.

This research uses the same methods of Lorains and MacMahon (2009) by investigating speeded video clips, but builds upon it by testing more ART speeds and applying time pressure on decisions. This has resulted in testing of a more 'game-like' video-based simulation with the elite target group.

The difference in decision times was interesting, in that the elite athletes recorded faster decisions on the slower speeded clips. While these results do go against the findings of Johnson and Raab (2003) who found decisions made quickly or when the first option was taken, were more accurate, the authors don't believe these results reflect any processing methods or substantial findings, but is a design matter that could be considered in future research. The findings could be explained by the fact that decision times were taken from the point at which the video paused to the time of decision. As the slower speeded clips played out for longer, athletes seemed to track the player and had already made their decision before the video paused.

From a coaching point of view, the use of ART video to improve decision based simulation training has many practical advantages. Video-based decision making is not physically demanding as it is 'off the feet' training, coaches are not needed to be present and the set up is simple and inexpensive, using generally easily accessible game-based film. This method of training is also something athletes can do in their own home, while the ART aspect maintains the 'game-like' features. Future research should investigate the 'optimal' ART training speed, which is fast enough to elicit automatic behavior, but is still perceived to be game-like.

# References

Araujo, D. *et al.*, 2006, The ecological dynamics of decision making in sport, *Psychol Sport Exerc*, **7**, 653–676.

Johnson, J. and Raab, M., 2003, Take the first: Option-generation and resulting choices, *Organiz Behav Hum Decision Processes*, **91**, 215–229.

Lorains, M. and MacMahon, C., 2009, Adapting the functional overreaching principle to cognitive skills: Expertise differences using speed manipulations in a video-based decision-making task, In *Proceedings of the 12th World Congress of Sport Psychology (ISSP)*, Marrakesh, Morocco.

Starkes, J.L. and Lindley, S., 1994, Can we hasten expertise by video simulation? *Quest*, **46**, 211–222.

Vidulich, M. *et al.*, 1983, Time compressed components for air intercept control skills, In *Proceedings of the 27th Meeting of the Human Factors Society*, pp. 161–164.

# CHAPTER THIRTY-NINE

# Area covered by diving actions performed by male college soccer goalkeepers

K. Matsukura[1] and T. Asai[2]

[1]Doctoral Program of Comprehensive Human Sciences,
University of Tsukuba, Japan
[2]Comprehensive Human Sciences, University of Tsukuba, Japan

## 1. INTRODUCTION

In soccer, the goalkeeper is not always able to respond to a shot just by shifting his standing position. It is sometimes necessary for him to dive to defend the goal (which is 2.44 m high and 7.32 m wide) from a shot that has a shooting speed of 100 km per hour or more (Nunome *et al.*, 2002). There are a few studies conducted to date on diving motions (Suzuki *et al.*, 1988; Graham-Smith and Lees, 1999; Spratford *et al.*, 2009). Suzuki *et al.* (1988) referred to the relationship between the diving motion and the ability of the goalkeeper, in which skilled goalkeepers have a faster diving speed and reach for the ball in a straighter line than unskilled goalkeepers. Graham-Smith and Lees (1999) conducted biomechanical studies of diving motion, finding that it varies according to the course and distance of the incoming ball, requiring various necessary and important element forces to be generated by the rotational movement of the trunk and the extension of joints.

To clarify the area covered by the goalkeeper's diving motion, Kerwin and Bray (2006), using diving motion and vertical jump data recorded on video, studied the goalkeeper's reaching area at the time of a penalty kick taken by the opponent, presenting a diagram showing a concentric shape of the range of motion.

Therefore, in this study, we compared the reaching times and trajectories of the diving motion according to the height and distance of the balls. In addition, by creating a diagram depicting the various areas covered by the diving motion at fixed intervals of time, we attempted to clarify the reachable areas covered by the goalkeeper's diving motion in response to balls at different heights and distances.

## 2. METHODS

Subjects were 13 goalkeepers from a college soccer team whose average height was 179.8±5.5cm, average weight was 73.0±5.3kg, and average age was 20.5±1.5years. They were smaller and lighter than the subjects in previous research (185.2±3.8cm, 80.2±3.3kg in Spratford *et al.*, 2009). As the subjects were college students, they can be considered physically fully developed. They were asked their goalkeeping experience before the trial. The average number of years of goalkeeper experience was 10.5±3.5, none of the players was conspicuously immature in terms of diving technique. To avoid the goalkeepers from colliding with the goalpost during dives and encouraged them to dive forward, pendulum balls were positioned 50 cm in front of the goal line for high and middle height target and soccer balls were also positioned on the ground 50 cm in front of the goal line for low height target (Figure 1).

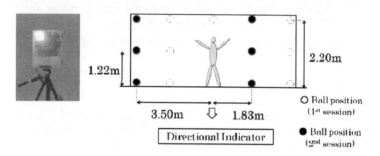

**Figure 1** Positions of balls in the experiment (photo refers to the directional indicator used in the experiment). Reproduced from Matsukura and Asai (2009), with permission.

The subject stood ready in the middle of the soccer goal (2.44 m × 7.32 m) on the assumption of receiving real shots, looking at the directional indicator held by an experimental assistant. In response to the timing indicated by the directional indicator, the subject dove to reach the balls, each placed as shown in Figure 1 in accordance with the directional indicator's signal.

The central portion of the directional indicator was composed of green and yellow LEDs, showing the timing for directional indications by gradually narrowing the central rectangular form over approximately 1s. After the central rectangular form disappeared, any one of the eight directions was displayed. The signal was programmed at random to minimize possible learning effects. Attempts were photographed twice for each ball position for recording and measurement. The entire experiment was implemented in two sessions. In the first session, out of the 13 locations, three balls (upper, middle, and lower) were positioned on one side farther from the subject, and another three were positioned on the other side close to the subject. This ensured that the subject was ready to dive a longer or shorter distance. Of the two attempts that were made for each of the 13 positions for measurement, we analysed the one with the shorter reaching time from the directional indication to the time the subject touched the ball.

In this experiment, because the subjects differed in body size and were comparatively high in competition level, all were assumed to be good at ball-reaching motions such as side steps and cross steps. Thus, they were given only the instruction 'You are to reach the ball as quickly as possible by diving'.

Using the images photographed by a high-speed camera (250 fps), the number of frames from the moment of the directional indication to the time the subject touched the ball was counted and then converted into time.

The bottom-left edge of the goal viewed from behind was set to be the co-ordinate origin of the *X*- (horizontal) and *Y*- (vertical) co-ordinates. We acquired the trajectories of the motion and the position (measured every 0.1s) of the point of the subject's hand that touched the ball (the third metacarpophalangeal joint) during the reaching time. The co-ordinate values of these points were obtained by calibrating the two-dimensional images based on the standard of the goal frame (2.44 m × 7.32 m) and converting them into actual lengths.

The five co-ordinate values positioned outermost for the same reaching time were selected out of the co-ordinate values of the hand touching the ball. These values were extrapolated by conducting a secondary fitting of them on a polar co-ordinate system to acquire an approximate curve.

To compare reaching times, the time needed to reach the ball was made a dependent variable, and a repeated-measurement three-factor dispersion analysis was conducted, which included the distance factor from the goalkeeper to the balls farther- and nearer-positioned (two standards), the right and left factor under the two standards, and the height factor of upper-, middle-, and lower-positioned balls. As a result, if the interactions were significant, a repeated-measurement two-factor dispersion analysis was conducted, and the Bonferroni method was employed for the subordinate test thereafter. The significance level of the statistical tests was 5%.

## 3. RESULTS AND DISCUSSION

The average values and standard deviations of the reaching times for all subjects by ball direction are shown in Table 1. The repeated-measurement three-factor dispersion analysis of distance, right vs. left, and height revealed that, although no significant difference appeared in the main effect of the right vs. left factor, the main effect of the distance factor (F $[1,12]$ = 1427.9, $p < 0.05$) and the main effect of the height factor (F $[2,24]$ = 102.9, $p < 0.05$), and the interaction between the distance and height factors (F $[2.24]$ = 68.7, $p < 0.05$) were significant. Because the interaction between the distance and height factors was significant, a repeated-measurement two-factor dispersion analysis was conducted with the distance factor divided into longer and shorter. Because the result revealed that only the main effect of the height factor (F $[2.24]$ = 49.8, $p < 0.05$; F $[2.24]$ = 142.3, $p < 0.05$) in both longer and shorter distances is significant, multiple comparisons by the Bonferroni method were conducted to demonstrate that significant differences in reaching time for the three height standards were observed. In summary, in attempts at balls positioned at greater distances from the goalkeeper, the time needed to reach the ball became significant and was longer in the order of middle, lower, and upper heights, whereas the time needed to reach the ball in attempts at nearer distances became significant and longer in the order of middle, upper, and lower heights.

The results of the reaching time suggest that the chance of saving by the goalkeeper varies according to the height of the ball even for shots horizontally the same distance from him. Our results also suggest that there is an opposite trend for the chance of saving by the goalkeeper between short and long horizontal distances to the ball, in which the goalkeeper has less chance for a lower shot than higher shot at the short distance and has a higher shot than lower shot at the long distance.

**Table 1** Average reaching time by direction.

| | Left | | Centre | Right | |
|---|---|---|---|---|---|
| | Far | Near | | Near | Far |
| Upper | 1.42(0.06) | 1.00(0.08) | 0.76(0.10) | 1.00(0.08) | 1.38(0.07) |
| Middle | 1.27(0.07) | 0.81(0.05) | | 0.85(0.08) | 1.28(0.06) |
| Lower | 1.34(0.07) | 1.06(0.10) | | 1.04(0.11) | 1.34(0.06) |

Note: Values are mean (sd) in second. *Significant difference between each condition.

Figure 2 depicts the centre position of the hand (the third metacarpophalangeal joint) photographed every 0.1 s for a period of 1.5 s after the directional indication for all subjects. The five most externally positioned marks for the same reaching time are selected from among the marks for the same reaching time in Figure 2 to undergo a second fitting in the polar co-ordinate system in order to obtain an approximate curve. This curve is connected by curved interpolations to create an estimated diagram of reaching area, as shown in Figure 3. Because no significant movement of the hand from the initial ready position was seen for a period of 0.7 s after the directional indication, as in the result of analysis (Figure 2), this diagram was displayed using data acquired from 0.8 s onward after the directional indication. Furthermore, the data for 1.4 s onward revealed that delays occurred in reaching the ball, and there are marks for data before the data for 1.3 s. Therefore, the data for 1.4 s and earlier are also excluded.

Kerwin and Bray (2006) described the estimated reaching area at the time of a penalty kick in a concentric form around the central position of the ground based on a penalty kick-reproducing experiment. They indicated that reaching area varies if the height of the ball differs, even if the horizontal distance to the ball from the centre is the same. Furthermore, the reaching area in the same period of time for a higher ball becomes narrower than for a ball positioned in the middle, which corresponds to the result of our experiment shown in Figure 3. However, if we look at the reaching area for low balls, because it is described as a concentric form around the central position of the ground, it is found to be the most widespread area. This result differs from ours, in which the reaching area for low balls is not wider than that for medium-height balls, as shown in Figure 2.

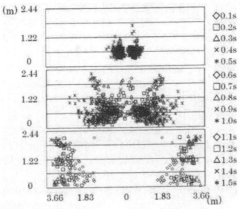

**Figure 2** Temporal positions of the hand touching the ball every 0.1 s after the directional indication for a period of 1.5 s are collectively recorded for all subjects for shorter and longer distances. Reproduced from Matsukura and Asai (2009), with permission.

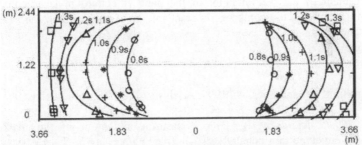

**Figure 3** This diagram is based on temporal moving trajectories of the hand every 0.1 s for a period of 0.8 to 1.3 s after the directional indication. External frame is based on the size of a soccer goal (2.44 m × 7.32 m).
Reproduced from Matsukura and Asai (2009), with permission.

In the diagram of an estimated reaching time reported by Kerwin and Bray (2006), the theoretically acquired reaching area is applied to the range where the goalkeeper does not reach for the ball. Under the experimental conditions of our study, the goalkeeper could predict a timing indication and then needs to reach for the ball in the direction indicated by the directional indicator, which seems to be similar to a real shooting situation where the goalkeeper is ready for the shot and starts to move after judging the course of the kicked ball. The results of our study provide useful information to improve the goalkeeper's training method, for example, the need to improve diving technique to unreachable zones. From the viewpoint of the attacking side of soccer, these results would provide several insights into the unavoidable weak areas of goalkeepers.

## 4. CONCLUSION

Through an experiment in which a goalkeeper dives toward a ball in response to a directional indicator that electronically displays a randomly chosen direction, this study sought to clarify the reaching area of the goalkeeper's diving motion by considering the differences in diving motions according to differences in ball position (height and distance) in terms of reaching time and hand trajectory. The results are summarised below:

- To compare reaching times for various ball heights (upper, middle, and lower), in the attempts by the goalkeeper to reach a ball positioned at shorter distances, the time needed to reach the ball becomes significantly longer in the order of middle, upper, and lower height on both the right and left sides. In contrast, in the attempts by the goalkeeper to reach a more distant ball, the reaching time becomes significantly longer in the order of middle, lower, and upper height.

- A diagram of estimated reaching area was created on the basis of the temporal movement of the central point of the hand (the third metacarpophalangeal joint), clarifying the goalkeeper's reachable areas according to the height and distance of the ball.

## References

Graham-Smith, P. and Lees, A., 1999, Analysis of technique of goalkeepers during the penalty kick. *J Sports Sci*, **19**, 910–916.

Kerwin, D. G. and Bray, K., 2006, Measuring and modeling the goalkeeper's diving envelope in a penalty kick. In *The Engineering of Sport 6*, New York: Springer, pp. 321–326.

Matsukura, K. and Asai, T., 2009, Reaching area of diving actions performed by soccer goalkeepers. *J Phys Educ, Health Sport Sci*, **54**, 317–326.

Nunome, H. *et al.*, 2002, Three-dimensional kinetic analysis of side-foot and instep soccer kicks. *Med Sci Sports Exerc*, **34**, 2028–2036.

Spratford, W. *et al.*, 2009, The influence of dive direction on the movement characteristics for elite football goalkeepers. *Sports Biomech*, **8**, 235–244.

Suzuki, S. *et al.*, 1988, Analysis of the goalkeeper's diving motion. In *Science and Football*, London: E. & F. N. Spon, pp. 468–475.

# CHAPTER FORTY

# The processes underlying 'game intelligence' skills in soccer players

A. Roca, P. R. Ford and A. M. Williams

Research Institute for Sport and Exercise Sciences,
Liverpool John Moores University, UK

## 1. INTRODUCTION

The ability of players to *anticipate* the actions of others and to select appropriate *decisions* under time pressure is essential to expert performance in soccer. These 'game intelligence' skills appear to be dependent on perception and cognition (Williams *et al.*, 2011). Over the last two decades or so, researchers have sought to better understand the perceptual-cognitive characteristics that differentiate experts from less skilled athletes (e.g., see Starkes and Ericsson, 2003). Sophisticated eye movement registration techniques have provided information on individual and group differences in visual search behaviours. For example, Williams *et al.* (1994) demonstrated that experienced soccer players search the display more extensively and pick up early arising visual information to guide their performance when compared with less experienced counterparts.

The majority of researchers studying perceptual-cognitive expertise have tended to collect eye movement recordings in isolation in order to identify the sources of information that experts use to guide their performance. There is a lack of research focusing on how performers process and translate the information extracted from the visual display into appropriate strategic/tactical decisions. Verbal protocol analysis techniques can provide this information by assessing the nature of the cognitive (thought) strategies used during actual performance. Ward *et al.* (2003) provided one of the few attempts to record verbal reports during a film-based recognition task involving soccer. The elite players elicited more extensive and detailed verbal reports of thoughts when compared with their sub-elite peers, probably indicating they have more advanced memory representations (e.g., long-term working memory, LTWM, Ericsson and Kintsch, 1995). Moreover, although there have been a few successful attempts to identify important discriminating characteristics between experts and novices in soccer, the majority of researchers have focused on examining anticipation exclusively, with relatively few attempts to measure other aspects of performance such as decision making (for exceptions, see Helsen and Starkes, 1999; Vaeyens *et al.*, 2007). Thus, since anticipation and decision making are considered crucial to performance in soccer, well-controlled efforts are needed to integrate and examine both judgments concurrently (i.e., what is going to happen next and what is the appropriate response).

We examine the underlying perceptual-cognitive processes mediating anticipation and decision making judgements in skilled and less skilled players during a dynamic, representative soccer task. We expect the skilled players to outperform their less skilled peers, with systematic between-group differences being apparent in the underlying perceptual and cognitive processes employed.

## 2. METHODS

### 2.1. Participants

A total of 48 male outfield soccer players participated across two experiments. In Experiment 1, 12 skilled and 12 less skilled players participated, whereas in Experiment 2, a new set of 12 skilled and 12 less skilled participants took part. Skilled participants (age 23.5 ± 3.3 years; mean ± *s*) were professional and semi-professional soccer players with an average of 14.5 ± 3.4 years playing experience. Less skilled participants (age 24.2 ± 3.1 years) were amateur or recreational players and had taken part in soccer irregularly for an average of 11.2 ± 3.6 years.

### 2.2. Procedure and task

In both experiments, participants were presented with a representative video-based task simulation involving four warm-up and 20 test clips of life-size 11 versus 11 dynamic situations filmed from a central defender's perspective. The action sequences lasted approximately 5 s, with each one being occluded at a key moment in the action (e.g., player in possession of the ball about to make an attacking pass, shoot at goal, or maintain possession of the ball by dribbling forward). The test film was back projected onto a 2.7 m (h) x 3.6 m (w) widescreen using a video projection system (Hitachi ED-A101, Yokohama, Japan). Participants were required to take the place of the central defender and move and interact with the footage as if playing in a competitive match. The accuracy of anticipation and decision making judgments at occlusion were recorded across the two experiments.

Process tracing measures comprising of visual gaze characteristics (Experiment 1) and retrospective verbal reports of thoughts (Experiment 2) were recorded. In Experiment 1, a mobile eye tracking system (Applied Science Laboratories, Bedford, MA, USA) was used to collect visual search data. This is a video-based monocular system that measures eye point-of-gaze with respect to a head-mounted scene camera. In Experiment 2, a wireless microphone system (Sennheiser EW 112-P G3, Wedemark, Germany) was employed to collect verbal reports. Participants were given instruction and training on how to think aloud and provide retrospective verbal reports prior to testing (see Ericsson and Simon, 1993). Each individual training and test session was completed in around 60 min.

## 2.3. Data analysis

### Experiment 1

Anticipation accuracy was defined as whether or not the participant correctly verbalised the next action of the player in possession of the ball. Decision making accuracy was defined as whether or not the participant decided on/executed and verbalised the most appropriate action, which was pre-determined by a panel of UEFA qualified soccer coaches. Both anticipation and decision making accuracy were calculated as the mean number of trials (%) in which the participant selected the correct response. The two measures were analysed separately using independent $t$ tests.

Two visual search measures were recorded. Search rate data included the mean fixation duration (in milliseconds), the mean number of fixations, and the mean number of fixation locations per trial, which were analysed separately using independent $t$ tests. Percentage viewing time data were analysed using a Group (skilled, less skilled) x Fixation Location (player in possession of the ball x ball x opponent x teammate x space) ANOVA. This latter measure was the percentage of total viewing time spent fixating each of the various areas of the display. Tukey's post-hoc tests were applied to explore significant interaction effects and a level of $P<.05$ was set for statistical significance.

### Experiment 2

The measures of anticipation and decision making accuracy were the same as in Experiment 1. Verbal reports were classified according to a structure adapted from Ericsson and Simon (1993) and further developed by Ward *et al.* (2003). Four types of verbal statement categories were coded: monitoring; evaluations; predictions; and planning. The mean number of statements per trial in each category was calculated for both groups. Verbal report data were analysed using a Group (skilled, less skilled) x Type of Verbal Statement ANOVA. Statistical significance was set at $P<.05$.

## 3. RESULTS

### 3.1. Experiment 1

Skilled players were more accurate than less skilled in anticipating the actions of opponents (68.3 ± 7.2 vs. 37.5 ± 6.5%), $t_{22} = 10.98$, $P<.001$, and in selecting an appropriate action to execute (80.6 ± 5.2 vs. 49.2 ± 9.6%), $t_{16.71} = 9.96$, $P<.001$.

There were significant skill-based differences in the mean fixation duration, $t_{22} = -8.24$, $P<.001$, the mean number of fixations, $t_{22} = 9.31$, $P<.001$, and the mean number of fixation locations per trial, $t_{22} = 9.27$, $P<.001$. Skilled players employed a more exhaustive search strategy than less skilled counterparts involving more fixations (12.33 ± 1.79 vs. 6.86 ± 0.97 fixations) of shorter duration (394 ± 83 vs. 766 ± 131 ms) and on significantly more areas of the display (6.67 ± 1.08 vs. 3.47 ± 0.50 fixation locations).

The mean data for percentage viewing time are presented in Figure 1. There was a significant Group x Fixation Location interaction, $F_{2.10,46.29} = 18.90$, $P<.001$. Post-hoc testing revealed that skilled players spent significantly more time fixating on the opponents' movements and areas of 'free space' in comparison with their less skilled counterparts. In contrast, less skilled players spent significantly more time fixating the player in possession of the ball and ball itself compared with the skilled players.

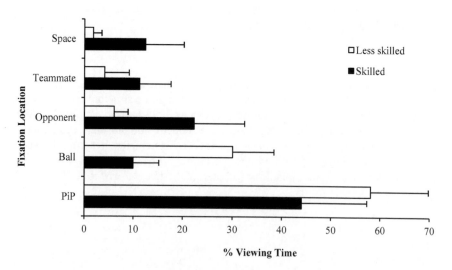

**Figure 1** Mean ± *s* percentage time spent viewing each fixation location across groups. (*PiP* player in possession of the ball).

## 3.2. Experiment 2

Skilled players were more accurate than less skilled counterparts in anticipating the actions of opponents ($69.2 \pm 7.7$ vs. $34.9 \pm 9.0\%$), $t_{22} = 10.02$, $P<.001$, and in selecting and executing appropriate tactical decisions ($83.0 \pm 8.9$ vs. $50.6 \pm 6.2\%$), $t_{22} = 10.32$, $P<.001$.

There was a significant skill-based difference for the total number of verbal statements generated per trial, $F_{1,22} = 23.18$, $P<.001$. Skilled players ($7.58 \pm 1.25$ statements) verbalised significantly more statements than the less skilled players ($5.25 \pm 1.12$ statements). The Group x Type of Thought Statement interaction was not significant, $F_{2.16,47.43} = 1.81$, $P = .17$. The greater number of statements generated by skilled players compared with the less skilled may have affected this interaction. Thus, frequency scores were subsequently normalised into proportional data. Less skilled players were found to make a higher percentage of monitoring statements compared with the skilled players ($67.4 \pm 9.8$ vs. $47.3 \pm 8.4\%$). In contrast, skilled players made a higher proportion of evaluation, prediction, and planning statements than their less skilled peers ($52.7 \pm 8.4$ vs. $32.6 \pm 9.8\%$).

## 4. DISCUSSION AND CONCLUSION

The skill-based differences in anticipation and decision making judgments were underpinned by quantitatively different underlying perceptual and cognitive processes. Skilled players made a greater number of fixations for shorter duration and towards more informative areas of the display, most likely increasing their awareness of the positions and movements of opponents/teammates and any potential areas of free space that may be uncovered or exploited. In contrast, less skilled players spent longer periods of time watching the ball or the player in possession of the ball. These data suggest that a more exhaustive search strategy and analysis of the display appears to be crucial for facilitating superior anticipation and decision making performance in soccer. Findings support previous research showing skill-based differences in visual search strategy (Williams *et al.*, 1994).

Furthermore, when compared with their less skilled counterparts, skilled players engaged in a greater proportion of evaluation, prediction, and planning thoughts, suggesting they employed more advanced soccer-specific memory representations to solve the task-situations. As predicted by Ericsson and Kintsch's (1995) LTWM theory, skilled players likely possess and activate more complex and superior task-specific memory representations permitting them to easily access and retrieve specific information in current scenarios and, therefore, facilitate better anticipation and decision making compared with less skilled peers.

Our findings support and extend previous work (e.g., Williams *et al.*, 2011) and highlight the perceptual-cognitive processes underpinning superior anticipation and decision making performance in soccer. The development of these 'game intelligence' skills may be facilitated through relevant practice and training interventions (Stratton *et al.*, 2004). In future researchers should seek to examine the nature and type of practice (conditions) that lead to the acquisition of superior judgements and their underlying processes in soccer players. Such research would provide a principled basis for practitioners involved in talent identification and development to design the most appropriate learning, training, and practice environments.

## Acknowledgements

The investigation was funded by the Portuguese Foundation for Science and Technology (FCT) – Ministry of Education and Science.

## References

Ericsson, K.A. and Kintsch, W., 1995, Long-term working memory. *Psychological Review*, **102**, 211–245.

Ericsson, K.A. and Simon, H.A., 1993, *Protocol Analysis: Verbal Reports as Data*, Cambridge, MA: Bradford Books/MIT Press.

Helsen, W.F. and Starkes, J.L., 1999, A multidimensional approach to skilled perception and performance in sport. *Applied Cognitive Psychology*, **13**, 1–27.

Starkes, J.L. and Ericsson, K.A., 2003, *Expert Performance in Sports: Advances in Research on Sport and Expertise*, Champaign, IL: Human Kinetics.

Stratton, G. *et al.*, 2004. *Youth Soccer: From Science to Performance*, London: Routledge.

Vaeyens, R. *et al.*, 2007, Mechanisms underpinning successful decision making in skilled youth soccer players: An analysis of visual search behaviors. *J Motor Behav*, **39**, 395–408.

Ward, P. *et al.*, 2003, Underlying mechanisms of perceptual-cognitive expertise in soccer. *J Sport Exerc Psychol*, **25**, S136.

Williams, A.M. *et al.*, 1994, Visual search strategies of experienced and inexperienced soccer players. *Res Quart Exerc Sport*, **65**, 127–135.

Williams, A.M. *et al.*, 2011, Perceptual-cognitive expertise in sport and its acquisition: Implications for applied cognitive psychology. *Applied Cognitive Psychology*, **25**, 432–442.

# CHAPTER FORTY-ONE

# Prior high-intensity intermittent running reduces exercise intensity and skill performance in small-sided rugby games

T. Kempton and A. J. Coutts

University of Technology, Sydney, Australia

## 1. INTRODUCTION

Small-sided games (SSGs) are commonly used to improve technical and tactical abilities in team sport athletes and have shown to provide a comparable aerobic stimulus to traditional interval training methods. It has been shown that the perceptual (rating of perceived exertion) and physiological load (heart rate, blood lactate) experienced during SSGs can be controlled by manipulating exercise prescription factors such as field size, player number, rule modifications and coach encouragement (Hill-Haas et al., 2011; Kennett et al., 2012). However, it is unclear whether SSGs provide a different training stimulus when completed in a fatigued or non-fatigued state. Acute fatigue has been reported during team sport competition play, typically following brief periods of high-intensity running (HIR) (Bradley et al., 2009, Mohr et al., 2003), and has been associated with declines in physical performance. While it is established that match-related physical fatigue may reduce exercise intensity during competitive play, further research is required to understand the influence of acute physical fatigue on exercise intensity during SSGs.

To date only one study has examined whether skill-related performance is affected by match-related fatigue in a similar manner as physical performance during professional soccer match play (Carling and Dupont, 2011). Carling and colleagues reported that while HIR distance declined between halves and during the final third of matches, it was not associated with a reduction in technical skill performance. However, the assessment of the influence of fatigue on technical performance during competition is problematic due to the possible impact of psychological, tactical and situational factors. To overcome this, recent studies have examined the influence of physical fatigue on skill tests in controlled match-simulations (Lyons et al., 2006; Rampinini et al., 2008; Royal et al., 2006; Sunderland, 2005; Young et al., 2010). Most (Lyons et al., 2006; Rampinini et al., 2008; Sunderland, 2005) of these studies have reported that skilled performance is impaired by match-related fatigue. At present it is not known if acute physical fatigue influences skill performance in SSGs.

If there is an effect of fatigue on skill performance in SSGs, there may be important implications for the placement of SSG training within whole training sessions. Therefore, to address this problem, the present study was designed to assess the influence of an acute intermittent training bout on exercise intensity and skill performance in rugby specific SSGs.

## 2. METHODS

Ten elite male rugby union players (age: 18.6 ± 0.7 y, mass: 98.4 ± 16.0 kg, stature: 185.2 ± 8.7 cm) from the same state academy program participated in the study. The testing procedures were approved by a Research Ethics Committee.

The 10-week pre-season training period served as a familiarisation with the SSGs. The head coach provided an overall subjective skill rating of each player using a 5-point (1 = 'below average', 5 = 'outstanding') Likert scale. Players were rated on their game sense, ball skills and evasiveness and completed the Yo-Yo intermittent recovery test (Yo-Yo IRT1) to assess aerobic performance. The three skill ratings and the fitness rating were combined to produce a composite score and overall ranking and to select evenly matched SSG teams.

The SSGs were conducted during the final two weeks of the pre-season. Players were required to perform both a bout of intermittent training and the SSG during each session. There were two randomised training sessions per week, separated by at least 48 h. For the 'fatigued' condition, participants completed a bout of intermittent training immediately followed by the SSG. The order was then reversed for the 'non-fatigued' state. The design was replicated during the second week so that the participants completed SSG twice under each condition. The SSGs were played at the beginning of the training session following a standardised 15 min warm up.

The SSG used in the study was 'offside touch' (Gabbett, 2010). Each match consisted of two seven-minute halves separated by a 60 s half-time period. The composition of teams, player number (6 v 6), and coach encouragement were standardised. The field was 70 x 50 m and was controlled by the same referee. The intermittent training session consisted of 8 x 180 m efforts, beginning every 90 s. The intermittent training was controlled by a coach with a stop-watch to ensure that participants completed 1440 m of high-intensity running in 12 min.

Global rating of perceived exertion (RPE) were recorded immediately after each intermittent training period and small-sided game using the CR10 scale. Heart rate was recorded at 5-s intervals during both the SSG and intermittent training (Polar, Polar Electro Oy, Finland). Heart rate monitors were also worn during the Yo-Yo IRT1 to determine maximum heart rate. Exercise intensity during the SSGs and intermittent training bouts was measured using heart rate and was expressed as a mean (HRmean) and percentage of maximum heart rate (%HRmax).

Player movements during the SSGs and intermittent training were measured using portable global position system (GPS) units (SPI-Pro, 5 Hz, GPSports, Canberra, ACT Australia). Following each match, the GPS data were downloaded to the TeamAMS proprietary software for detailed analysis. The total distance (TD), HIR (>14.5 km h$^{-1}$) and VHIR (>20 km h$^{-1}$) distance were calculated. The frequency of high-speed zone (sprints >23 km h$^{-1}$) entries during games was also collected.

Each SSG was recorded from an elevated aspect with a digital video camera (HDRXR350V, Sony, Tokyo Japan). The SSGs were then coded using manual notation to quantify the frequency for each of the following events:

1. Involvements with the ball: number of situations where the player is in contact with the ball.
2. Catching error: number of unsuccessful attempts to receive the ball.
3. Effective disposal: number of times a player successfully passes the ball to a teammate or scores a try when in possession of the ball.
4. Ineffective disposal: number of times a player fails to execute an effective disposal, often due to an inaccurate pass or being 'caught' in possession.

A dependent sample t-test was used to compare physical and technical performance between non-fatigued and fatigued SSGs. For skill, counts data was transformed and checked for Poisson distribution prior to applying the t-test. Data are presented as the mean (±SD). Statistical significance was set at p < 0.05.

## 3. RESULTS

The technical skill demands of fatigued and non-fatigued offside SSGs are shown in Table 1. There were reductions (p = 0.03) in the number of effective disposals, disposal efficiency (p = 0.019) and an increase in percentage error (p = 0.036) in SSGs completed in the fatigued state.

**Table 1** Skill demands for SSG under non-fatigued and fatigued conditions (mean ± SD).

|  | Non-fatigued | Fatigued | Mean difference (±90 CI) |
|---|---|---|---|
| Receives (n) | 19.5 ± 4.9 | 14.8 ± 6.3 | 4.7 (3.4 to 6.6) |
| Catching errors (n) | 0.4 ± 0.5 | 0.1 ± 0.3 | 0.3 (-0.2 to 0.7) |
| Effective disposals (n) | 17.4 ± 4.4 | 11.9 ± 5.9† | 5.5 (4.2 to 7.3) |
| Ineffective disposals (n) | 2.1 ± 1.6 | 2.9 ± 1.4 | -0.8 (-1.9 to 0.4) |
| Disposal efficiency (%) | 89.4 ± 7.1 | 79.1 ± 8.9† | 10.3 (3.2 to 18.4) |
| Total involvements (n) | 19.9 ± 4.9 | 14.9 ± 6.2 | 5 (3.6 to 6.9) |
| Total errors (n) | 2.5 ± 1.7 | 3.0 ± 1.3 | -0.5 (1.6 to 0.6) |
| Percentage error (%) | 12.4 ± 7.1 | 21.7 ± 9.1† | -9.3 (-16.6 to -3.1) |

†Significant differences (p < 0.05) between non-fatigued and fatigued condition for SSGs. n – number.

The SSGs in a non-fatigued resulted in greater total distance covered; greater distance covered at HIR and VHIR intensity; and a greater number of sprint efforts (p = 0.007, p = 0.002, p = 0.015 and p = 0.032, respectively). In contrast, the internal load (HRmean, %HR$_{max}$ and RPE) did not differ between conditions (p = 0.548 and p = 0.505, respectively).

**Table 2** Physiological demands for SSG under non-fatigued and fatigued conditions (mean ± SD).

|  | Non-fatigued | Fatigued | Mean Difference (±90 CI) |
|---|---|---|---|
| Total distance (m) | 2031 ± 200 | 1786 ± 128† | 245 (127 to 363) |
| Relative distance (m·min$^{-1}$) | 133 ± 13 | 115 ± 7† | 18 (11 to 26) |
| HIR distance (m) | 494 ± 141 | 293 ± 83† | 201 (134 to 269) |
| VHIR distance (m) | 121 ± 73 | 51 ± 25† | 70 (38 to102) |
| Sprint efforts (n) | 4.6 ± 3.1 | 2.0 ± 0.9† | 2.6 (1 to 4) |
| HR mean (beats·min$^{-1}$) | 162 ± 21 | 167 ± 11 | -5 (-17 to 7) |
| Percentage HR max (%) | 0.83 ± 0.10 | 0.86 ± 0.06 | -0.03 (-0.09 to 0.03) |
| RPE (AU) | 8.2 ± 0.6 | 8.7 ± 0.8 | -0.5 (-0.8 to -0.2) |

†Significant differences (p < 0.05) between non-fatigued and fatigued condition for SSGs. n – number. AU – arbitrary units.

## 4. DISCUSSION

This study is the first to compare the technical and physical demands of rugby based SSGs in a fatigued and non-fatigued state. Previous research has examined the effect of field size, player number and coach encouragement on the physiological and technical demands of SSGs (Hill-Haas *et al.*, 2011; Kennett *et al.*, 2012). These studies have shown that by manipulating these factors the aerobic training stimulus and skill demands of SSGs can be altered significantly. The results of the present study demonstrate that prior high-intensity intermittent training contributes to acute fatigue which may cause significant changes in the physiological and skill demands of SSGs.

The players in the non-fatigued state exhibited an overall higher level of technical skill proficiency compared to SSGs completed under fatigued conditions. Specifically, the number of effective disposals and disposal efficiency was significantly higher, while the error percentage was lower for non-fatigued players when compared to the fatigued state. The present results indicate that while the participants experienced a reduction in the proficiency of skill executions (e.g. effective disposals and disposal efficiency) there was no significant reduction in the number of involvements. These results are in contrast to previous studies of technical performance during elite soccer match-play (Carling and Dupont, 2011; Rampinini *et al.*, 2009). The difference between the present results and these previous studies may be due to differences in game structure between professional soccer match-play and the rugby-based SSG performed in the current investigation.

The offside SSG used in this study is not typical of rugby union. This lack of familiarity with the offside game structure may have also contributed to the large reductions in skill-performance in the fatigue condition. The combination of an unfamiliar game structure and increased physical and technical demands in the present study may have compounded the fatigue induced reduction of technical skill proficiency. These findings indicate that there may be an acute fatigue influence on some technical skill abilities.

There was greater total (and relative) distance, HIR and VHIR distance and frequency of sprint efforts observed in the non-fatigued state compared to the fatigued state. These findings are similar to the reductions in physical performance observed during motion analyses of competitive match play for various team sports (Bradley *et al.*, 2009; Coutts *et al.*, 2009a). Research has shown that match-related fatigue may result in a reduction in measures of exercise intensity such as total distance and HIR distance during the final stages of the match (Bradley *et al.*, 2009) and following brief periods of HIR (Mohr *et al.*, 2003).

The relative distance during the non-fatigued SSGs is comparable to that reported in offside SSGs involving elite rugby league players (Gabbett *et al.*, 2010), but greatly exceeded movement intensity reported for elite rugby union match-play (Roberts *et al.*, 2008). The greater movement demands observed in the SSGs may be attributable to the absence of physical collisions, which contribute significantly to the physical demands of competitive rugby union match-play; reduced player numbers and the 'offside' format of the SSG. On the basis of these observations, we suggest that 'offside' SSGs can be used in training to provide an overloaded aerobic stimulus and the opportunity to execute a variety of rugby specific technical skills in a modified game environment.

Despite the higher movement demands during the non-fatigued state, measures of internal load such as HRmean, %HRmax and RPE did not differ between conditions. Previous research has reported that %HRpeak accounted for approximately 42% of variance of RPE following SSGs. It has been suggested that other factors including blood lactate, metabolic acidosis, ventilatory drive, respiratory gases and body temperature may also contribute to RPE in SSGs (Coutts *et al.*, 2009b). Therefore, the lack of difference in HR and RPE between conditions (despite the lower external load in the fatigued condition) may be attributable to other factors such as metabolic inertia from the preceding high-intensity intermittent session.

These findings show that potentiating HR and RPE responses with a priming bout of high-intensity intermittent training can achieve a greater aerobic training stimulus. However, if the goal of the SSG is to complete high quality, fast paced skills then SSGs should be completed without prior high-intensity training. Conversely, players may benefit from developing skill performance under fatigue when intermittent training is completed before SSGs within the same session.

## References

Bradley, P. *et al.*, 2009, High-intensity running in English FA Premier League soccer matches. *J Sports Sci*, **27**, 159–168.

Carling, C. and Dupont, G., 2011, Are declines in physical performance associated with a reduction in skill-related performance during professional soccer match-play? *J Sports Sci*, **29**, 63–71.

Coutts, A.J. *et al.*, 2009a, Match running demands of elite Australian Rules Football. *J Sci Med Sport*, **13**, 543–548.

Coutts, A.J. *et al.*, 2009b, Heart rate and blood lactate correlates of perceived exertion during small-sided soccer games. *J Sci Med Sport*, **12**, 79–84.

Gabbett, T.D. *et al.*, 2010, Physiological and skill demands of 'onside' and 'offside' games. *J Strength Cond Res*, **24**, 2979–2983.

Hill-Haas, S. *et al.*, 2011, Physiology of small-sided games training in football. *J Sports Med*, **41**, 199–220.

Kennett, D. *et al.*, 2012, Factors affecting exercise intensity in rugby-specific small-sided games. *Journal of Strength and Conditioning Research*, in press.

Lyons, M. *et al.*, 2006, Performance of soccer passing skills under moderate and high-intensity localised muscle fatigue. *J Strength Cond Res*, **20**, 197–202.

Mohr, M. *et al.*, 2003, Match performance of high-standard soccer players with special reference to development of fatigue. *J Sports Sci*, **21**, 519–528.

Rampinini, E. *et al.*, 2008, Effect of match-related fatigue on short-passing ability in young soccer players. *J Med Sci Sport Exerc*, **40**, 934–942.

Rampinini, E. *et al.*, 2009, Technical performance during soccer matches of the Italian Serie A league: Effect of fatigue and competitive level. *J Med Sport*, **12**, 227–233.

Roberts, S. *et al.*, 2008, The physical demands of elite English rugby union. *J Sports Sci*, **26**, 825–833.

Royal, K. *et al.*, 2006, The effects of fatigue on decision making and shooting skill performance in water polo players. *J Sports Sci*, **24**, 807–815.

Sunderland, C. and M. Nevill, 2005, High-intensity intermittent running and field hockey skill performance in the heat. *J Sports Sci*, **23**, 531–540.

Young, W. *et al.*, 2010, Acute effect of exercise on kicking accuracy in elite Australian football players. *J Sci Med Sport*, **13**, 85–89.

# CHAPTER FORTY-TWO

# Video self-modeling and kicking accuracy on the non-preferred side

K. Steel[1], R. Adams[2], S. Coulson[2], P. Clothier[1] and D. Walker[2]

[1]School of Biomedical and Health Science, University of Western Sydney, Sydney, Australia, [2]Discipline of Physiotherapy, School of Biomedical and Health Science, University of Sydney, Sydney, Australia

## 1. INTRODUCTION

Video-self-modeling (VSM) in skill acquisition (Dowrick, 2007) involves observational learning where learners view instances of their best skill performance. As learners improve, successive best performance tapes can be made (Dowrick and Dove, 1980). VSM incorporates both positive self-review (PSR), where only the individual's best instances of the target skill are depicted, and feed-forward (FF), where special effects video editing is used to show individuals video of themselves performing at a level they have not in fact achieved. PSR-VSM can generate substantial improvements, from training more confident behavior in a swimming pool (Dowrick and Dove, 1980), to training better quality smiling (Coulson et al., 2006). To date, applications of PSR in sports settings have had varying success (Feltz et al., 2008; Law and Ste-Marie, 2005; Starek and McCullagh, 1999), and applications of FF in sports settings are limited to single-case reports, e.g. Franks and Maile (1991). Here a power lifter was shown tapes of herself apparently lifting more weight than she had previously attempted. Over 25 weeks of intervention, she achieved a 26% improvement in weight lifted. The possibility of providing FF to players exists in several football codes where it can often be observed that although the code nominally requires bilateral motor skills, even elite players may still show an evident side preference (Grouios, 2004).

Mirror reversing video of preferred-side skills permits the construction of a feed-forward self-model tape where the individual can observe themselves producing a skill, apparently with their non-preferred limb, at a performance level beyond that which they could normally achieve with that limb. According to Massen and Prinz (2007) a motor plan for the non-preferred side would be constructed upon viewing the movement sequence, so even if the difference in the motor pattern for the two sides was a subtle one, the superior preferred-side pattern could be translated into motor planning for the non-preferred side and enable it to achieve the observed outcome. FF-VSM was achieved in the present study by showing the players mirror-reversed footage of their preferred side skill performance, such that the clip observed was apparently of their non-preferred foot.

## 2. METHODS

N=8 Australian Football League (AFL) players aged 16–54 years volunteered to participate in this study. All participants were current players in the Sydney metropolitan club competition, training for two sessions during the week, with one competition game on weekends. Approval for the study was obtained from the University Human Research Ethics Committee and all participants gave written informed consent prior to commencement.

Testing short (25m) punt kicks for accuracy was conducted in an indoor sports court (35m in length x 15m in width). The target was a team-mate standing 25metres from the kicker. A video camera was placed directly in front of the kicker at 8metres from the ball contact point, and additional video cameras were placed to each side of the kicking line (Figure 1). A fourth digital video camera was directed toward the target in order to score accuracy for each trial, measured as distance from the centre of the target. The participants were instructed to kick a standard AFL match ball as accurately as possible toward the target, who was asked to try to catch the ball without moving their feet from their original position. A total of 25 kicks were performed by each participant. Kicks were randomly allocated, and 'right' or 'left' was called out to the participant before he began his approach.

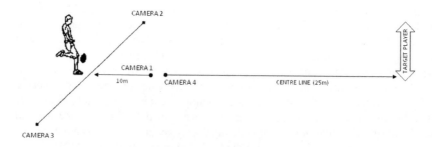

**Figure 1** Experimental set-up for recording kicks and kick accuracy.

The frontal video footage was then mirror-reversed using Adobe Premier Pro CS3 software (Adobe Systems Inc.), with this edited product recorded onto a DVD for each player. The individual DVDs contained footage of that player's three best (i.e. most direct) preferred-foot kicks which had been mirror reversed, and thus the footage displayed apparent non-preferred foot kicks. Each clip was repeated twice on the DVD and the six kicks formed a sequence lasting one minute. All participants were instructed to watch their DVD three times a day for three weeks. A post-test was conducted after two weeks, with a retention-test completed two weeks after. Players also recorded each session of viewing in a training diary which was collected at the end of the three week training intervention, with their DVDs.

Swinger™ software was used to measure the distance between the centre of the chest of the target and the point of ball contact for each kick. Using SPSS Windows v.16, repeated-measures analysis of variance and matched-pair t-tests were conducted on these error scores, or distances from the target, achieved by the preferred foot and the non-preferred foot at pre-test, post-test and retention-test. Chi-square analysis was conducted on the classifications of the kick biomechanics. For optimum punt kicking biomechanics the ball should be guided down to the foot with the ipsilateral hand, which then swings back while the contralateral hand swings forward to provide balance during kick follow-through (Ball, 2008). However, if the contralateral hand is used to release the ball, it can only be delivered at an angle across the front of the body, rather than directly down.

## 3. RESULTS

Overall, 53% of kicks were close enough to be caught by the target. Figure 2 shows the mean error distances from the target receiver for kicks made by both feet at the three test occasions. From analysis of variance, preferred foot kicks were found to have significantly lower error overall than non-preferred foot kicks (*diff* = 28.5 cms, $p = 0.003$). Contrast analysis showed that the magnitude of the preferred foot accuracy advantage over the non-preferred foot was relatively greater at the retention test than at the mean of the previous two test occasions (*diff* = 22.7cms, $p = 0.04$), but that when occasions were compared within each of the preferred and non-preferred sides separately, the error distances at retention were not significantly different from distances at the previous tests ($p = 0.22$ and $0.16$ respectively).

When examined for each test occasion, kicking accuracy was significantly greater for the preferred foot than for the non-preferred foot at the pre-test (*diff* = 21.3 cms, $p = 0.034$), while at the immediate post-test after watching their FF DVD, the difference was 20.5 cms and not significant ($p = 0.055$). Later, at the retention-test, a return to significant superiority of the preferred foot for kick accuracy was observed (*diff* = 43.6 cms, $p<0.01$). Frequency of use of different hands for ball delivery to the preferred and non-preferred feet on the three test occasions was collated (Table 1a). The most obvious feature of this tabulation was that while the non-preferred hand was never used to deliver the ball to the preferred foot, the preferred hand was sometimes used to drop the ball onto the non-preferred foot.

Chi-square analysis showed an association between use of the single hand or both hands and whether the kick was from the preferred and non-preferred foot, with relatively more ipsilateral hand use for preferred foot kicks, and this was significant at all three test occasions (all $p< 0.01$). When the pattern of hand use for only the non-preferred foot was examined, three matrices could be constructed (Table 1b) one with Pre-Test and Post-Test as the column headings, another with

Pre-Test and Retention Test, and a final matrix with Post-Test and Retention Test. Considering the pattern of hand use for just the non-preferred foot, there was no significant change from the Pre-Test to the Post-Test ($\chi^2_{2df}$ = 5.77, $p$= 0.056). At the retention test, however, there were relatively fewer releases made by the contralateral hand, and the hand used for ball release and test occasion were now significantly associated ($\chi^2_{2df}$ = 6.41, $p$= 0.04). The pattern at retention testing was not significantly different from hand use at the post-test ($\chi^2_{2df}$ = 0.06, $p$=0.97). Thus hand use for the non-preferred foot changed after DVD viewing, and the change was retained. At the final debriefing, players reported that after the post-test, they had found out indirectly about the mirror reversal technique used to create the FF DVDs.

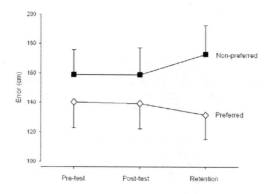

**Figure 2** Mean error of the kicks from the centre of the chest of the target (receiver) for the three test sessions. Error bars show the 95% confidence interval for the means.

**Table 1a** Frequency of use of ipsilateral hand, both hands, and the contralateral hand in ball release for the preferred and non-preferred foot over the three test occasions.

| Delivery Hand | Pre-Test | | Post-Test | | Retention-Test | |
|---|---|---|---|---|---|---|
| | N-P Foot | P-Foot | N-P Foot | P-Foot | N-P Foot | P-Foot |
| Ipsilateral | 49 | 90 | 63 | 88 | 64 | 88 |
| Both | 25 | 12 | 24 | 13 | 25 | 12 |
| Contralateral | 24 | 0 | 12 | 0 | 11 | 0 |

**Table 1b** Frequency of hand use for ball delivery to the non-preferred foot only at Pre-Test, Post-Test and Retention-Test.

| Delivery Hand | Non-Preferred Foot only | | | | | |
|---|---|---|---|---|---|---|
| | Pre-Test | Post-Test | Pre-Test | Retention-Test | Post-Test | Retention-Test |
| Ipsilateral | 49 | 63 | 49 | 64 | 63 | 64 |
| Both | 25 | 24 | 25 | 24 | 24 | 25 |
| Contralateral | 24 | 12 | 24 | 11 | 12 | 11 |

## 4. DISCUSSION

Support for the view that players can acquire improved motor patterns from watching individually prepared FF DVDs was found in the significant change in the pattern of releasing hand use evident at the retention-test, and this change was already apparent at the post-test. When the ipsilateral releasing hand was employed more often at the post-test, there was no longer a significant difference between sides in kick accuracy, so these players had, in the non-preferred hand, the motor control needed for an accurate ball drop. However, even though this pattern continued to be used at the retention-test, there was a marked deterioration in accuracy in kicks made with the non-preferred foot compared with the preferred foot. In the absence of a control group who simply did the three tests without an intervention, an unambiguous account of this result cannot be proposed. The asymmetry of the change in accuracy of kicks for the preferred and non-preferred sides at retention testing makes it unlikely, however, that the effect arose from the testing constituting a more concentrated practice of short kicks than the players would normally undertake. Equivalent amounts of testing took place on both sides, but at retention testing the accuracy changes were in different directions. Our interpretation of this result is that it represents a reversion to a greater degree of cognitive control of action on the non-preferred side, a phenomenon that Masters and Maxwell (2008) term 'reinvestment'.

The relative deterioration in non-preferred foot kick accuracy corresponded in time with the players becoming aware that the good quality non-preferred foot kicks that they had been watching were in fact their preferred foot, mirror-reversed, so any concerns players had about lower quality with their non-preferred side performance may have been confirmed. Further, it is likely that foot preference in football players is associated with differences in the amount of kicking practice, with thus a relatively lower level of automaticity of movement control for kicks on the non-preferred side. Under such circumstances, reversion to conscious control of non-preferred side kicking would become likely if players were given information that created doubts. There is also some similarity here to the effect noted by Law and Ste-Marie (2005) where the participants were critical of the performances on their personal 'highlights' clips, searching for execution errors. Criticism of non-preferred side performance may arise more readily if players already see it as being at a lower level.

There are limitations to the present study that may have affected the results at retention, and these include the relatively small sample size, the lack of a 'no video' control group, and the fact that the participants found out about the reversal manipulation used to make the FF DVDs. Although the intention with FF DVD here was to bypass conscious processes and directly influence automatic motor control processes, in the current research unintended discovery of the stratagem that had been used to produce the FF DVDs may have led the participants to use conscious skill control during final testing, and consequently to a worse non-preferred side performance. In future work, a self-report instrument such as the

Movement Specific Reinvestment Scale (Masters *et al.*, 2005) could provide specific information about how players think about their non-preferred side during skill execution. Further work is needed to identify the optimal way of presenting to players the video training experiences that may lead to improved performance in kicking with the non-preferred foot.

## 5. CONCLUSIONS

The use of FF VSM to train non-preferred foot kicking by Australian Football League players showed promising results, but also suggested that what athletes think they are watching, and what they think they are watching it for, may be important determinants of outcome of FF VSM in sport.

### References

Ball, K., 2008, Biomechanical considerations of distance kicking in Australian Rules football. *Sports Biomechanics*, **7**, 10–23.

Coulson, S.E., *et al.*, 2006, Physiotherapy rehabilitation of the smile after long-term Facial Nerve Palsy using Video Self-Modelling and implementation intentions. *Otolaryngology: Head and Neck Surgery*, **134**, 48–55.

Dowrick, P.W., 2007, Community-driven learning activities, creating futures: 30,000 people can't be wrong – Can they? *Am J Community Psych*, **39**, 13-19.

Dowrick, P.W. and Dove, C., 1980, The use of self-modeling to improve swimming performance of spina bifida children. *J Appl Behav Anly*, **13**, 51–56.

Feltz, D. *et al.*, 2008, The effect of self-modeling on shooting performance and self-efficacy with intercollegiate hockey players. In M. Simmons, L. Foster, *Sport & Exercise Psychology Research Advances*, NY: Nova Sci, pp. 9–18.

Franks, I.M., and Maile, L.J., 1991, The use of video in sport skill acquisition. In *Practical Guide to Using Video in the Behavioural Sciences*, New York: Wiley and Sons, pp. 231–243.

Grouios, G., 2004, Motoric dominance and sporting excellence: Training versus heredity. *Percep Motor Skill*, **98**, 53–66.

Law, B. and Ste-Marie, D.M., 2005, Effects of self-modeling on figure skating jump performance and psychological variables. *Eur J Sport Sci*, **5**, 143–152.

Massen, C. and Prinz, W., 2007, Activation of action rules in action observation. *J Exper Psychol: Learning, Memory, and Cognition*, **33**, 1118–1130.

Masters, R.S.W. *et al.*, 2005, Development of a movement specific Reinvestment Scale. In *Proceedings of the ISSP 11th World Congress of Sport Psychology*, Sydney, Australia.

Masters, R. and Maxwell, J., 2008, The theory of reinvestment. *Int Rev Sport Exerc Psychol*, **1**, 160–183.

Starek, J. and McCullagh, P., 1999, The effect of self-modeling on the performance of beginning swimmers. *The Sport Psychologist*, **13**, 269–287.

# CHAPTER FORTY-THREE

# Passing ability of adolescent soccer players during 4-day tournament play

W. Sinclair and J. Artis

Institute of Sport and Exercise Science, James Cook University, Australia

## 1. INTRODUCTION

Characterizing soccer skill performance has previously incorporated a variety of methodologies assessing cognitive, perceptual and motor skills (Ali, 2011). As fatigue increases throughout the course of a game, significant reductions in match performance occurs, including distances covered and high-intensity intervals (Mohr et al., 2003). Similarly in adolescent soccer players, the number of sprints decline towards the end of a game (Buchheit et al., 2010). Therefore, as many goals are scored towards the end of a game and result from short-passing (Rampinini et al., 2008), a player's ability to execute the short-pass in a game-like environment is imperative to team performance. Previous research has shown adolescent soccer players have a reduced short-passing ability following the second half of a match compared to the first as a result of match-related fatigue and high-intensity running (Rampinini et al., 2008). With many representative soccer teams contesting tournaments that consist of many games over a number of consecutive days, managing match-related fatigue is critical to tournament performance.

Previously during tournament play, reduced match performance including distances covered (total and high-intensity running) and increased perceptions of fatigue have been identified in adolescent soccer players (Rowsell et al., 2011). Predominantly as a result of insufficient recovery periods and strategies between games, this match-related fatigue has been reported to have significant implications on the short-passing ability as well as technical proficiency during simulated game-play (Stone et al., 2009; Rowsell et al., 2011). Due to the complexities of soccer match-play, tests that allow game specific proficiencies (such as accuracy and ball control) and techniques (such as dribbing and passing) should be utilized to assess any influence of fatigue on skill performance. Therefore the aim of the present study was to investigate the influence of match-related fatigue on the technical execution of adolescent soccer player's short-passing ability across a 4-day tournament.

## 2. METHODS

### Participants

Male regional Academy representative soccer players (n=12; mean ±SD; age 13.7 ± 0.5 yr; body mass 50.1 ± 6.3 kg; height 161.3 ± 7.6 cm) participating in a 4-day representative tournament volunteered for this study. All players and their parents or guardians provided written consent prior to commencement of the study which was approved by both the Academy and the Institutional Human Ethics Committee.

Players undertook a balanced structured training program which incorporated speed, agility, aerobic conditioning as well as strategic play development as part of their inclusion in the Academy. The team in the present study progressed through the 4-day tournament against other regional representative Academies undefeated in their 4 games. All games were contested on professionally manicured, open-air fields with fine weather and average environmental conditions throughout the games of 26.1 ± 0.64°C and 47.4 ± 8.1% relative humidity.

In the 3 weeks prior to the tournament, players underwent 3-5 familiarization sessions for the Loughborough Soccer Passing Test (LSPT) prior to a training session (Ali *et al.*, 2007; Ali, 2011). Each familiarization was conducted at the tournament venue on an adjacent field in order to familiarize players with the match-day routine. All familiarization and testing sessions were conducted by the same researcher controlling the test and another researcher recording any penalties incurred. The LSPT requires a player to rebound the ball off one of four benches (2.5 x 0.3 m), placed in a rectangular testing area (12 x 9 m) via a designated passing area (Ali *et al.*, 2007; Ali, 2011). Players were required to rebound the ball off the bench corresponding to an audible instruction from the administrator and this was completed 16 times (8 long passes and 8 short passes in a randomized order) as fast and accurately as possible. Players were allocated 43 sec to complete the LSPT with time penalties accrued for hitting the wrong bench (decision making, 5 sec); missing the bench (accuracy, 5 sec) or target (coloured, 0.6 x 0.3 m area on each bench) but still hitting the bench (accuracy, 3 sec); passing the ball outside the designated area or the ball hit a marker cone (ball control, 2 sec); and time adjustments per 1 sec over (time, 1 sec) or under (time, -1 sec) the allocated 43 sec (Ali *et al.*, 2007).

During the tournament, each test was conducted away from team-mates, coaching staff and parents: once immediately following the standardized team warm-up protocol and again straight after each match. Time was recorded by the administrator calling out the randomized passing order while the other administrator recorded the accuracy of all passing attempts. Final time for the LSPT therefore represents the total time to complete the LSPT plus the time penalties accrued. Throughout the tournament testing sessions, players and coaches were not informed of their performance time or penalties incurred. The LSPT has been shown to have high validity and repeatability following familiarization (Ali *et al.*, 2007) with comparable ICCs in the current study (0.55 to 0.67) for total time (including accrued penalties) and time taken to complete the LSPT, respectively.

A two-way (day x time) repeated measures ANOVA was used to analyze the LSPT time variables (time taken to complete; final time; total time penalties and time penalties accrued for time, ball control, accuracy and decision making) with *post hoc* comparisons via Tukey's test. All results are presented mean ± SD and an alpha level set at 0.05.

## 3. RESULTS

Time to complete the LSPT was slower for the players following their games compared to pre-game ($p = 0.025$; Table 1). Additionally, there was a main effect of time for ball control, accuracy, decision-making and resultant combined penalties post-game compared to that of pre-game ($p<0.001$; Table 1).

Differences were identified for final time (time plus time penalties accrued) across the 4 days of the tournament (Figure 1). There were no differences between pre-game results for any of the time variables assessed ($p > 0.05$).

**Table 1** Mean (±SD) times and penalties for the Loughborough Soccer Passing Test prior to (pre-) and following (post-) games during a 4-day tournament.

| Variable | Pre-game | Post-game | *p*-value |
|---|---|---|---|
| Time to complete | 49.51 ± 0.70 | 50.71 ± 0.86 | 0.025 |
| Penalties: | | | |
|   –  Time | 6.57 ± 0.67 | 7.74 ± 0.84 | 0.022 |
|   –  Ball control | 2.17 ± 0.27 | 3.23 ± 0.47 | 0.027 |
|   –  Decision-making | 0.63 ± 0.19 | 1.31 ± 0.32 | 0.044 |
|   –  Accuracy | 4.31 ± 1.19 | 12.71 ± 0.95* | <0.001 |
| Total time penalties | 13.68 ± 1.49 | 24.98 ± 1.08* | <0.001 |
| Final time | 63.19 ± 2.04 | 75.69 ± 1.73* | <0.001 |

\* $p$ <0.001, greater than pre-game.

Total time penalties incurred during the LSPT were greatest post-game on day 4 (Post d4) with pre-game penalties being less than those incurred post-game for days 2 to 4 ($p<0.01$; Figure 1).

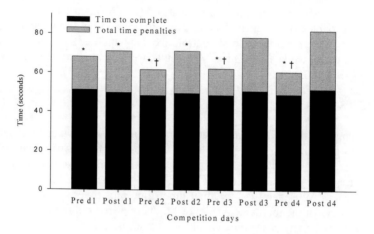

**Figure 1** Final time (time to complete + total time penalties) pre- and post-games to complete the Loughborough Soccer Passing Test during a 4-day tournament.
\* < post d4 time penalties, p<0.01; † < same day post-game, *p*<0.01.

## 4. DISCUSSION

Results of the present study support those previously identifying a decline in the short-passing ability of adolescent soccer players following a game (Rampinini *et al.*, 2008). Although significantly different across all penalty classifications, accuracy appeared to be the most significant aspect influenced by match-induced fatigue due to the greater time penalties post-game. When taken into consideration with the timing of the post-game LSPT (immediately after the game), match-related fatigue appears to be the most likely cause. Interestingly though, other motor skills assessed (such as time taken to complete the LSPT and ball control) were also greater post-game but were comparatively smaller in magnitude compared to the accuracy penalties. Additionally, results of the decision making (psychomotor) skill component were also much smaller in magnitude compared to accuracy time penalties. Previous research has proposed physiological mechanisms influencing match-related fatigue and performances as causative of the deterioration in a player's passing ability (Bangsbo *et al.*, 2006; Rampinini *et al.*, 2008).

With inferior recovery strategies between matches, performances may become impaired as a result of the potential cumulative influence of multiple matches played over consecutive days (Rowsell *et al.*, 2009). Reduced distances and running intensities between halves have been identified in professional players (Mohr *et al.*, 2003), with match running performances during a 4-day junior soccer tournament also shown to decline over consecutive matches (Rowsell *et al.*, 2011).

Although match running was not observed in the present study, there appears to be no influence of any previous match-related fatigue on subsequent pre-game LSPT results. However, the significantly greater time penalties incurred by the players for the post-game LSPT on the final day of competition may suggest a cumulative influence of the previous games.

In previous research, decrements in soccer skill performance have been observed as early as half time (Mohr *et al.*, 2003; Rampinini *et al.*, 2008; Stone *et al.*, 2009). In one study using older adolescent players than those in the current study (17.6 ± 0.5 yr), the short-passing abilities of players assessed, as determined by LSPT performance, were comparable to those of the players in the current study (Rampinini *et al.*, 2008). This previous study identified significantly reduced short-passing ability after the first half of the game with further decrements following the second half suggesting an early onset of match-related fatigue in adolescent players. In a study of professional players, Mohr and colleagues (2003) identified more tackles made per player in the first half compared to the second. The cumulative influence of match-related fatigue on post-game LSPT results in the present study were observed throughout the tournament with time penalties incurred each day increasing between days 2 to 4 (Post d2 to Post d4; Figure 1). The substantial time penalties incurred during the final LSPT of the tournament (Post d4) may be reflective of both match-related fatigue as well as a potentially reduced motivation after a physically demanding and mentally fatiguing tournament.

## 5. CONCLUSION

This study identified a match-induced decline in the short-passing ability of adolescent soccer players across a 4-day tournament primarily due to a decline in technical proficiency. Such results suggest that assessing soccer skills performance is complex, however, once evidence is obtained, coaching strategies can then be implemented to address such deficiencies.

## References

Ali, A., 2011, Measuring soccer skill performance: A review. *Scand J Med Sci Sports*, **21**, 170–183.

Ali, A. *et al.*, 2007, Reliability and validity of two tests of soccer skill. *J Sports Sci*, **25**, 1461–1470.

Bangsbo, J. *et al.*, 2006, Physical and metabolic demands of training and match-play in the elite football player. *J Sports Sci*, **24**, 665–674.

Buchheit, M. *et al.*, 2010, Repeated-sprint sequences during youth soccer matches. *Int J Sports Med*, **31**, 709–716.

Mohr, M. *et al.*, 2003, Match performance of high-standard soccer players with special reference to development of fatigue. *J Sports Sci*, **21**, 519–528.

Rampinini, E. *et al.*, 2008, Effect of match-related fatigue on short-passing ability in young soccer players. *Med Sci Sports Exerc*, **40**, 934–942.

Rowsell, G.J. *et al.*, 2009, Effects of cold-water immersion on physical performance between successive matches in high-performance junior male soccer players. *J Sports Sci*, **27**, 565–573.

Rowsell, G.J. *et al.*, 2011, Effect of post-match cold-water immersion on subsequent match running performance in junior soccer players during tournament play. *J Sports Sci*, **29**, 1–6.

Stone, K.J. *et al.*, 2009, The effect of 45 minutes of soccer-specific exercise on the performance of soccer skills. *Int J Sports Physiol Perf*, **4**, 165–175.

# Part V
# Performance profiling

# CHAPTER FORTY-FOUR

# Relationship between Draft Camp test scores and career success by position in the Australian Football League

S. J. Anderson[1], B. Dawson[1] and P. Peeling[1,2]

[1]School of Sport Science, Exercise and Health, The University of Western Australia, Crawley, Australia; [2]Western Australian Institute of Sport, Mt Claremont, Australia

## 1. INTRODUCTION

The Australian Football League (AFL) National Draft Camp annually screens approximately 70 of the most talented young players in the country on a variety of measures, such as basic anthropometry, physical fitness, psychomotor ability and psychological aptitude. To date, some association between an athlete's performance during the Draft Camp and their subsequent likelihood of being drafted has been established (Pyne et al., 2005). Additionally, it is also recognised that playing position may influence the Draft Camp test performance (Pyne *et al.*, 2006). With such predictors evident, Weston *et al.*, (2007) examined whether test performances during the Draft Camp may also predict future career success (determined as playing >40 games in the AFL); with only weak associations evident. Despite this, Weston *et al.*, (2007) did not consider positional roles when assessing the relationship between Draft Camp performance and subsequent career success. As such, this investigation aimed to assess the association between AFL Draft Camp test scores and being drafted, draft position, number of games played and career success of drafted players (including those still playing), with players separated into positional categories.

## 2. METHODS

The test results of 588 players (age ~17–18 years) attending the AFL National Draft Camp for the years 2001–2008 were analysed. In some instances, players with a pre-existing injury were excluded from one or more assessments in the testing protocol; therefore, some degree of sample size variability existed between tests.

For this investigation, only the anthropometry and physical fitness test scores from the National Draft Camp were considered. These test protocols included: *Anthropometry:* measures of stature (cm), body mass (kg), sum of seven skinfolds (mm), hand span (cm), and arm length (cm). *Physical Fitness:* tests of power (standing vertical jump and running vertical jump using both right and left foot for take-off), speed (20 m sprint), planned agility (AFL specific agility test), aerobic capacity (20 m multi-stage shuttle run and 3 km time trial) and repeated sprint ability (6 x 20 m repeat sprint test on a 20 s departure time).

Data obtained from eight years of AFL Draft Camp testing was pooled and analysed as one data set. The data was also analysed with players separated according to playing position; determined according to standing height (small <180cm, medium 181–190cm, tall >191cm), and functional playing position (midfield, forward and defender). These positions include Small Midfielder (SM), Medium Midfielder (MM), Medium Forward (MF), Medium Defender (MD), Tall Forward (TF), Tall Defender (TD) and Ruckmen (RM). Next, all attendees were further categorised by draft status (drafted or not-drafted); with drafted players ranked according to their draft position for the year they were drafted (i.e. 1, 2, 3 etc). Subsequently, the number of games played to the end of the 2009 season was registered against players who had made an AFL debut; with players then grouped as having achieved career success (>40 AFL games to the end of the 2009 season) or not. Only players drafted up to, and including the 2006 AFL Draft were considered for career success, since subsequent draftees had inadequate time to play >40 games, which is the approximate average career length in the AFL (Weston *et al.*, 2007).

Frequencies were used to show the number of National Draft Camp attendees drafted, and the number of players that achieved career success. Descriptive statistics were generated for each testing variable, across all Draft Camp years. A principal component factor analysis was conducted on Draft Camp test scores (pooled data), grouped into the categories of anthropometry and physical fitness for rotated components factor analysis to cluster like scores. This was repeated for each positional category. With each factor analysis conducted, factor z scores were calculated for each individual player test score. These factor z scores were then used for multiple regression calculations related to the combined data for 2001-2008, and for each positional category. Multiple stepwise regression analysis was conducted for the test results of anthropometry only (Model 1) or the combination of anthropometry and physical fitness (Model 2). The regression equations were used as predictors of draft status, draft position, number of AFL games and AFL success. This was performed on the pooled data, as well as for each positional category. Statistical significance was accepted at $p<0.05$.

## 3. RESULTS

Table 1 presents the total number of players (by position) who were drafted, their draft position, if they made an AFL debut, and their number of games played. The number of players achieving AFL career success is also shown here. In this period, 64% of attendees were drafted by an AFL club. This pooled percentage is similar to that per positional category, ranging from 60% (MF) to 69% (TF). Of the drafted players, 65% went on to make an AFL debut. This is again similar across positional categories, ranging from 59% (RM) to 70% (MM). It was found that 49% of the players making an AFL debut achieved AFL career success. This differed across positional categories, ranging from 38% (TF and RM) to 71% (MM). A comparison of Draft Camp test scores and achievement of AFL career success is presented in Table 2. Successful players were significantly ($p < 0.05$) shorter, and had a shorter arm length. Table 2 also presents differences in test scores between successful and non-successful AFL players by positional category. Successful SM had significantly ($p < 0.05$) higher running VJ scores (left-sided), and faster agility run times. Successful MM were significantly ($p < 0.05$) lighter. Successful RM were significantly ($p < 0.05$) slower in the sprint tests. Successful TD had significantly ($p < 0.05$) lower running VJ (right-sided) scores.

**Factor analysis**

The factor analysis (pooled data) indicated that anthropometry, height (0.912), arm length (0.864), weight (0.796) and handspan (0.674) loaded together for one component, with skinfolds (0.975) loading by itself. Additionally, the sprint tests (5 m: 0.923, 10 m: 0.947, 20 m: 0.900) and the agility run (0.589) loaded together for one component. Right and left running VJ (0.837 and 0.814) loaded with the standing VJ test (0.740), whilst the 20 m shuttle run (-0.937) and 3 km time trial (0.934) loaded together for another component. When repeated for different positions, the factor analyses displayed similar results to that of the pooled data.

**Multiple regression**

These results are summarised in Table 3. For pooled data, the overall predictive value of the Draft Camp test scores was very low; with a maximum of 11% of shared variance being accounted for. However, Draft Camp test scores did show significant predictive ability for the likelihood of being drafted and for draft position ($p < 0.05$). No significant predictors were found for number of games played or for achievement of AFL success.

When considered by player position, Draft Camp test scores had significant predictive value for the likelihood of MM (28% of variance, $p < 0.05$), MF (27% of variance, $p < 0.05$) and TF (25% of variance, $p < 0.05$) being drafted. Additionally, it was found that test scores had significant predictive value for the draft position of SM (36% of variance, $p < 0.05$) and MF (45% of variance, $p < 0.01$). The only position to suggest that Draft Camp test scores were predictive of number of games played was MF, with 40% of variance being accounted for ($p < 0.01$). However, this was only with anthropometry (Model 1) used in the regression analysis. Draft Camp test scores of MM and RM were found to have significant predictive value in predicting AFL career success; accounting for 33% (MM: $p < 0.05$) and 43% (RM: $p < 0.01$) of shared variance respectively, when anthropometric and fitness testing data were combined (Model 2).

**Table 1** Player Draft and AFL Status from AFL Draft Camps 2001-2008 (ranges in parentheses).

| Position | Frequency | Drafted | | Mean (±SD) | AFL Debut | | Mean (±SD) | |
| --- | --- | --- | --- | --- | --- | --- | --- | --- |
| | | Yes | No | Draft Position | Yes | No | AFL Games Played^ | AFL Success* |
| Small Midfield | 83 | 54 (65%) | 29 | 29(±18) (1-77) | 37 (69%) | 17 | 53(±48) (1-142) | 20 (54%) |
| Medium Midfield | 98 | 64 (65%) | 34 | 23(±21) (1-83) | 45 (70%) | 19 | 66(±47) (1-178) | 32 (71%) |
| Medium Forward | 83 | 50 (60%) | 33 | 31(±18) (1-80) | 33 (66%) | 17 | 38(±41) (1-166) | 13 (39%) |
| Medium Defender | 82 | 52 (63%) | 30 | 33(±19) (2-67) | 31 (60%) | 21 | 38(±37) (1-145) | 16 (52%) |
| Tall Forward | 90 | 62 (69%) | 28 | 27(±20) (1-74) | 39 (63%) | 23 | 32(±35) (1-117) | 15 (38%) |
| Tall Defender | 84 | 51 (61%) | 32 | 29(±19) (3-80) | 33 (65%) | 19 | 34(±34) (1-119) | 13 (39%) |
| Ruck | 68 | 44 (65%) | 24 | 26(±18) (1-79) | 26 (59%) | 18 | 29(±29) (1-102) | 10 (38%) |
| **Total (2001-2008)** | **588** | **377** | **211** | | **244** | **134** | | **119**[#] |
| **%** | | **64%** | **36%** | | **65%** | **35%** | | **49%** |

* Defined as > 40 games; ^ To end of 2006 season;
# Of the players making an AFL debut 2001-2006 (2007-2008 not included).

**Table 2** Comparison of Draft Camp test scores (pooled data) and achievement of AFL career success (>40 games) and by positional category.

| Category | Test | Successful | Unsuccessful |
| --- | --- | --- | --- |
| Pooled Data | Height (cm) | 187.1 (±6.1) | 189.8 (±6.9)* |
| | Arm Length (cm) | 81.5 (±3.8) | 83.0 (±3.8)* |
| Small Midfielder | Running VJ (left) (cm) | 79 (±7) | 74 (±7)* |
| | Agility Run (s) | 8.32 (±0.23) | 8.55 (±0.29)* |
| Medium Midfielder | Weight (kg) | 79.16 (±4.87) | 80.65 (±5.60)** |
| Tall Defender | Running VJ (Right) (cm) | 64 (±12) | 72 (±10)* |
| Ruck | 5 m Sprint (s) | 1.16 (±0.06) | 1.10 (±0.06)* |
| | 10 m Sprint (s) | 1.91 (±0.08) | 1.85 (±0.07)* |

* Signifies $p<0.05$; ** Signifies $p<0.01$; VJ = Vertical Jump.

**Table 3** Multiple regression analysis summary for being drafted,
draft position, games played and career success.

| Variable | Data Pool | Model | R | R Square | Adjusted R Square |
|---|---|---|---|---|---|
| **Drafted** | Medium Midfield | 2 | 0.532 | .283** | 0.214 |
| | Medium Forward | 2 | 0.522 | .272** | 0.188 |
| | Tall Forward | 2 | 0.498 | .248** | 0.186 |
| | 2001-2008 (All Positions) | 2 | 0.332 | .110** | 0.089 |
| **Draft Position** | Small Midfield | 2 | 0.599 | .359* | 0.23 |
| | Medium Forward | 2 | 0.67 | .448** | 0.326 |
| | 2001-2008 (All Positions) | 2 | 0.283 | .080* | 0.045 |
| **Games Played** | Medium Forward | 1 | 0.636 | .404** | 0.323 |
| **AFL Success** | Medium Midfield | 1 | 0.424 | .180* | 0.127 |
| | | 2 | 0.571 | .326* | 0.205 |
| | Ruckmen | 1 | 0.577 | .332* | 0.272 |
| | | 2 | 0.653 | .427* | 0.276 |

* Signifies p<0.05; ** Signifies p<0.01: Model 1 = Anthropometry only;
Model 2 = Anthropometry + Physical Fitness.

## 4. DISCUSSION

The results suggest that similar percentages of players attending the AFL National Draft Camp are successfully drafted, and then make an AFL debut, even across positional categories. However, it appears that a greater percentage of midfield players achieve career success when compared to athletes drafted under other positional categories. Such an outcome might seem surprising given the greater physical demand placed on these playing positions throughout a competitive game, but it must also be acknowledged that there are more of this type of player in teams than for other positions. Caution should be applied in interpreting this result, since the position of a player may change throughout their career, as a result of factors such as improved skills and game sense, team requirements, increased fitness or body changes likely to occur within a maturing athlete. As such, the initial categorisation of Draft Camp attendees to a playing position may not reflect the predominant position in which they may achieve career success.

When making associations between Draft Camp test scores and eventual career success, it is apparent that there is no consistent trend in successful attributes, either throughout the pooled data or by positional category. In fact, for TD and RM, successful players were out-performed by their non-successful counterparts on a number of tests. To this end, such an outcome would likely suggest that the test performance differences that do exist between drafted and non drafted players are of no practical significance. As might have been expected, the factor analysis showed that within both pooled data and positional categories, tests of speed and agility shared a relationship, as did the two endurance tests and the three tests of jump-specific power. These outcomes suggest that the testing protocols used within the AFL National Draft Camp are specific enough to isolate and individually assess the different components of fitness.

The results of the regression analysis suggest that the predictive nature of the Draft Camp test results is quite low for pooled data, but somewhat improved when positions are considered. It was established that the pooled Draft Camp test scores may predict the chance of being drafted and at which draft position the player is selected. However, this may reflect the emphasis that recruiting scouts place on drafting talented athletes rather than any association these scores have to playing ability or the likelihood of achieving career success. This trend was also evident when considering playing position; however, some predictive ability of Draft Camp test scores on career success was found in MM and RM. Despite these significant outcomes, it is still evident that a maximum of only 43% of shared variance was accounted for, thus suggesting that other factors are important and not considered when using AFL Draft Camp test results to predict how well an athlete will progress in the AFL.

In summary, these results show that athlete selection into the AFL should not be based solely on test performances recorded during the AFL National Draft Camp. It is evident that Draft Camp tests of anthropometry and physical fitness do not account for enough variance to be heralded as predictors of player success in the AFL, as was reported previously (Weston *et al.*, 2007). This is likely due to the multi-faceted nature of the game, with many other factors involved (skill, game sense, mental toughness, drive to win, etc) that are not accounted for with the tests implemented during this camp. Finally, it should be considered that the test performances recorded by athletes at the Draft Camp are only reflective of their current state of fitness, and for the most part, these are probably the most trainable aspects of a potential draftee. As such, a larger emphasis should be placed on the game sense, skill and playing ability of an athlete.

### References

Pyne, D.B. *et al.*, 2005, Fitness testing and career progression in AFL football. *J Sci Med Sport*, **8**, 321–332.

Pyne, D.B. *et al.*, 2006, Positional differences in fitness and anthropometric characteristics in Australian football. *J Sci Med Sport*, **9**, 143–150.

Weston, E. *et al.*, 2007, Australian Football League draft camp scores and career success. Proceedings of the Sixth World Congress on Science and Football, *J Sports Sci Med*, **6**, 67–68.

# CHAPTER FORTY-FIVE

# Sports-specific anthropometry in Japanese soccer players analyzed by three-dimensional photonic scanning

Y. Hoshikawa[1], N. Ii[1], T. Iida[1], M. Muramatsu[1], Y. Nakajima[1], K. Chuman[2] and T. Ikoma[2]

[1]Sports Photonics Laboratory, Hamamatsu Photonics K.K., Japan
[2]Yamaha Football Club Co. Ltd., Iwata-City, Japan

## 1. INTRODUCTION

Whole-body three-dimensional (3D) photonic scanners for measuring the human body surface were initially developed for the clothing industry. However, they can now be used for multiple anthropometric measurements in athletes: body size, shape, circumference, volume and composition (Stewart, 2010). We applied this technology to Japanese elite soccer players from youth to professional. The first purpose of the study was to describe soccer-related anthropometry according to age and playing position. The second was to compare Japanese soccer players with soccer players from other countries and athletes in other sports.

## 2. METHODS

A total of 277 Japanese elite soccer players from the ages of 12 to 30 yrs participated in the study. The players were divided into 5 age groups; under 13 (U-13), 15 (U-15), 17 (U-17), 21 (U-21) and over 22 (O-22) yrs. All of the O-22 players were professional players. Forwards (FW), Midfielders (MF), and Defenders (DF) were grouped together as outfield players (FD) except when analyzing player position differences. Goalkeepers were expressed as GK. The study further included 5 Brazilian and 4 Korean soccer professionals in the FD as well as 12 sprinters, 10 canoeist, 21 rowers and 20 untrained control subjects (Table1). Body composition was measured by the Bod Pod system (LMI, Inc.). Circumferences in cm (Cir) of upper arm, chest, hip, middle of thigh and calf were measured by a 3D scanner (Hamamatsu Photonics). Cir on both sides of the body were averaged for the arms and legs. Because of difference in height between the groups, Cir divided by height x 100 (%Cir) were also used for analyses. ANOVA and Kruskal-Wallis tests were used to examine the differences between groups.

## 3. RESULTS

The Cir are included in Table 1. Differences between playing positions, between age-groups, between events, and between players from Japan and foreign countries were analyzed based on the data.

**Table 1** Subject characteristics and circumferences.

| | | | Number | Age | Height | Body mass | Upper-arm | Chest | Hip | Mid-thigh | Calf |
|---|---|---|---|---|---|---|---|---|---|---|---|
| | | | | yrs | cm | kg | cm | cm | cm | cm | cm |
| Japanese | GK | U-13 | 6 | 13.1(0.3) | 169.9(5.6) | 59.3(7.1) | 25.9(1.8) | 82.4(5.8) | 92.8(3.9) | 48.5(3.3) | 36.1(1.5) |
| | | U-15 | 7 | 14.8(0.6) | 178.3(4.9) | 69.6(4.8) | 27.9(1.5) | 88.1(5.7) | 98.4(3.3) | 52.1(2.6) | 37.8(1.4) |
| | | U-17 | 4 | 17.1(0.2) | 182.0(5.2) | 72.7(4.3) | 28.7(0.8) | 91.5(2.2) | 98.5(1.3) | 53.0(1.2) | 38.0(1.1) |
| | | U-21 | 4 | 20.8(1.2) | 183.6(3.7) | 77.2(3.8) | 30.6(0.5) | 94.7(1.2) | 100.6(1.8) | 52.6(2.1) | 37.4(1.3) |
| | | O-22 | 7 | 25.2(2.8) | 183.3(3.3) | 77.0(7.5) | 30.7(2.1) | 93.9(4.1) | 100.9(1.9) | 53.0(3.1) | 38.9(2.5) |
| Japanese | FD (FW,MF, DF) | U-13 | 58 | 13.1(0.2) | 160.2(7.3) | 48.2(7.6) | 23.1(2.0) | 77.5(5.0) | 85.8(5.3) | 44.3(3.4) | 33.7(2.3) |
| | | U-15 | 63 | 15.0(0.5) | 169.1(5.7) | 58.3(8.0) | 25.1(2.3) | 83.5(5.0) | 93.0(5.5) | 48.5(3.5) | 36.0(2.4) |
| | | U-17 | 46 | 17.0(0.5) | 171.8(4.6) | 66.1(5.2) | 27.6(1.4) | 88.5(3.5) | 97.1(3.5) | 52.4(2.4) | 38.0(1.8) |
| | | U-21 | 28 | 20.2(1.2) | 175.0(6.4) | 70.3(6.8) | 28.7(1.7) | 91.4(3.3) | 98.3(3.8) | 53.4(2.8) | 38.4(1.9) |
| | | O-22 | 54 | 25.1(2.2) | 175.9(5.0) | 70.7(5.3) | 28.7(1.5) | 92.1(3.0) | 98.7(3.1) | 53.4(2.1) | 38.5(1.6) |
| Brazilian | FD | | 5 | 25.9(2.6) | 176.3(5.3) | 75.0(5.4) | 30.2(1.7) | 95.5(3.5) | 99.5(3.5) | 55.0(2.6) | 38.4(1.6) |
| Korean | FD | | 4 | 23.5(0.7) | 177.0(4.1) | 74.4(3.3) | 30.0(0.8) | 93.2(2.5) | 100.4(1.1) | 55.5(0.9) | 38.9(0.5) |
| Japanese | Sprinters | | 12 | 17.3(0.5) | 175.9(6.2) | 63.9(6.0) | 26.8(2.0) | 87.2(4.3) | 96.0(3.4) | 50.7(2.6) | 37.2(2.0) |
| | Rowers | | 21 | 17.1(1.5) | 171.8(6.7) | 63.6(8.2) | 27.3(2.0) | 88.0(5.1) | 95.3(4.6) | 51.1(3.1) | 36.2(2.2) |
| | Canoeists | | 10 | 19.1(4.9) | 167.3(4.2) | 64.5(10.2) | 30.1(3.0) | 93.2(7.8) | 95.7(5.6) | 51.2(5.1) | 36.3(2.6) |
| | Controls | | 20 | 17.2(0.4) | 167.4(4.7) | 57.3(6.7) | 25.8(2.5) | 83.6(4.8) | 94.5(4.3) | 48.4(4.1) | 35.3(2.9) |

mean(s.d.)

### 3.1. Comparison between playing positions

Data from the U-21 and O-22 were used in the analyses. There were no significant differences among the DF, MF, and FW in any %Cir. Although not a significant difference, the upper-arm (Figure 1) and chest %Cir were higher in GK than in other positions. In contrast, the hip, mid-thigh and calf %Cir were lower in GK. The mid-thigh %Cir for GK was found to be lower significantly from all other player positions (Figure 1).

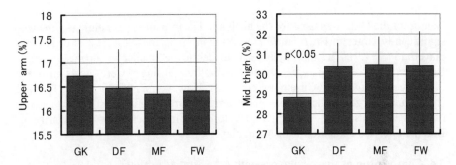

**Figure 1** Differences in upper-arm and mid-thigh %Cir by player position in U-21 and O-22.

## 3.2. Comparison between age groups

All measurements for %Cir increased with age until U-17 for both GK and FD. Upper-arm and chest Cir for GK and FD, and mid-thigh Cir for FD were developed larger than the hip or calf Cir in O-22 relative to U-13 (Figure 2). Hip, mid-thigh and calf Cir reached levels similar to O-22 at U-17 although upper-arm and chest Cir increased with age until U-22 regardless of position. These results suggest that not only hip and leg but also upper-body muscularity is an important characteristic among professional soccer players.

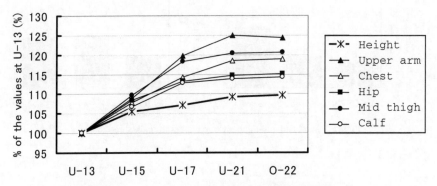

**Figure 2** Relative changes in height and Cir for FD from U-13 onwards.

### 3.3. Comparisons of Japanese players with other country players

Data from the O-22 was used for the analyses. Fat-free mass per height (kg/m) was significantly larger in Brazilian (39.0±1.8) than in Japanese (37.1±2.0) or Korean players (37.3±1.9). The mid-thigh %Cir tended to be smaller in Japanese than in Brazilian or Korean players (Figure 3) although there were no significant differences in any leg %Cir among countries. However, Brazilian players showed significantly larger %Cir for the upper-arm (Figure 3) and chest than Japanese players, which suggest distinctive development in upper-body muscularity in Brazilian players compared with Asian players.

### 3.4. Comparison of soccer players with other sports athletes

Data from the U-17 was used for the analyses. Soccer players showed a significantly larger value only for calf %Cir compared to other sports athletes, which was significantly larger in soccer players than in sprinters (Figure 4). The upper-arm and chest %Cir (Figure 4) were larger in canoeists than in all other athletes, although soccer players also showed a significantly larger chest %Cir than the untrained controls.

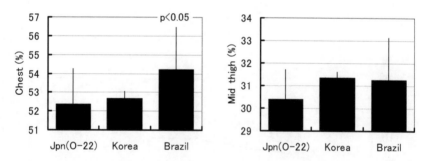

**Figure 3** Chest and mid-thigh %Cir in players from the three countries.

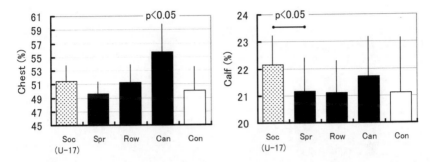

**Figure 4** Chest and calf %Cir in athletes and untrained controls. Soc, soccer players; Spr, sprinters; Row, rowers; Can, canoeists; Con, untrained controls.

## 4. DISCUSSION AND CONCLUSIONS

Reilly, *et al.* (2000) reported that the mesomorphic somatotype was dominant among elite soccer players. Results for Japanese players in this study were in line with those of Reilly *et al.* (2000). Measurements for young and professional soccer players differed not only in body size but also in body shape. All circumferences from U-13 to professionals increased more than height although the extent of the increase varied depending on the circumferences. Hip, mid-thigh and calf circumferences levelled off at U-17 while upper-arm and chest circumferences continued to increase from U-17 to U-21. These results suggest upper-body muscularity as well as hip and leg muscularity is an important characteristic in professional soccer players. This tendency was much more evident in Brazilian than Japanese soccer players. The 3D scanning could be a useful tool for identifying differences in players' kinanthropometry.

## References

Reilly, T. *et al.*, 2000, Anthropometric and physiological predispositions for elite soccer. *J Sports Sci*, **18**, 669–683.
Stewart, A.D., 2010, Kinanthropometry and body composition: A natural home for three-dimensional photonic scanning. *J Sports Sci*, **28**, 455–457.

## CHAPTER FORTY-SIX

# Longitudinal changes in sprint performance in relation to fitness development in U-14 soccer players

T. Iida[1], Y. Hoshikawa[1], K. Chuman[2], T. Ikoma[2],
M. Muramatsu[1] and Y. Nakajima[1]

[1]Sports Photonics Laboratory, Hamamatsu Photonics K.K., Japan
[2]Jubilo Iwata, Yamaha Football Club Co., Ltd., Japan

## 1. INTRODUCTION

Sprint ability is generally accepted as an essential element in modern soccer. Many previous studies indicate that sprint ability over short distances serves as a discriminator for higher level performance in young soccer players (Reilly, *et al.*, 2000; Vaeyens, *et al.*, 2006; Gil, *et al.*, 2007). Philippaerts, *et al.* (2006) have shown that maximal development in running speed in soccer players at puberty occurs coincidently with the peak growth velocity in height. Mendez-Villanueva, *et al.* (2011) suggested that development of fat-free mass could be a factor related to faster sprinting in post-pubertal soccer players. Therefore, information that correlates sprinting to physical development in young soccer players is important for designing effective training at this age. Despite many studies on improving sprinting in young soccer players there is little longitudinal data which enables us to examine speed development directly with physical development. In this study we investigated longitudinal changes in 20 m sprint times as well as anthropometric and fitness profiles of U-14 players for two consecutive years. The purpose of the study is to identify the particular anthropometric and fitness characteristics relating to sprint development in players during early adolescence. Towards that end, the first approach taken was to examine correlations between sprint speed and variables relating to anthropometry and fitness. The second approach taken was to compare the magnitude of developments in physique and fitness between players showing different improvements in sprinting during those two years.

## 2. METHODS

Fifty players from the U-14 squad of a club belonging to the Japan Professional Football League Division 1 participated in the study. Table 1 shows the characteristics of the subjects. During a period of two years, each subject was coached at nearly the same weekly training schedule which was 1.5 to 2 hours per day, 5 days per week and 1 game on the weekend. Physical training was conducted approximately two times per week and was mainly long distance running, interval training and circuit training using the player's own body mass as a load. Neither high-resistance training nor plyometric training were included.

The 20 m sprint times of the players were measured by infrared photocell sensors (Optical Laptime Watcher, Hamamatsu Photonics K.K.) placed at distances of 5, 10, 15, and 20 m. As described in Kubo, *et al.* (2011), the sensors detected the release of the subject's rear foot at the start and the passage of the subject's trunk through the respective sensors. Each subject performed 3 sprinting trials with a 5-min interval rest and the best time taken to cover the 20 m distance was used for data analysis. All measurements were conducted on the same grass soccer field using the same equipment. Body composition was measured using the BODPOD system (LMI, Inc.). Leg length and circumference were measured by a three-dimensional photonic scanner (Hamamatsu Photonics K.K.). Muscle cross-sectional area (CSA) for trunk and thigh muscles were determined using magnetic resonance imaging (0.2-T Signa Profile, GE) in the same way as earlier studies (Hoshikawa, *et al.*, 2006, 2009). The CSA of the psoas majors, gluteus maximus and thigh muscles at upper(70%), middle(50%) and lower(30%) femur levels were determined on the images. Vertical height of squat jump (SJ) and countermovement jump with the arm swing (CMJ) were measured by filming with height calibration. The top of the head was digitized to measure the vertical jump height for each test performance. The onset of blood lactate accumulation (OBLA) and $\dot{V}O_{2max}$ were measured by an incremental test on a treadmill. The test protocol was a 3-minute submaximal run followed by a 1-minute rest repeated for 4 to 6 times with the running speed increased from 180 to 280 m/min. Blood lactate was measured immediately after each submaximal run to determine OBLA, which was defined as the speed at 4mmol/L lactate concentration. After that, a final run to exhaustion was performed to determine $\dot{V}O_{2max}$ by using a calibrated Meta Max metabolic system (Cortex Biophysic GmbH).

Although all subjects were examined four times at intervals of 6 months for a period of 2 years, only the data from the first (M1) and last (M2) measurements were included in statistical analyses. Pearson-product correlations between sprint times for 20 m (20-m ST) and variables of anthropometry and fitness at M1 and between changes during the 2 years were calculated to examine their association. The 10 respective players showing the largest (L; -0.22±0.03 sec) and the smallest (S; -0.01±0.03 sec) improvements in 20-m ST from M1 to M2 were compared by a non-pared t-test. The statistical software SPSS ver.11.5 was used for analyses. Statistical significance was set at p<0.05.

**Table 1** Characteristics of the subjects.

|      | Age (years) | Height (cm) | Weight (kg) | Percent body fat (%) | Fat-free mass (kg) |
|------|-------------|-------------|-------------|----------------------|--------------------|
| M1   | 12.8±0.5    | 163.2±8.6   | 51.0±9.1    | 11.4±3.4             | 45.3±8.4           |
| M2   | 14.5±0.6 †  | 170.2±6.8 † | 59.0±9.0 †  | 10.3±2.9 †           | 52.9±7.7 †         |

mean±SD    † : p<0.05

## 3. RESULTS

Table 2 shows mean sprint times, leg length, thigh circumference, muscle CSA, vertical jump height and aerobic ability at M1 and M2. All sprint times at M2 were significantly faster than those at M1 (p<0.05). Length, circumference, muscle CSA, vertical jumps and aerobic ability also improved significantly from M1 to M2 (p<0.05).

Significant negative correlations were observed between the 20-m ST and height, weight, leg length, circumference, fat-free mass, muscle CSA and vertical jumps at M1 while a significant positive correlation was found between the 20-m ST and percent body fat (Table 3). The correlation coefficients at M1 were relatively higher in fat-free mass, muscle CSA and vertical jumps and peak at upper thigh muscle CSA (r=-0.71; p<0.05). There was also a significant negative correlation between the 20-m ST and absolute $\dot{V}O_{2max}$ at M1; although the correlation coefficients for relative $\dot{V}O_{2max}$ and the OBLA were not significant (p>0.05). Correlation coefficients between the 20-m ST and these longitudinal changes were reduced compared to those at M1 (Table 3). However, fat-free mass and muscle CSA at M1 and these longitudinal changes showed relatively higher correlation coefficients to the 20-m ST than the other variables.

Longitudinal increments in height, weight, leg length, upper and middle thigh circumference, fat-free mass, muscle CSA and absolute $\dot{V}O_{2max}$ were significantly larger in L than in S (p<0.05, Table 4). The longitudinal decrement in percent body fat and increment in SJ showed tendencies for L to be larger than S, although the differences did not reach a significant value (p=0.06, 0.10).

The longitudinal changes expressed in percentage were greater in muscle CSA than in any other variables except absolute $\dot{V}O_{2max}$. Differences in percentage changes between L and S were greatest in CSA for the gluteus maximus and psoas major which were almost twice those in S (Table 4).

**Table 2** Sprint times and other variables.

|  |  | M1 | M2 |
|---|---|---|---|
| Sprint times (sec) | 5m | 1.07±0.05 | 1.04±0.04 † |
|  | 10m | 1.86±0.08 | 1.80±0.06 † |
|  | 15m | 2.57±0.11 | 2.48±0.08 † |
|  | 20m | 3.24±0.14 | 3.13±0.11 † |
| Leg length (cm) |  | 78.7±4.6 | 81.3±3.7 † |
| Circumference (cm) | Upper thigh | 50.6±4.1 | 53.6±4.0 † |
|  | Middle thigh | 45.5±3.9 | 48.8±3.8 † |
| Muscle CSA (cm$^2$) | Psoas major | 12.7±2.8 | 15.2±3.0 † |
|  | Gluteus maximus | 84.2±17.3 | 105.1±17.7 † |
|  | Upper thigh | 124.4±21.4 | 150.7±22.4 † |
|  | Middle thigh | 114.3±20.6 | 136.8±22.3 † |
|  | Lower thigh | 77.4±15.3 | 92.4±16.1 † |
| Vertical jump (cm) | SJ | 33.2±4.0 | 36.5±4.4 † |
|  | CMJ | 45.3±4.4 | 51.1±4.3 † |
| Aerobic ability | VO$_2$max (ml/min) | 3396±555 | 4124±567 † |
|  | VO$_2$max/weight (ml/kg/min) | 66.8±5.5 | 70.2±5.8 † |
|  | OBLA speed (m/min) | 245±18 | 256±17 † |

mean±SD   † : p<0.05

**Table 3** Correlation coefficients among 20-m ST and fitness variables.

|  | M1 | Changes |
|---|---|---|
| Height (cm) | -0.43† | -0.36† |
| Weight (kg) | -0.47† | -0.34† |
| Leg length (cm) | -0.37† | -0.35† |
| Upper thigh circumference (cm) | -0.48† | -0.31† |
| Middle thigh circumference (cm) | -0.46† | -0.27 |
| Percent body fat (%) | 0.49† | 0.32† |
| Fat-free mass (kg) | -0.55† | -0.46† |
| Muscle  CSA (cm$^2$) |  |  |
| Psoas major | -0.57† | -0.41† |
| Gluteus maximus | -0.59† | -0.46† |
| Upper thigh | -0.71† | -0.56† |
| Middle thigh | -0.67† | -0.54† |
| Lower thigh | -0.61† | -0.53† |
| Vertical jump (cm) |  |  |
| SJ | -0.62† | -0.29† |
| CMJ | -0.58† | 0.03 |
| Aerobic ability |  |  |
| VO$_2$max (ml/min) | -0.54† | -0.42† |
| VO$_2$max/weight (ml/kg/min) | -0.08 | -0.26 |
| OBLA speed (m/min) | -0.01 | 0.09 |

† : P<0.05 Indicating the correlation coefficients

**Table 4** Longitudinal changes in L and S over 2 years.

| | Changes | | | | | |
|---|---|---|---|---|---|---|
| | L | | | S | | |
| | M1 | M2 | Δ(%) | M1 | M2 | Δ(%) |
| 20-m ST (sec) | 3.425±0.1 | 3.202±0.1 | -6.5† | 3.136±0.1 | 3.123±0.1 | -0.5 |
| Height (cm) | 157.2±9.2 | 167.4±8.9 | 6.5† | 163.8±6.8 | 168.9±5.7 | 3.2 |
| Weight (kg) | 44.9±7.5 | 54.9±8.7 | 22.5† | 51.1±8.1 | 57.7±9.3 | 13.2 |
| Leg length (cm) | 76.0±5.2 | 80.8±4.5 | 6.5† | 78.5±3.7 | 80.0±3.4 | 1.9 |
| Upper thigh circumference (cm) | 47.7±3.4 | 52.1±3.3 | 9.2† | 50.3±3.9 | 53.2±4.2 | 5.7 |
| Middle thigh circumference (cm) | 43.0±3.4 | 46.9±3.2 | 9.2† | 45.8±4.2 | 48.5±4.0 | 6.0 |
| Calf circumference (cm) | 32.7±2.2 | 34.8±2.1 | 6.5 | 34.5±2.6 | 36.2±2.8 | 4.9 |
| Body fat (%) | 13.4±3.5 | 10.4±2.0 | -20.6 | 9.7±2.7 | 9.3±2.7 | -3.17 |
| Fat-free mass (kg) | 38.8±6.4 | 49.2±7.8 | 26.9† | 46.1±7.3 | 52.4±8.5 | 13.7 |
| Muscle CSA (cm²) | | | | | | |
| Psoas major | 10.1±1.3 | 13.2±2.3 | 30.6† | 13.4±2.4 | 15.4±3.5 | 14.2 |
| Gluteus maximus | 70.4±10.0 | 95.1±11.5 | 35.7† | 85.3±13.6 | 101.1±16.4 | 18.7 |
| Upper thigh muscle | 106.1±12.3 | 136.6±16.7 | 28.8† | 129.3±19.9 | 152.5±25.3 | 17.8 |
| Middle thigh muscle | 97.0±13.3 | 123.2±17.4 | 26.9† | 120.4±21.4 | 138.5±25.8 | 15.0 |
| Lower thigh muscle | 64.6±8.8 | 82.5±12.0 | 27.7† | 81.8±16.9 | 94.3±19.1 | 15.4 |
| Vertical jump (cm) | | | | | | |
| SJ | 29.7±2.6 | 34.1±4.4 | 14.6 | 34.9±3.0 | 37.2±4.1 | 7.0 |
| CMJ | 43.0±3.6 | 48.6±5.6 | 13.1 | 47.3±4.4 | 53.6±4.0 | 13.7 |
| Aerobic ability | | | | | | |
| VO₂max (ml/min) | 3019±491 | 3986±609 | 32.8† | 3362±514 | 3902±608 | 16.6 |
| VO₂max/weight (ml/kg/min) | 67.6±7.9 | 72.6±4.4 | 8.2 | 66.1±6.4 | 67.7±4.7 | 3.0 |
| OBLA speed (m/min) | 241±22.4 | 251±16.2 | 4.3 | 236±20.0 | 251±20.6 | 6.7 |

†:$p<0.05$ Significantly different from S

## 4. DISCUSSION

As noted in earlier studies (Mendez-Villanueva, *et al.*, 2011; Kubo, *et al.*, 2011), we confirmed positive correlations between development of muscularity (fat-free mass and muscle CSA) and sprint speed in young soccer players. These results provide insight that muscular development is an important factor for faster sprinting in early adolescent players. It is likely that increases in muscle CSA facilitate development of strength and power in the players. The higher correlations of the 20-m ST with vertical jumps as well as muscle CSA at M1 were also indicative of higher power in players having larger muscle CSA. Previous studies (Hoshikawa, *et al.*, 2006, 2009; Kubo, *et al.*, 2011) have provided evidence that junior track sprinters and professional soccer players who have faster sprint ability also have larger CSA for trunk and thigh muscles. The results for the U-14 group in this paper were in agreement with those studies.

Also worth noting is that the percentage of body fat had a negative impact on the 20-m ST in this study. This result suggests that increased fat mass can be disadvantageous in sprinting. This may prove particularly true for the U-14 group, since boys during early adolescence generally have a higher percentage of body fat compared with boys in their post adolescent stage.

Players whose 20-m ST results improved to a greater extent during the 2 years (L) exhibited a larger development in physique (height, weight, leg length, thigh circumference, fat-free mass and muscle CSA) and body composition (percent body fat) compared to their less improved counterparts (S). The extent of changes in L was relatively large in fat-free mass and muscle CSA with percentage increases between 27 to 36%. These results support the above suggestion that muscular development is important for faster sprinting. Moreover, the changes in percentage increase were higher in muscle CSA for gluteus maximus and psoas major than for thigh muscles. These results suggest that greater size development, particularly in hip-related muscles, may prove important for attaining sprint ability in early adolescent players.

The players in L were in their adolescent growth spurt period so their height increased by more than 10 cm during the 2 years. This is a period of large muscular development in males. It is therefore possible that differences observed between L and S can be ascribed simply to individual variations in growth spurt timing. One element worth noting is that the increase in leg length was larger in L than in S. Longer legs with stronger hip-related muscles enable a long stride in sprinting. Since leg length exhibits large growth during the earlier phase of adolescent growth spurt, a large improvement in sprint ability is likely to appear during this period when accompanied by sufficient muscular development. Further analysis of how muscular development contributes to sprint ability in U-14s is needed at the same level of biological maturity.

In conclusion, sprint ability in U-14s is largely affected by greater development in fat-free mass and muscle CSA. Hip-related muscles may prove more important in sprint ability. U-14 players undergo large changes in physique and muscularity within a short biological period. The high level of sprinting required for successful players may be achieved by a synergy of biological maturation and concomitant systemic training. In view of these facts, we suggest that training that promotes specific and appropriate muscularity can be effective in early adolescent soccer players seeking to attain high sprint ability.

# References

Gil, S. *et al.*, 2007, Selection of young soccer players in terms of anthropometric and physiological factors, *J Sports Med and Phys Fitness*, **47**, 25–32.

Hoshikawa, Y. *et al.,* 2006, Influence of the psoas major and thigh muscularity on 100-m times in junior sprinters, *Med Sci Sports Exerc*, **38**, 2138–2143.

Hoshikawa, Y. *et al.*, 2009, Differences in muscularity of psoas major and thigh muscles in relation to sprint and vertical jump performances between elite young and professional soccer players, In *Science and Football VI*, London: Routledge, pp.149–154.

Kubo, T. *et al.*, 2011, Contribution of trunk muscularity on sprint run, *Int J Sports Med*, **32**, 223–228.

Mendez-Villanueva, A. *et al.*, 2011, Age-related differences in acceleration, maximum running speed, and repeated-sprint performance in young soccer players, *J Sports Sci*, **29**, 477–484.

Philippaerts, R.M. *et al.*, 2006, The relationship between peak height velocity and physical performance in youth soccer players, *J Sports Sci*, **24**, 221–230.

Reilly, T. *et al.*, 2000, A multidisciplinary approach to talent identification in soccer, *J Sports Sci*, **18**, 695–702.

Vaeyens, R. *et al.*, 2006, A multidisciplinary selection model for youth soccer: The Ghent youth soccer project, *Br J Sports Med*, **40**, 928–934.

# CHAPTER FORTY-SEVEN

# Anthropometrics of elite senior male Italian rugby union players

S. Pogliaghi, G. Da Lozzo and G. De Roia

Faculty of Human Movement Sciences, University of Verona, Italy

## 1. INTRODUCTION

Rugby is a collision team sport, classified as an interval aerobic-anaerobic activity involving great muscle masses and force efforts of both upper and lower extremities (Duthie *et al.*, 2003, 2005 and 2006).

Game analysis and functional and anthropometric evaluation of players of different skill, gender and/or age are classical approaches to the understanding of the physical demands of rugby (Reilly, 2003; Duthie *et al.*, 2003 and 2005; Scott, 2003; Deutsch, 2007). Anthropometric evaluation of athletes is essential to assist talent selection, guide training, monitor seasonal variations and quantify the evolving demands of the game. Evaluation requires a specific normative database that accounts for different geographical, technical and age contexts. Yet, while anthropometric evaluation is carried out on a regular basis by national federations as well as by individual clubs, data are kept confidential and/or are collected in a non-standardized mode.

Furthermore, scientific data on rugby union players are relatively scarce and mainly referred to the southern hemisphere (Duthie *et al.*, 2003, 2005 and 2006). Finally, due to the evolution of rugby union in the most recent years (Duthie *et al.*, 2003), the data that are currently available might not be actual (Scott *et al.*, 2003). All the above factors limit the availability/usefulness of anthropometric data to different contexts both in the sport and in the scientific community.

To fill in this gap, this descriptive study was aimed at providing reference data on anthropometric characteristics of elite senior male rugby players of the southern European region.

## 2. METHODS

To obtain an homogeneous sample of elite senior players we selected only subjects who were regularly engaged in elite training and international competitions. As a result, 127 male players from the National Senior and 'A' Italian rugby union teams (60 forwards and 67 backs) were measured between 2006 and 2009, before the Six Nations Championship.

In the morning, before breakfast, body weight (digital scale, Seca 877, Seca, Leicester, UK) and stature (vertical stadiometer, Seca, Leicester, UK) were determined to the nearest 0.1 kg and 0.5 cm. Skinfold thicknesses were measured, in triplicate, by a single skilled investigator (pectoral, scapular, triceps, iliac, abdominal and thigh) using a pincer type caliper (Holtain T/W skinfold caliper, Holtain limited, UK). For each skinfold, an average value was calculated (after having discarded possible aberrant values, i.e. difference > 1mm). Thereafter % body fat was estimated based on the sum of the 6 skin fold thicknesses (SS, in mm) with the formula (Golding *et al.*, 1982):

$$\% \text{ body fat} = (0.2 * (SS)) - (0.0003 * SS2) + (1.133 * age) - 5.7$$

and lean body mass was calculated as:

$$LBM = \text{body weight} - (\text{body weight} * \% \text{ body fat})$$

The within subject coefficient of variation of measures taken on the same day was 0.2 % for all parameters.

The average and standard deviation (SD) were calculated in forwards (FW) and backs (BK) and in positional subgroups (Deutsch, 2007). Groups were compared using un-paired *t*-test followed by Bonferroni correction and the significant level was set at < 0.05.

## 3. RESULTS

Athletes were 26±5 years old, with a rather homogeneous playing experience (16±5 years). Forwards (FW) were significantly heavier (108±8 vs 91±6 kg), taller (190±7 vs 183±5 cm), had a larger % body fat (16±4 vs 11±4%) and fat free mass (91±5 vs 80±6 kg) compared to backs (BK).

Significant differences in all the measured parameters were detected among FW subgroups (Table 1) yet not between BK subgroups (Table 2).

**Table 1** Antropometric characteristics of forwards (FW) subgroups.
*, ° and § indicate, respectively, a significant difference *vs* props, hookers and locks.

| Group | FW | | | |
|---|---|---|---|---|
| Role | Props (#18) | Hooker (#6) | Locks (#14) | 3rd row (#22) |
| Age (yrs) | 27±5 | 26±3 | 24±3 | 25±3 |
| Mass (kg) | 116±7 | 103±1* | 109±6*° | 103±6*°§ |
| Height (cm) | 185±3 | 181±1* | 197±2*° | 190±5*°§ |
| Body fat (%) | 20±3 | 17±2* | 17± 3* | 13±3*°§ |
| Fat Free Mass (kg) | 93±5 | 86±3* | 90±4 | 90±4*° |
| FFM/height (kg/m) | 50.3±2.5 | 47.4±1.5* | 45.6±2.4* | 47.1±1.9*°§ |

**Table 2** Anthropometric characteristics of backs (BK) subgroups.
BK subgroups are significantly different from FW yet no differences were detected among them.

| Group | BK | | |
|---|---|---|---|
| Role | Half scrum (#10) | Fly-half, centre (#30) | Wings, full back (#27) |
| Age (yrs) | 26±5 | 24±3 | 24±3 |
| Mass (kg) | 87±4 | 92±6 | 90±6 |
| Height (cm) | 178±3 | 183±5 | 185±5 |
| Body fat (%) | 12±3 | 11±4 | 11±3 |
| Fat Free Mass (kg) | 77±4 | 81± 5 | 80±6 |
| FFM/height (kg/m) | 43.2±2.0 | 44.5± 2.0 | 43.5±2.3 |

## 4. DISCUSSION

Our study provides a large and updated reference database for elite male rugby union players in the southern European region. In accordance with the literature, our data document significant role differences in anthropometric parameters between FW and BK and between FW subgroups and no differences within BK positional subgroups. This confirms the specificity in the physical requirements of rugby union in individual playing positions in senior males at the elite international level.

Furthermore, our data report very similar values in stature and lean body mass compared to the existing literature on southern (Duthie *et al.*, 2003 and 2006) and northern hemisphere (Scott, 2003). On the contrary, our players, specially the first and second row FW, appear to have a larger fat mass compared to previous work. Such difference may be due to the fact the rugby players in this study were selected mainly based on their playing performance in a country where rugby is a minor sport and the physical characteristics required to play in first and second row are present in a very limited fraction of the population (>90° percentile).

In conclusion, our study provides updated anthropometric data for elite professional rugby union players. This reference database can assist talent selection, addressing individual athletes to the role for which they are more gifted and guide individualized training to match the demands of the game. Furthermore, periodic monitoring of a variety of playing populations is necessary to quantify and compare the evolving demands of the game.

### References

Deutsch, M.U. *et al.*, 2007, Time-motion analysis of professional rugby union players during match-play. *J Sports Sci*, **25**, 461–472.

Duthie, G. *et al.*, 2003, Applied physiology and game analysis of rugby union. *Sports Med*, **33**, 973–991.

Duthie, G. *et al.*, 2005, Time motion analysis of 2001 and 2002 super 12 rugby. *J Sports Sci*, **23**, 523–530.

Duthie, G.M. *et al.*, 2006, Anthropometry profiles of elite rugby players: quantifying changes in lean mass. *Br J Sports Med*, **40**, 202–207.

Golding, L. *et al.*, 1982, *The Y's Way to Physical Fitness*. Rosemont, IL: National Board of the YMCA.

Scott, A.C. *et al.*, 2003, Aerobic exercise physiology in a professional rugby union team. *Int J Cardiol*, **87**, 173–177.

# CHAPTER FORTY-EIGHT

# Effects of sex, game format, and skill type on ball possession in Norwegian youth soccer

A. Tenga[1], L. T. Ronglan[2] and E. Sigmundstad[1]

[1]Department of Coaching and Psychology, Norwegian School
of Sport Sciences, Oslo, Norway
[2]Research Centre for Training and Performance, Norwegian School
of Sport Sciences, Oslo, Norway.

## 1. INTRODUCTION

Small-sided games are commonly used as a training strategy as well as a competition form in children and youth soccer. The benefits of the game-centered approach which include promoting players' game understanding (McMorris, 1998), ability to make good choices in different game situations (Alexander and Penny, 2005), and development of relational skills (McPhail *et al.*, 2008) have been well documented in the literature.

However, a full benefit naturally presupposes a modification in games to match players' experience and skill level in order to create optimal learning environment with both meaningful successes as well as realistic challenges (Ronglan, 2008). Hill-Haas *et al.* (2011) reported that small-sided games may facilitate the development of technical and tactical awareness within the appropriate context of a game, but its realization depends on game design. Therefore, the knowledge obtained from the comparative analyses between match performances in different game formats is considered useful for enhancing more skill learning and development for youth players (Griffin and Butler, 2005). In addition, factors such as sex and skill type are thought to have influence on the performance also in youth soccer. Sex differences in game-related statistics have been reported earlier in basketball (Sampaio *et al.*, 2004) and in volleyball (Joao *et al.*, 2010). These differences in game performance were attributed to anthropometric and physiological differences between women and men.

The aim of this study is to assess the influence of sex, game format, and skill factors on retaining ball possession and on stopping opponent's ball possession in Norwegian youth soccer.

## 2. METHODS

Boys and girls soccer teams with 13 years old players from Norwegian amateur soccer clubs participated in this study. Five 35-minute matches were organized in seven a side (two matches; one for each sex) and eleven a side (three matches; two for girls and one for boys) and video-recorded for post event analysis. A total of 2130 (1813 offensive and 317 defensive) ball involvements from these matches were registered and analyzed.

A ball involvement was used as a basic unit of analysis. It was defined as a deliberate offensive action on the ball by a player from the attacking team (offensive ball involvement) and a deliberate defensive action on the ball or in the vicinity of the ball by a player from the defending team (defensive ball involvement), assessed qualitatively based on the player's intention in the specific match situation.

Four categorical variables were analyzed. These included two independent variables (offensive skill and defensive skill) and two dependent variables (offensive outcome and defensive outcome). Offensive skill *dribbling*, including running with the ball in 1vs.1 situations, was operationally defined as advancing past opponent player(s) in the direction towards the opponent's goal while maintaining control over the ball. Offensive skill *running with the ball* included all runs with the ball that do not involve 1vs.1 situations. The kappa correlation coefficient values ($\kappa$) for inter-observer reliability (Altman, 1991) for the four categorical variables used ranged between $\kappa=0.84$ to $\kappa=0.95$.

The association between the independent variables and the dependent variables were tested first by chi-square analysis and then by univariate and multivariate logistic regression analyses in which the dependent variable was whether a ball possession was retained or not, and whether an opponent's ball possession was stopped or not. An alpha value of $< 0.05$ was used.

## 3. RESULTS AND DISCUSSION

More ball involvements per outfield player were registered in 7vs.7 (mean=37.8; range=19-60) game format compared to 11vs.11 (mean=22.3; range=5-54). Further, in 11vs.11, both sex groups showed a reduction in ball involvements and an increase in variation in the number of ball involvements per outfield player. However, boys (mean=47 in 7vs.7; mean=24.1 in 11vs.11) showed a larger reduction in mean ball involvements compared to girls (mean=28.6 in 7vs.7; mean=21.4 in 11vs.11). The results also showed girls (range=19-42 in 7vs.7; range=5-45 in 11vs.11) had a larger increase in variation of number of ball involvements compared to boys (range=37-60 in 7vs.7; range=12-54 in 11vs.11).

Differences were observed between proportions of retained and lost ball possessions. The proportion of retained ball possessions for boys (57.7%) was higher than for girls (42.3%), while for the lost ball possessions the proportion for girls (63.4%) was higher than for boys (36.6%) (Table 1), irrespective of game format. There were differences (P<0.001) in the probability of retaining ball possession between categories in all three factors (Table 1). For example, the proportion of ball possessions retained when passing the ball (54.9%) was higher than when dribbling (16.5%) or receiving (10.6%) or when running with the ball (10.0%). Similarly, differences were also observed between proportions of stopped and unstopped opponent's ball possessions. The proportion of stopped ball possessions for girls (59.0%) was higher than for boys (41.0%), while for the unstopped opponent's ball possessions the proportion for boys (51.6%) was higher than for girls (48.4%) (Table 2), irrespective of game format. Similar probability results with differences for the factors of game format (P=0.004) and defensive skill (P<0.001) and a strong tendency for the factor of sex (P=0.06) were registered for stopping opponent's ball possession (Table 2). For example, tight pressure with tackling (83.8%) was clearly more successful in stopping opponent's ball possessions than either tight pressure without tackling (39.1%) or loose pressure (30.0%).

No differences in the odds ratio (OR) for retaining a ball possession were found between univariate and multivariate analyses. There were differences in the odds ratio from multivariate analyses for retaining a ball possession between categories for all three factors. For offensive skill, higher odds ratio was registered when passing the ball compared with when running with the ball, while no differences were found between dribbling or receiving and running with the ball (Table 3). There was a difference in odds ratio (OR) for stopping an opponent's ball possession between univariate and multivariate analyses. Girls registered a higher odds ratio than boys in multivariate analysis (OR=2.87; 95% confidence interval: 1.64 to 5.01; P<0.001) but not in univariate analysis (OR=1.53; 95% confidence interval: 0.98 to 2.39; P=0.06) (Table 4). There were differences in the odds ratio from multivariate analyses for stopping an opponent's ball possession between categories for all three factors. For defensive skill, higher odds ratio was registered when employing tight pressure with tackling compared with loose pressure (> 2 m), while no differences were found between tight pressure without tackling and loose pressure (> 2 m) (Table 4).

The multivariate analyses results for sex reflect observed difference in the flow of match play, with girls' matches having more shifts of ball possession between the two opposing teams. Further, the 7vs.7 game format produced higher odds ratios for favorable performances on ball possession, both offensively and defensively, compared with 11vs.11. For skills, the results show that running with the ball, receiving, and dribbling were the least effective skills on retaining ball possession, while loose pressure and tight pressure without tackling were the least effective skills on stopping opponent's ball possession.

**Table 1** Number of retained (n=847) and lost (n=966) ball possessions and percentage of retained ball possessions by different categories according to sex, game format, and offensive skill (N=1813).

| Variable | N (%) | Possession retained | Possession lost | Possession retained % | P |
|---|---|---|---|---|---|
| **Sex** | | | | | <0.001* |
| Boys | 843 (46.5) | 489 | 354 | 58.0 | |
| Girls | 970 (53.5) | 358 | 612 | 36.9 | |
| **Game format** | | | | | <0.001* |
| 7 vs. 7 | 716 (39.5) | 373 | 343 | 52.1 | |
| 11 vs. 11 | 1097 (60.5) | 474 | 623 | 43.2 | |
| **Offensive skill** | | | | | <0.001** |
| Dribbling | 79 (4.4) | 13 | 66 | 16.5 | |
| Passing | 1461 (81.8) | 802 | 659 | 54.9 | |
| Receiving | 216 (12.1) | 23 | 193 | 10.6 | |
| Running with the ball | 30 (1.7) | 3 | 27 | 10.0 | |

*Fisher's Exact Test.          **Pearson Chi-square.

**Table 2** Number of stopped (n=156) and unstopped (n=161) opponent's ball possessions and percentage of stopped opponent's ball possessions by different categories according to sex, game format, and defensive skill (N=317).

| Variable | N (%) | Possession stopped | Possession unstopped | Possession stopped (%) | P |
|---|---|---|---|---|---|
| **Sex** | | | | | 0.06 |
| Girls | 170 (53.6) | 92 | 78 | 54.1 | |
| Boys | 147 (46.4) | 64 | 83 | 43.5 | |
| **Game format** | | | | | 0.004* |
| 7 vs. 7 | 127 (40.1) | 75 | 52 | 59.1 | |
| 11 vs. 11 | 190 (59.9) | 81 | 109 | 42.6 | |
| **Defensive skill** | | | | | <0.001** |
| Tight pressure (within 2m) | 230 (73.2) | 90 | 140 | 39.1 | |
| Tight pressure + tackling | 74 (23.6) | 62 | 12 | 83.8 | |
| Loose pressure (> 2m) | 10 (3.2) | 3 | 7 | 30.0 | |

* Fisher's Exact Test.          **Pearson Chi-square.

**Table 3** Odds ratio (OR) for retaining a ball possession by different categories according to sex, game format, and offensive skill.

| Variable | Univariate analysis | | Multivariate analysis | |
|---|---|---|---|---|
| | OR (95% CI) | P | OR (95% CI) | P |
| **Sex** | | | | |
| Boys | 2.36 (1.96-2.85) | <0.001 | 2.20 (1.79-2.71) | <0.001 |
| Girls[a] | 1 | | 1 | |
| **Game format** | | | | |
| 7 vs. 7 | 1.43 (1.18-1.73) | <0.001 | 1.24 (1.00-1.53) | 0.049 |
| 11 vs. 11[a] | 1 | | 1 | |
| **Offensive skill** | | | | |
| Dribbling | 1.77 (0.47-6.72) | 0.40 | 1.68 (0.44-6.47) | 0.45 |
| Passing | 10.95 (3.31-36.27) | <0.001 | 10.62 (3.18-35.51) | <0.001 |
| Receiving | 1.07 (0.30-3.81) | 0.91 | 1.05 (0.29-3.76) | 0.95 |
| Running with the ball[a] | 1 | | 1 | |

Note: The odds ratio (OR) reflects the chance of retaining ball possession, compared with the reference category[a].

**Table 4** Odds ratio (OR) for stopping an opponent's ball possession by different categories according to sex, game format, and defensive skill.

| Variable | Univariate analysis | | Multivariate analysis | |
|---|---|---|---|---|
| | OR (95% CI) | P | OR (95% CI) | P |
| **Sex** | | | | |
| Girls | 1.53 (0.98-2.39) | 0.06 | 2.87 (1.64-5.01) | <0.001 |
| Boys[a] | 1 | | 1 | |
| **Game format** | | | | |
| 7 vs. 7 | 1.94 (1.23-3.06) | 0.004 | 1.76 (1.01-3.09) | 0.048 |
| 11 vs. 11[a] | 1 | | 1 | |
| **Defensive skill** | | | | |
| Tight pressure (within 2 m) | 1.50 (0.38-5.95) | 0.56 | 1.86 (0.43-8.06) | 0.41 |
| Tight pressure + tackling | 12.06 (2.73-53.34) | 0.001 | 17.19 (3.52-83.96) | <0.001 |
| Loose pressure (> 2 m)[a] | 1 | | 1 | |

Note: The odds ratio (OR) reflects the chance of stopping an opponent's ball possession, compared with the reference category[a].

## 4. CONCLUSION

The 7vs.7 game format incorporated more ball involvements compared with 11vs.11. All three factors had an effect on ball possession; with sex and skill type appearing to be the strongest. In specific, boys appeared to be more successful in retaining ball possession than girls, while girls were more successful in stopping opponent's ball possession than boys. Compared to 11vs.11, 7vs.7 seems to be a more favorable game format to enhance skill development for 13-years old players of both sexes. *Passing* skill was the most effective skill for retaining ball possession, while *tight pressure with tackling* was the most effective skill for stopping opponent's ball possession.

## References

Alexander, K. and Penny, D., 2005, Teaching under the influence: Feeding games for understanding into the sport education development-refinement cycle, *Phys Educ Sport Pedagogy*, **10**, 287–301.

Altman, D.G., 1991, Some common problems in medical research. In *Practical Statistics for Medical Research*, London: Chapman & Hall, pp. 403–409.

Joao, P.V. *et al.*, 2010, Sex differences in discriminative power of volleyball game-related statistics. *Percep Motor Skills*, **111**, 893–900.

Griffin, L.L. and Butler, J.L., 2005, *Teaching Games for Understanding: Theory, Research and Practice*, Champaign, IL: Human Kinetics.

Hill-Haas, S.V. *et al.*, 2011, Physiology of small-sided games training in football: A systematic review, *Sports Med*, **41**, 199–220.

McMorris, T., 1998, Teaching games for understanding: I's contribution to the knowledge of skill acquisition from a motor learning perspective, *European J Phys Educ*, **3**, 65–74.

McPhail, A. *et al.*, 2008, Throwing and catching as relational skills in game play: Situated learning in a modified game unit. *J Teach Phys Educ*, **27**, 100–115.

Ronglan, L.T., 2008, *Lagspill, læring og ledelse: Om lagspillenes didaktikk,* Oslo: Akilles Forlag.

Sampaio, J. *et al.*, 2004, Discriminative power of basketball game-related statistics by level of competition and sex. *Percep Motor Skills*, **32**, 1231–1238.

# CHAPTER FORTY-NINE

# Adapting the competition model in youth football: a comparison between 5-a-side and 7-a-side football with U10-players

J. Castellano and I. Echeazarra

University of the Basque Country (UPV-EHU), Spain

## 1. INTRODUCTION

Association football, similar to other sports, has been modified to make sport practice easier for children and youngsters. Some authors (Lapresa *et al.*, 2010) give relevance to the structural adaptation of training by changing the size of the field of play, the amount of players, the duration of the match and by varying the interaction between the space and the players.

Modification of the playing rules changes the *internal logic* of the game (Parlebas, 2001) and the behavior of players. Therefore, it is important to evaluate how these changes influence the game. The aim is to find the rules that generate best behaviors in order to advance sport learning.

A specifically *ad hoc* observation tool, designed according to the framework of the observational methodology (Anguera, 1990), was used to evaluate the *playing action* (Parlebas, 2001) of these football modalities. Assuming the fact that football is a *collaboration-opposition game*, the designed tool was used to search motor responses and strategic behaviors of interaction between players in the real context (place and time) where it takes place. Data quality was analyzed to validate the reliability of the data, in order to validate the reliability of the designed taxonomical system.

The designed observation tool was used to compare 5-a-side football and 7-a-side football for youth players whose ages are under 10 years old (U10). The aim of the current study was to determine the effects that these two competition models present in young football players' ways of playing.

## 2. METHODS

### 2.1. Sample

Football players from three top football clubs, with an age between 9 and 10 years old, participated in the study (n=36). Six matches of both 5-a-side football and 7-a-side football were recorded. In Table 1, 5- and 7-a-side football playing rules such as pitch dimensions, ball size, number of players, duration of the match and offside are specified.

**Table 1** 5- and 7-a-side football playing rules.

|  | **5-a-side football** | **7-a-side football** |
|---|---|---|
| Pitch dimensions | 50x28 m | 60x35 m |
| Ball size | Size 4 | Size 4 |
| Number of players | 4 vs. 4 plus goalkeepers | 6 vs. 6 plus goalkeepers |
| Duration of the match | 25 minutes | 25 minutes |
| Offside | None | Yes (12 m from the target) |

### 2.2. Taxonomic system

Similar to other studies (Casamichana and Castellano, 2010; Gabbett and Mulvey, 2008; Kelly and Drust, 2009; Mallo and Navarro, 2008; Tessitore *et al.*, 2006), an *ad hoc* observation tool was used to observe, analyze and evaluate players' behaviors. Our taxonomic system was developed combining *category systems* and *field formats* (Anguera, 1990). That implies putting the different categories into groups (macrocategories or criteria). The unit of observation was the player's individual ball possession (Psotta and Bunc, 2009). The taxonomic system was performed under five criteria: how the ball possession starts (14 levels), where the ball possession starts and finishes (8 levels each zone), who has the ball possession (12 levels), how many contacts with the ball are done per player (8 levels) and how players finish the individual ball possession (6 levels). The criteria and levels are shown in Table 2.

### 2.3. Software

The *Measuring and Observation Tool in Sport* (MOTS) software (Castellano *et al.*, 2008) was used to observe code and register players' behaviors.

### 2.4. Analysis of the quality of data

One match codified twice was used to estimate the data reliability. The estimated values for within-observer reliability (*Cohen's kappa*) may be considered as optimum, since *kappa* was above 0.9 for each criterion and 0.95 for the session as a whole.

## 2.5. Statistical analysis

Firstly, a Levene's test was performed to analyze the homogeneity of variances. This property was confirmed (p>0.05). The normality of variables was tested by a Shapiro-Wilk test for all the studied categories. Except for penalty (PLTY), zones 2 and 8 (Z2, Z8) and from 5 to 8 ball touches (T5, T6, T7 and T8,) this property was confirmed for all the categories. Therefore, goalkeeper (POR) PLTY, Z2 and Z8 categories were excluded from the analysis. About contact balls, T5, T6, T7 and T8 categories, the normality was not achieved. Therefore, they were grouped into only one variable and were recoded as T5+ (5 or more than 5 ball touches). The normality of the rest of the variables was confirmed.

Secondly, once six matches were registered (three to 5-a-side football and three to 7-a-side football), the variance components and the accuracy of generalizations were analyzed by means of a design comprizing three facets: model (M), criterion (C) an category (K) [M*C*(K:C)], where the category facet was nested to the criterion category (K:C). Generalizability Theory (GT) can be used, for any type of measurement, to separate the real variability from the error variability. A common characteristic in the Observational Methodology is the fact that behaviors can only be partly observed. Because of this fact, it becomes necessary to investigate if the observed variance is related with the individuals, the measuring tools, the place or other facets. A Generalized Lineal Model (type III data) was performed to obtaining the results, as the data were not taken randomly (Table 2). A generalizability analysis was also conducted to assess the variability of each facet and their interactions (percentage of variance). Furthermore, the analysis was configured for the K(C)/M measurement method, and relative and absolute generalizability coefficients were determined.

Finally, a Student's t-test test for independent samples was used to compare the results of the two competition models (2 levels). Significance level was set at *p<0.05*.

## 3. RESULTS AND DISCUSSION

Table 2 shows the coefficients of determination ($r^2$) were almost 1 and this indicates that the chosen facets explain almost all the variability of the models. That gives an explanation about the variability of the model, where the combination of the selected facets is the responsible of that variability. It is noteworthy to mention that the used model is significant in its whole, and also in all the facets and the interactions between them (level of significance *Pr>F=<.001*).

In respect of the variability observed in each facet and their interactions, we can observe that the criterion facet and its linked category contributed to most of the observed variability. On the other hand, the model facet explained just 3% of the variance explained. That means that there is no significant difference between the two competition systems compared. Just a very few of the total variability could not be explained through the three facets considered in the study, as the residual value was less than 1%.

**Table 2** Type III variance component analysis in the three facet model M*C*(K:C) [*Model*Criterion*(Category:Criterion)*] for the set of the six matches.

|  | Df | SC type III | Pr > F | % |
|---|---|---|---|---|
| Model (competition model) [M] | 1 | 1470.1 | <.0001 | 3.3 |
| Criterion [C] | 5 | 51580.1 | <.0001 | 74.6 |
| Model*Criterion | 5 | 570.8 | <.0001 | 1.7 |
| Category(Criterion) [K] | 35 | 16064.5 | <.0001 | 20.0 |
| Model*Category(Criterion) | 35 | 164.5 | 0.0007 | 0.4 |
| $r^2 = 0.985$ | | Pr > F = <.001 | | |
| Measure plan = K(C)/M | | e2= 0.99 | $\Phi = 0.97$ | |

*Note.* $r^2$ is the coefficient of determination, Df are the liberty degrees, SC type III is the sum of squares for type III data, Pr > F is the level of significance and the variability % of each facet and their interactions, $e^2$ is the relative coefficient and $\Phi$ represents the absolute coefficient generalizability.

Finally, Table 3 shows means and standard deviation for the different categories. Significant differences were observed only for 8 of the 58 categories studied: POR INT, Z1, Z6, J1, J2, J4 and T1 (level of significance $p<0.05$).

## 4. CONCLUSION

There were less than 5% of differences for the analyzed categories between 5 and 7-a-side football. Likewise, the model of competition explained 3% of the variance only. These results suggest that both football modalities demand similar technical and tactical football skills for U10 children.

In spite of the essential similarity, slight differences were found between the 5-a-side and the 7-a-side football competition models. Therefore, we could conclude that: 1) the goalkeeper participates more in the 5-a-side model, it means that teams end more times the attacks; 2) the players touch the ball more times in the 5a-side model; and 3) individual ball possessions with only one touch (including here the interception of the ball) were higher in 5-a-side football compared to 7-a-side football modality.

### Acknowledgements

We gratefully acknowledge the support of the Álava Football Federation and Álava Provincial County in the project 'Formando en el fútbol de formación'.

**Table 3** Means and ±SD (Standard Deviation) for the observed motor behaviors of the players in the different football models.

| Criterion | Categories | Description | Competition Model | | | |
|---|---|---|---|---|---|---|
| | | | F5 | | F7 | |
| | | | Mean | ±SD | Mean | ±SD |
| Starting | REC | regain possession of the ball | 68 | 10 | 58 | 10 |
| | CON | continue possession | 172 | 17 | 191 | 19 |
| | **POR*** | **goalkeeper with hands** | **14** | **2** | **10** | **1** |
| | TRE | take the ball after an INT | 27 | 6 | 26 | 3 |
| | **INT*** | **intercept the ball** | **50** | **3** | **41** | **2** |
| | SdP | goal kick | 10 | 2 | 6 | 2 |
| | SdC | kick off | 5 | 3 | 6 | 2 |
| | SdBm | throw in | 27 | 6 | 21 | 6 |
| | CORNp | corner kick | 5 | 2 | 4 | 2 |
| | FAL | free kick | 2 | 3 | 5 | 2 |
| | PLTY | penalty kick | 0 | 1 | 0 | 1 |
| Zone | **Z1*** | **right defensive zone** | **64** | **5** | **46** | **10** |
| | Z2 | left defensive zone | 42 | 10 | 39 | 9 |
| | Z3 | right defensive-medium zone | 59 | 13 | 64 | 15 |
| | Z4 | left defensive-medium zone | 53 | 11 | 60 | 15 |
| | Z5 | right medium-ofensive-zone | 55 | 5 | 49 | 7 |
| | **Z6*** | **left medium-ofensive zone** | **59** | **2** | **76** | **2** |
| | Z7 | right offensive zone | 20 | 4 | 14 | 3 |
| | Z8 | left offensive zone | 30 | 4 | 21 | 8 |
| Player | **J1*** | **goalkeeper** | **58** | **6** | **30** | **2** |
| | **J2*** | **defender** | **83** | **11** | **64** | **3** |
| | J3 | right midfielder | 91 | 21 | 71 | 15 |
| | **J4*** | **left midfielder** | **79** | **9** | **44** | **8** |
| | J5 | forward | 69 | 8 | 59 | 1 |
| Ball touches | **T1*** | **one touch** | **240** | **11** | **213** | **6** |
| | T2 | two touches | 66 | 22 | 76 | 8 |
| | T3 | three touches | 37 | 8 | 45 | 12 |
| | T4 | four touches | 21 | 7 | 21 | 9 |
| | T5+ | five and more touches | 33 | 11 | 21 | 5 |
| Finalization | PAS | pass | 170 | 14 | 190 | 20 |
| | TIRO | shoot | 27 | 4 | 12 | 8 |
| | PER | loss of the ball | 70 | 8 | 66 | 14 |
| | GOLP | kick the ball | 31 | 4 | 26 | 7 |
| | GOL | goal | 4 | 3 | 5 | 2 |
| | ROBO | steal the ball | 16 | 4 | 12 | 3 |

Note: * Significant difference: $p < 0.05$.

## References

Anguera, M.T., 1990, Metodología observacional, In *Metodología de la investigación en ciencias del comportamiento*, Murcia: Universidad de Murcia, pp. 125–236.

Casamichana, D. and Castellano, J., 2010, Time–motion, heart rate, perceptual and motor behaviour demands in small-sides soccer games: Effects of pitch size. *J Sports Sci*, **28**, 1615–1623.

Castellano, J. *et al.*, 2007, Optimising a probabilistic model of the development of play in soccer. *Quality and Quantity*, **41**, 93–104.

Gabbett, T.J. and Mulvey, M.J., 2008, Time-motion analysis of small-sided training games and competition in elite women soccer players. *J Strength Cond Res*, **22**, 543–552.

Jonsson, G.K. *et al.*, 2006, Hidden patterns of play interaction in football using SOFT-CODER. *Behavior Research Methods Instruments and Computers*, **38**, 372–381.

Kelly, D. and Drust, B., 2009, The effect of pitch dimensions on heart rate responses and technical demands of small-sided soccer games in elite players. *J Sci Med Sport*, **12**, 475–479.

Lapresa, D. *et al.*, 2010, Adaptando la competición en la iniciación al fútbol: Estudio comparativo de las modalidades de fútbol 3 y fútbol 5 en categoría prebenjamín. *Apunts, Educación Física y Deportes*, **101**, 43–56.

Mallo, J. and Navarro, E., 2008, Physical load imposed on soccer players during small-sided training games. *J Sports Med Phys Fitness*, **48**, 166–171.

Parlebas, P., 2001, *Juegos, deporte y sociedad. Léxico de praxiología motriz*. Barcelona: Paidotribo.

Psotta, R. and Bunc, V., 2009, Heart rate response and game-related activity of younger school-age boys in different formats of soccer game. *Science, Movement and Health*, **9**, 69–73.

Tessitore, A. *et al.*, 2006, Physiological and technical aspects of '6-a-side' soccer drills. *J Sports Med Phys Fitness*, **46**, 36–43.

# CHAPTER FIFTY

# The relationships between change of direction speed, sprint speed and jump ability in collegiate soccer players

S. Sasaki[1], Y. Nagano[2], T. Sakurai[1] and T. Fukubayashi[3]

[1]Tokyo Ariake University of Medical and Health Sciences, Tokyo, Japan
[2]Niigata University of Health and Welfare, Niigata, Japan
[3]Waseda University, Saitama, Japan

## 1. INTRODUCTION

Changes of direction are required in all football games, e.g., Soccer, Rugby Football and American Football. Some researchers have stated that the ability to change direction while sprinting is a determinant of field sports performance (Sheppard and Young, 2006) or a prerequisite for successful participation in modern-day field sports (Brughelli et al., 2008). Moreover, the ability to change direction is a key factor in developing elite soccer players as it is the strongest predictor for talent identification (Reilly et al., 2000).

Some factors have been proposed as being related to the ability to change direction (Young et al., 2002). Sheppard and Young (2006) have described factors that are considered important in determining changes in direction ability, which include straight sprint speed and leg muscle qualities. Some researchers have reported on the relationship between an agility test and sprint or jump test. However, such previous research has failed to examine which combinations of sprint speed and jump ability can predict differences in change of direction speed. Thus, the purpose of this study was to investigate the relationships between various change of direction speeds, straight sprint speeds and vertical jump heights in Japanese collegiate soccer players.

## 2. METHODS

### Subjects

One hundred and seventy-five male collegiate soccer players participated in this study (Table 1). All participants were free of lower extremity pain, a history of serious injury or operative treatment, or subjective symptoms which could interfere with sports activities. The study was approved by the Faculty of Sport Sciences Ethics Committee, Waseda University. All subjects and, if necessary, their parents, received an explanation of all experimental procedures, and informed consent was obtained before the testing began. The investigations were conducted in accordance with the Declaration of Helsinki.

**Table 1** Physical characteristics (mean ± SD).

| total | 2005–2010 (n = 175) | | |
|---|---|---|---|
| year | 2005–2006 | 2007–2008 | 2009–2010 |
| (number of subjects) | (n = 103) | (n = 96) | (n = 88) |
| age (yrs) | 20.4 ± 1.3 | 20.9 ± 1.2 | 20.5 ± 1.2 |
| height (m) | 1.74 ± 0.05 | 1.75 ± 0.06 | 1.75 ± 0.06 |
| weight (kg) | 67.4 ± 5.9 | 68.2 ± 6.2 | 67.5 ± 5.8 |

## Procedures

Following a standardized warm-up, subjects were required to perform the agility test, the sprint test and the jump test on an artificial turf pitch. They were allowed to perform several preparatory trials so as to understand the appropriate technique. All tests were performed duplicate; with at least 2 min or more rest provided between all efforts. The best score was used for statistical analysis

Straight sprint performance was evaluated using a 20m sprint test. Infrared timing gates (Brower timing gate, USA) were positioned at the start line and at 5m, 10m, and 20m at height of approximately 1m. Flying 10m sprint time was defined as the section time between the 10m and 20m marks in a 20m sprint test. The participants were instructed to run at maximum speed through the final pair of sensors. Timing started when the laser of the starting gate was broken.

Jump ability was evaluated using vertical jump (VJ) test with backward and forward arm swing, which was used to measure leg muscle power (Everett and John, 2008). A digital vertical jump meter (Jump MD, Japan) was used in this test. A measuring tape was fastened to the abdomen of the participant and a string was tied from the measuring tape to the center of the jumping board. The participant then jumped as high as possible. Jumping performance was recorded as the distance between standing and jumping heights determined from the tape measure. This method was used in some previous studies (Clark *et al.*, 2011; Tsimeas *et al.*, 2005).

Change of direction speed was evaluated using three types of agility test (Figure 1). The pro-agility test was conducted in 2005–2006, which consisted of a 5m sprint, 10m sprint, and two direction changes of 180 degrees. A 10m agility shuttle test was conducted in 2007–2008, which consisted of a 10m sprint and one 180 degrees direction change. A zigzag agility test was conducted in 2009–2010, which consisted of a 5m sprint and three direction changes of 90 degrees. For all agility tests, timing gates were placed at the start and finish lines. If the subjects slipped during a direction change, the trials were excluded.

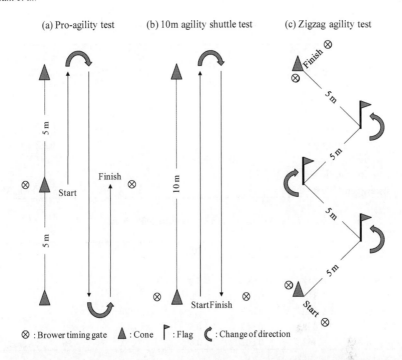

**Figure 1** Diagram of the agility tests. Reproduced from Sasaki *et al.*, 2011, with permission.

## Statistical analysis

All the data is expressed as mean ± standard deviation. Pearson product-moment correlation coefficients were calculated and used to determine the relationships among performance variables for each two years. In addition, variable screening was performed using stepwise multiple regression analysis for each of the three agility tests. All statistical procedures were performed using SPSS software (ver. 14.0 for Windows), and the statistical significance of all tests was set at $p < 0.05$.

## 3. RESULTS

Descriptive and performance characteristics are presented in Table 2. Tables 3, 4 and 5 display the Pearson product-moment correlation coefficients for each two years. The performance on all sprint speeds, counter-movement jumps and agility tests were correlated to a statistical significance ($p < 0.05$). With each agility test as the response variable, a significant relationship was found to exist among two of the five variables (Tables 6, 7 and 8). The obtained regression equations were: Pro-agility test (sec) = $0.805 \times 10\text{m sprint} - 0.006 \times \text{VJ} + 4.099$ ($R^2 = 0.280$, $p < 0.01$); 10m agility shuttle test (sec) = $0.331 \times 20\text{m sprint} - 0.007 \times \text{VJ} + 3.544$ ($R^2 = 0.222$, $p < 0.01$); Zigzag agility test (sec) = $1.405 \times \text{flying 10m sprint} + 0.668 \times 5\text{m sprint} + 3.144$ ($R^2 = 0.283$, $p < 0.01$).

**Table 2** Descriptive and performance characteristics (mean ± SD).

| year (number of subjects) | 2005-2006 (n = 103) | 2007-2008 (n = 96) | 2009-2010 (n = 88) |
|---|---|---|---|
| 5m sprint (sec) | 0.98 ± 0.06 | 1.01 ± 0.06 | 1.06 ± 0.08 |
| 10m sprint (sec) | 1.71 ± 0.07 | 1.75 ± 0.09 | 1.79 ± 0.09 |
| 20m sprint (sec) | 2.98 ± 0.11 | 3.04 ± 0.12 | 3.07 ± 0.14 |
| Flying 10m sprint (sec) | 1.27 ± 0.05 | 1.28 ± 0.05 | 1.28 ± 0.06 |
| Vertical jump (cm) | 60.8 ± 5.3 | 62.9 ± 5.1 | 62.2 ± 6.3 |
| Pro-agility test (sec) | 5.08 ± 0.15 | - | - |
| 10m agility shuttle test (sec) | - | 4.12 ± 0.13 | - |
| Zigzag agility test (sec) | - | - | 5.65 ± 0.23 |

**Table 3** Correlation coefficients in 2005–2006.

| | 5m | 10m | 20m | Flying 10m | VJ | Pro-agility |
|---|---|---|---|---|---|---|
| 5m | 1.000 | | | | | |
| 10m | 0.847 | 1.000 | | | | |
| 20m | 0.842 | 0.943 | 1.000 | | | |
| Flying 10m | 0.680 | 0.693 | 0.894 | 1.000 | | |
| VJ | −0.458 | −0.522 | −0.514 | −0.411 | 1.000 | |
| Pro-agility | 0.463 | 0.502 | 0.499 | 0.403 | −0.436 | 1.000 |

* All correlations are significant ($p < 0.05$)

**Table 4** Correlation coefficients in 2007–2008.

| | 5m | 10m | 20m | Flying 10m | VJ | 10m shuttle |
|---|---|---|---|---|---|---|
| 5m | 1.000 | | | | | |
| 10m | 0.873 | 1.000 | | | | |
| 20m | 0.864 | 0.927 | 1.000 | | | |
| Flying 10m | 0.484 | 0.401 | 0.715 | 1.000 | | |
| VJ | −0.207 | −0.312 | −0.360 | −0.298 | 1.000 | |
| 10m shuttle | 0.340 | 0.379 | 0.413 | 0.302 | −0.392 | 1.000 |

* All correlations are significant ($p < 0.05$)

**Table 5** Correlation coefficients in 2009–2010.

| | 5m | 10m | 20m | Flying 10m | VJ | Zigzag |
|---|---|---|---|---|---|---|
| 5m | 1.000 | | | | | |
| 10m | 0.928 | 1.000 | | | | |
| 20m | 0.884 | 0.943 | 1.000 | | | |
| Flying 10m | 0.608 | 0.631 | 0.854 | 1.000 | | |
| VJ | −0.345 | −0.358 | −0.459 | −0.508 | 1.000 | |
| Zigzag | 0.464 | 0.418 | 0.501 | 0.513 | −0.289 | 1.000 |

* All correlations are significant ($p < 0.05$)

**Table 6** Best model of pro-agility test.

|  | β-coefficients | p value |
|---|---|---|
| Intercept | 4.099 | |
| 10m sprint time | 0.805 | 0.001 |
| Vertical jump height | −0.006 | 0.017 |

**Table 7** Best model of 10m agility shuttle test.

|  | β-coefficients | p value |
|---|---|---|
| Intercept | 3.544 | |
| 20m sprint time | 0.331 | 0.002 |
| Vertical jump height | −0.007 | 0.005 |

**Table 8** Best model of zigzag agility test.

|  | β-coefficients | p value |
|---|---|---|
| Intercept | 3.144 | |
| Flying 10m sprint time | 1.405 | 0.002 |
| 5m sprint time | 0.668 | 0.038 |

## 4. DISCUSSION

The primary purpose of this study was to determine the relationships between various change of direction speeds, sprint speed and jump ability in collegiate soccer players. Sprint, jump and agility performances were all correlated with each other (Tables 3–5). These results were consistent with the previous study conducted by Vescovi and McGuigan (2008). Little and Williams (2005) suggested that acceleration, maximum speed and agility shared common physiological and biomechanical determinants. Therefore, it is considered that sprint speed and jump ability would be common attributes related to different change of direction speeds.

On the other hand, multiple regression analysis which combined different types of performances, succeeded in demonstrating significant predicting model for the pro-agility test, 10m agility shuttle test and zigzag agility test (Tables 6–8). These results suggest that specific physical factors would be necessary to influence change of direction speed. The character of an agility test is determined by a combination of the distance of sprint and the angles, or numbers of, direction change. A number of relevant agility tests and training protocols have been described by authors (Carling *et al.*, 2009; Everett and John, 2008; Sheppard and Young, 2006). Therefore, coaches in the field should select a suitable agility test or exercise for each sport and consider which attribute is important for each player or position. From this research, it would be suggested that side or middle position players who need middle to long sprint or leg muscle power should select a pro-agility test or 10m agility shuttle test, whilst attacking or offensive players who need short sprint or maximum speed should select zigzag agility tests. However, the participants in this study were all soccer players. Investigations of participants from other football codes would be necessary to determine how improvements in change of direction performance can be made in players of those sports.

The coefficients of determination in multiple regression analysis were at the low level between 0.222 and 0.283. A determining model of agility (Young *et al.*, 2002) was proposed using many factors, thus another some factors would relate to each change of direction performance in this study. In the future, it is our intention to consider the best model of various agility tests using some physical factors, such as sprint speed and muscle qualities, and kinematics data during change of direction from a technical aspect.

### References

Brughelli, M. *et al.*, 2008, Understanding change of direction ability in sport: A review of resistance training studies. *Sports Med*, **38**, 1045–1063.

Carling, C. *et al.*, 2009, Anaerobic and musculoskeletal performance. In *Performance Assessment for Field Sports*, 1st ed., Oxford, Routledge, pp. 133–169.

Clark, E.M. *et al.*, 2011, Children with low muscle strength are at an increased risk of fracture with exposure to exercise. *J Musc Neur Int*, **11**, 196–202.

Everett, H. and John, G., 2008, Administration, Scoring, and Interpretation of selected tests. In *Essentials of Strength Training and Conditioning*, Champaign, Human Kinetics, pp. 249–292.

Little, T. and Williams, A.G., 2005, Specificity of acceleration, maximum speed, and agility in professional soccer players. *J Strength Cond Res*, **19**, 76–78.

Reilly, T. *et al.*, 2000, A multidisciplinary approach to talent identification in soccer. *J Sports Sci*, **18**, 695–702.

Sasaki, S. *et al.*, 2011, The relationships between running with change of direction, straight sprint and counter-movement jump. *J Train Exerc Sport*, **23**, 143–144.

Sheppard, J.M. and Young, W.B., 2006, Agility literature review: Classification, training and testing. *J Sports Sci*, **24**, 919–932.

Tsimeas, P. *et al.*, 2005, Does living in urban or rural settings affect aspects of physical fitness in children? *Brit J Sport Med*, **39**, 671–674.

Vescovi, J.D. and McGuigan, M.R. 2008, Relationships between sprinting, agility, and jump ability in female athletes. *J Sports Sci*, **26**, 97–107.

Young, W.B. *et al.*, 2002, Is muscle power related to running speed with change direction? *J Sports Med Phys Fit*, **42**, 282–288.

# CHAPTER FIFTY-ONE

# Physical and technical differences between single-gender vs. mixed-gender small-sided training exercises for elite female soccer players

M. Tschopp[1, 2], R. Grand[1], K. Sonderegger[1] and B. von Siebenthal[2]

[1] Swiss Federal Institute of Sports Magglingen, Switzerland
[2] Swiss Football Association, Muri b. Bern, Switzerland

## 1. INTRODUCTION

Differences exist between male's and female's football (Kirkendall, 2007). For example, during match play, male players cover more distance in high intensity running than do women (Mohr *et al.*, 2008). It is assumed that male's football is also technically more advanced, although limited data support this assumption. In order to benefit from the higher physical and technical demands experienced by male athletes, women occasionally train with men. Yet, there is little evidence on what changes would occur when women train with men. Small-sided training games (SSG) have become popular in the recent years. SSG simulate the movement patterns of women's soccer competition (Gabbett and Mulvey, 2008). These games are equally effective at improving soccer specific endurance as interval training (Hill-Haas *et al.*, 2011). In addition, SSG also develop technical and tactical abilities. The present study aimed to evaluate the physical and technical-tactical differences between single-gender and mixed-gender training exercises for female elite soccer players.

## 2. METHOD

Eight female soccer players (age: 18.8±2.1 y; height: 1.68±0.04m; weight: 57.5±6.8kg; fitness level in Yo-Yo intermittent recovery test level 1:1436±320m), all members of a Swiss national team (U17, U19, and A-team, respectively), played a 6 vs. 6 SSG on two occasions: once with two all-female teams (SSG$_{fem}$) and once with two mixed-gender teams (SSG$_{mix}$) (one female player and five U16 boys, see Figure 1). All male players (age: 15.4±0.4 yrs) played at the highest national U16 level. The size of the field was 30x40m. After seven passes were completed, the team earned one point. The players engaged in two games, each lasting four minutes. The players had enough rest time between the games as the second game was not started before each player's individual lactate concentration was <2.5mmol/L (15-30 minutes pause). The mean of the two, four-minute games were determined for data analysis. During the game, heart rate (Polar Team[2] Pro) and distance covered (GPS Garmin Forerunner 305) were recorded. On the basis of the Yo-Yo intermittent recovery test level 1 (Bangsbo *et al.*, 2008) the mean of the individual % maximum heart rate ($\%HR_{max}$), between two and four minutes, was calculated. Immediately after each game, the rating of perceived exertion (RPE) (Borg, 1982) and lactate concentration (Arkray Lactate Pro LT-1710) were measured. Nine technical-tactical variables were measured using a video system and the results were compared between the two settings. The mean of the results of two video observers were used for data analysis. Technical error for inter-observer reliability was < 6.0%, except for the 'number of direct passes' variable (10.1%). The differences between the single- and mixed-gender games were determined using Student's paired t-test. The level of statistical significance was set at $p<0.05$. Cohen's effect sizes were calculated.

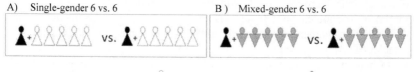

**Figure 1** Experimental setting. ⌾ Female player (black: subject); ⬇ U16 male player.

## 3. RESULTS

No significant differences were found in the physical parameters (Table 1). Lactate concentration and RPE tended to be higher in the $SSG_{mix}$. In the technical parameters, the biggest differences appeared in 'touches per ball possession', 'time in ball possession', and '% one-touch passes', which suggests higher technical demand in the $SSG_{mix}$ than in the $SSG_{fem}$. However, in the $SSG_{mix}$, fewer 'involvements with the ball', 'ball touches', and 'passes' also were recorded (Table 1 and Figure 2).

**Table 1** Differences in physical and technical performance between single- and mixed-gender 6 vs. 6 small-sided games (single: 6 ♀; mixed: 5♂+1♀). * Number or % per player. Values are mean±SD. † shows significant difference (p<0.05).

| Physical data | Single | Mixed |
|---|---|---|
| Distance (m) | 543.1±30.8 | 546.1±43.2 |
| %-H$_{rmax}$ | 92.1±1.9 | 91.8±2.8 |
| Lactate (mmol/l) | 4.6±1.1 | 5.4±1.8 |
| RPE | 13.1±1.7 | 13.6±0.9 |

| Technical data | Single | Mixed |
|---|---|---|
| Changes in team ball possession | 19.8±4.7 | 17.3±2.4 |
| Involvements with the ball* | 9.8±1.8 | 8.5±2.7 |
| Ball touches* | 20.9±7.4 | 15.1±6.2† |
| Touches per ball possession* | 2.2±0.4 | 1.7±0.3† |
| Mean time in ball possession (sec) | 1.2±0.4 | 0.9±0.4 |
| Passes* | 8.6±1.9 | 7.3±2.4† |
| One-touch passes* | 3.2±1.4 | 3.5±1.6 |
| % one-touch passes* | 36.2±16.3 | 47.2±18.7 |
| % successful passes* | 73.0±15.4 | 75.2±14.6 |

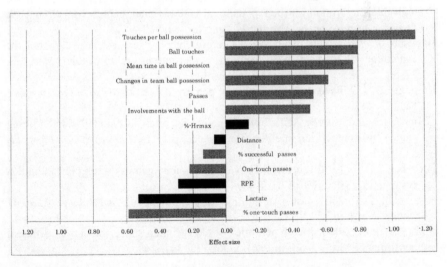

**Figure 2** Cohen's effect sizes for the differences between single- and mixed-gender 6 vs. 6 small-sided games (single: 6 ♀; mixed: 5♂+1♀). ■ Physical parameters, ■ Technical parameters. Positive effect sizes mean a higher value for single-gender, small-sided games.

## 4. DISCUSSION

Small-sided games are used as a means of improving skills and physical fitness in female players (Hill-Haas *et al.*, 2011). The present data suggest that, in a mixed-gender SSG, female players may benefit more from technical (skills proficiency) than from physical aspects. In the mixed-gender SSG group, the players had less time and touches per ball possession which allowed less time for ball control and decision-making. Interestingly, physical demands were only slightly higher in the mixed-gender SSG, although U16 male players have a notably higher fitness level than do female players of the same level in this study (unpublished data). However it can be assumed that physical demand could increase with increasing age or performance level of male players. This may be interesting for international female players as the physical demand in international games is higher in comparison to domestic league games (Andersson *et al.*, 2010). However, it should be cautioned when administering a mixed-gender SSG that skill acquisition of female players may be disturbed by lesser ball contact time compared to a single-gender SSG.

## References

Andersson, H.A. *et al.*, 2010, Elite female soccer players perform more high-intensity running when playing in international games compared with domestic league games. *J Strength Cond Res*, **24**, 912–919.

Bangsbo, J. *et al.*, 2008, The Yo-Yo intermittent recovery test: a useful tool for evaluation of physical performance in intermittent sports. *Sports Med*, **38**, 37–51.

Borg, GA., 1982, Psychophysical bases of perceived exertion. *Med Sci Sport Exerc*, **14**, 377–381.

Gabbett, T.J. and Mulvey, M.J., 2008, Time-motion analysis of small-sided training games and competition in elite women soccer players. *J Strength Cond Res*, **22**, 543–552.

Hill-Haas, S.V. *et al.*, 2011, Physiology of small-sided games training in football: A systematic review. *Sports Med*, **41**, 199–220.

Kirkendall, D.T., 2007, Issues in training the female player. *Brit J Sports Med*, **41** (Suppl I), i64–i67.

Mohr, M. *et al.*, 2008, Match activities of elite women soccer players at different performance levels. *J Strength Cond Res*, **22**, 341–349.

# Part VI

# Sports medicine

# CHAPTER FIFTY-TWO

# A prospective study of injuries sustained during a National Rugby League season

D. O'Connor

The University of Sydney, Sydney, Australia

## 1. INTRODUCTION

Rugby league is a collision sport with players involved in intermittent passages of play involving high intensity sprinting, passing, physical collisions and tackling, interspersed with low intensity walking and jogging throughout an 80 minute game period (Gabbett, 2005; O'Connor, 1996). Each team consists of 13 players on the field at any one time and four substitute players, with each team allowed 10 interchanges during the game. Rugby league has a high rate of injury. However, the majority of previously published papers report injuries from a small sample rather than all teams over an entire competition (Gibbs, 1993; Orchard, 2004; O'Connor, 2004). The aim of this study was to identify the incidence, site, nature and risk factors of injuries sustained by the three playing positional groups in the 2009 National Youth Competition (NYC) and National Rugby League (NRL) season.

## 2. METHOD

Sixteen clubs participating in the NRL and NYC competition were asked to prospectively collect data on the injuries sustained by their players during the 2009 season (26 rounds plus 'finals' matches). There were 459 players that participated in the NRL (first grade) and 559 players that participated in the NYC (Under 20 years) competition during the 2009 season. The injury definition used for this paper was: 'any injury that was sustained during a first grade NRL match (or NYC match) that resulted in missed match time'. Injury severity was classified as mild (0–1 missed games); moderate (2–4 missed games) or major (5 or more missed games) (Gibbs, 1993).

Players were categorised into three playing groups: outside backs (fullback, wing and centre); adjustables (five-eighth or stand-off, half-back and hooker; loose forward); and hit-up forwards (second-row and front-row or props) (King et al., 2011). Injury incidence was measured in units of injuries per 1000 player hours. Injuries that occurred during an NRL or NYC match were included in the numerator and only players participating in grade matches in each week were included in the denominator. The duration of each match was 80 minutes. This was calculated separately for NRL and NYC injuries.

## 3. RESULTS AND DISCUSSION

The data revealed that 287 (62.5%) NRL players sustained an injury during a game, with 479 injuries reported averaging 1.7 injuries per injured player, compared to 242 (43.3%) injured NYC players for 382 injuries. Table 1 depicts the incidence rate of match injuries for the three positional groups during the 2009 season. This trend of higher injury rates with age and level of competition is consistent with the literature (Brooks and Kemp, 2008). It is difficult to directly compare this to previous literature due to the variations in injury definitions and playing group definitions used in other studies. Two previous studies that analysed injuries at a single professional rugby league club recorded an incidence rate of 44.9/1000 hrs (Gibbs, 1993) and 39.8/1000 hrs (Orchard, 2004) indicating an increase in 2009 rates. It can be speculated that this may be due to an increase in the speed of today's match, rule changes, and also the increased sample size of this study. Previous studies have indicated that forwards (52.4–58%) have higher injury rates than backs (Gabbett, 2005; Gissane *et al.*, 1997; King *et al.*, 2010). The injury rate for hit-up forwards (NRL: 88.8/1000 hrs; NYC: 79/1000 hrs) was higher than outside backs and adjustables (Table 1).

**Table 1** Injury rate by playing position.

| Playing position | NRL injury rate/1000 hrs (95% CI) | | NYC injury rate/1000 hrs (95% CI) | |
|---|---|---|---|---|
| Outside backs | 63.2 | (53.7–72.7) | 46.7 | (38.6–55.0) |
| Adjustables | 56.1 | (46.1–66.1) | 40.2 | (31.7–48.7) |
| Hit-up forwards | 88.8 | (76.2–101.5) | 79.0 | (67.1–90.9) |

Lower limb injuries accounted for just over half of all injuries sustained at NRL and NYC level. Table 2 illustrates the incidence rate for each positional group per injury site. There was no significant difference between positional group and the site of injury for NRL or NYC players. The main injury sites for NRL and NYC backs were the ankle/foot and upper leg (groin, hamstring and quadriceps), each contributing 20–22% of the total injuries sustained by this group. Knee injuries contributed to 21.9% of NRL adjustables injuries and 17.9% of NRL hit-up forward injuries, although this is lower than previously reported (27.7%) at the professional level (Orchard, 2004). Head (including neck) injuries are also lower than previously cited in the literature (Alexander *et al.*, 1981; King *et al.*, 2010) with one study reporting an injury rate of 38/1000 hrs (Stephenson *et al.*, 1996). In the current study head/neck injuries were among the three main injury sites for NRL hit-up forwards (17.9%, 15.9/1000 hrs), NRL adjustables (17.5%, 9.8/1000 hrs) and NYC Hit-up forward (14.2%, 11.2/1000 hrs). The shoulder has also been identified as a common injury site among junior and semi-professional players (King and Gabbett, 2009). Interestingly, shoulder injuries were the most common injury for NYC adjustables accounting for 18.6% of their total injuries although incidence rates were 5.6–11.7/1000 hrs across all positions and grades. The lower incidence rates at the professional level may be linked to superior tackle technique but this requires further investigation.

Ligament sprains were found to be the most common type of injury for all positions in both grades (Table 2). Sprains contributed to 16.7–26% of total injuries in the NRL and 24.3–32.6% in the NYC with an injury rate of 19.5/1000 hrs for all hit-up forwards. Previous literature has indicated that ligament and joint injuries have been the most prevalent injury sustained at the professional rugby league level (Gissane *et al.*, 2001; Hoskins *et al.*, 2006) whereas muscular strains have the highest injury rate in amateur and semi-professional rugby league (Hoskins *et al.*, 2006; Gabbett, 2003; King and Gabbett, 2009). Muscle strains were the second most common injury in the NRL with the main contributor being hamstring strains. There was no significant difference between playing positions in each grade and the type of injury sustained.

The tackle contest has been identified as the dominant cause of rugby league injuries at all levels of competition (Gissane *et al.*, 1997; King *et al.*, 2010). The tackle contest accounts for approximately 57% of all injuries, which is within the range reported by Hoskins *et al.* (2006) although the incidence rates are lower than previously reported (Gissane *et al.*, 1997; Stephenson *et al.*, 1996). Supporting the findings of King *et al.* (2011), backs and hit-up forwards sustained more injuries when being tackled compared to executing the tackle while NYC adjustables had a higher injury rate when tackling rather than as the ball carrier. However, this trend was reversed for NRL adjustables. In the modern game the adjustables often execute the highest number of tackles in a game so it is unclear why this finding differs to King *et al.* (2011). The higher injury rates as ball carriers in the tackle may be a result of the force generated at the collision by the speed of the runner (particularly after a quick play-the-ball), the number of players in the tackle, the numerous directions of impact from the tacklers, and the lack of control the ball carrier has in falling when tackled.

Following the tackle, the main cause of injury for all positional groups was running and collision with a player/object (Table 3). Of the injuries classified, only 0.6% of injuries were sustained from illegal play.

Table 4 shows the severity of injuries obtained in the 2009 season. Mild (0–1 missed match) injuries registered as the most common for all positional groups in both the NRL and NYC. Hit-up forwards recorded the highest incidence rate for missing one game (see Table 2) during the NYC (224.4/1000hrs) and NRL (198.7/1000hrs) season with the adjustables registering the lowest injury rate (NYC: 89.3/1000hrs and NRL: 113.6/1000hrs). This may reflect the different roles of these two positional groups but warrants further investigation. On average, players missed 2–3 games per injury during the 2009 season.

**Table 2** Injury rates per 1000 hours (95% CI) for each body area and injury type by playing position.

| Injury Site | Backs | | Adjustables | | Hit-up forwards | |
|---|---|---|---|---|---|---|
| **Playing position NRL** | | | | | | |
| Head/neck | 7.1 | (3.9-10.3) | 9.8 | (5.6-14.0) | 15.9 | (10.6-21.2) |
| Shoulder | 7.1 | (3.9-10.3) | 7.0 | (3.5-10.6) | 11.7 | (7.1-16.3) |
| Arm/hand | 5.2 | (2.5-8.0) | 4.7 | (1.8-7.6) | 11.2 | (6.7-15.7) |
| Thorax/back | 4.9 | (2.2-7.5) | 6.1 | (2.8-9.4) | 7.9 | (4.2-11.7)) |
| Upper leg | 13.8 | (9.4-18.3) | 10.8 | (6.4-15.2) | 10.8 | (6.4-15.2) |
| Knee | 8.6 | (5.1-12.1) | 7.5 | (3.8-11.2) | 15.9 | (10.6-21.2) |
| Lower leg | 3.4 | (1.2-5.6) | 4.2 | (1.5-7.0) | 4.2 | (1.5-7.0) |
| Foot/ankle | 13.1 | (8.8-14.8) | 6.1 | (2.8-9.4) | 11.2 | (6.7-15.7) |
| | | | | | | |
| Concussion | 2.2 | (0.5-4.0) | 5.1 | (2.1-8.2) | 5.6 | (2.4-8.8) |
| Dislocation | 4.1 | (1.7-6.6) | 0.9 | (-0.4-2.2) | 4.7 | (1.8-7.6) |
| Fracture | 7.1 | (3.9-10.3) | 3.7 | (1.2-6.3) | 10.3 | (6.0-14.6) |
| Haematoma | 8.6 | (5.1-12.1) | 8.9 | (4.9-12.9) | 7.5 | (3.8-11.2) |
| Joint injury | 8.2 | (4.8-11.7) | 7.0 | (3.5-10.6) | 12.6 | (7.9-17.4) |
| Ligament sprain | 16.5 | (11.6-21.3) | 9.4 | (5.3-13.5) | 19.2 | (13.3-25.0) |
| Muscle strain | 12.3 | (8.1-16.6) | 9.8 | (5.6-14.0) | 14.0 | (9.0-19.0) |
| Other | 4.1 | (1.7-6.6) | 10.8 | (6.4-15.2) | 11.7 | (7.1-16.3) |
| | | | | | | |
| Injury rate for missing 1 match | 185.6 | (169-202) | 113.6 | (99-128) | 198.7 | (180-218) |

| Injury Site | Backs | | Adjustables | | Hit-up forwards | |
|---|---|---|---|---|---|---|
| **Playing position NYC** | | | | | | |
| Head/neck | 4.1 | (1.7-6.6) | 3.3 | (0.9-5.7) | 11.2 | (6.7-15.7) |
| Shoulder | 5.6 | (2.8-8.5) | 7.5 | (3.8-11.2) | 11.2 | (6.7-15.7) |
| Arm/hand | 3.7 | (1.4-6.1) | 4.7 | (1.8-7.6) | 7.9 | (4.2-11.7) |
| Thorax/back | 5.2 | (2.5-8.0) | 5.6 | (2.4-8.8) | 20.6 | (14.5-26.7) |
| Upper leg | 9.3 | (5.7-13.0) | 6.1 | (2.8-9.4) | 9.4 | (5.3-13.5) |
| Knee | 6.7 | (3.6-9.8) | 6.5 | (3.1-10.0) | 10.8 | (6.4-15.2) |
| Lower leg | 1.9 | (0.2-3.5) | 0.9 | (-0.4-2.2) | 6.5 | (3.1-10.0) |
| Foot/ankle | 10.1 | (6.3-13.9) | 5.1 | (2.1-8.2) | 12.6 | (7.9-17.4) |
| | | | | | | |
| Concussion | 1.9 | (0.2-3.5) | 1.4 | (-0.2-3.0) | 3.3 | (0.9-5.7) |
| Dislocation | 2.2 | (0.5-4.0) | 0.5 | (-0.5-1.4) | 4.7 | (1.8-7.6) |
| Fracture | 2.6 | (0.7-4.6) | 1.9 | (0.1-3.7) | 6.5 | (3.1-10.0) |
| Haematoma | 6.0 | (3.1-8.9) | 4.2 | (1.5-7.0) | 14.0 | (9.0-19.0) |
| Joint injury | 5.2 | (2.5-8.0) | 7.5 | (3.8-11.2) | 6.5 | (3.1-10.0) |
| Ligament sprain | 15.0 | (10.3-19.6) | 13.1 | (8.2-18.0) | 19.2 | (13.3-25.0) |
| Muscle strain | 9.7 | (6.0-13.5) | 5.1 | (2.1-8.2) | 8.4 | (4.5-12.3) |
| Other | 4.1 | (1.7-6.6) | 6.5 | (3.1-10.0) | 15.9 | (10.6-21.2) |
| | | | | | | |
| Injury rate for missing 1 match | 138.4 | (124-153) | 89.3 | (77-102) | 224.4 | (204-244) |

There was no significant difference between NRL backs (2.9, 2.2–3.6), adjustables (2.0, 1.4–2.6) and hit-up forwards (2.4, 1.8–2.9) or NYC backs (3.0, 2.3–3.6), adjustables (2.2, 1.7–2.7) and hit-up forwards (2.8, 2.2-3.5) for the number of missed games per injury. There was no significant difference between positional groups and the severity of the injury sustained, with the incidence rate for a major injury between 5.1–11.2/1000hrs for both grades. These results for major injuries are lower than those reported previously (Gabbett, 2005; Gibbs, 1993; Hodgson Phillips *et al.*, 1998; King *et al.*, 2011). For example, when analysing one NRL team over two seasons, King *et al.* (2011) reported an injury incidence rate of 12.5/1000 hrs (backs)–23.5/1000 hrs (adjustables) for injuries resulting in at least 5 missed matches. When major injuries were analysed further it was revealed that they predominantly occurred at the foot/ankle or knee and were sustained when being tackled. There was no difference between positional groups on whether a player was unable to complete a match due to injury or the rate at which they sustained a recurring injury (5–12/1000hrs).

**Table 3** Injury rates per 1000 hours (95% CI) for the main injury mechanisms for NRL and NYC players (by position).

| Injury | NRL | | | NYC | | |
|---|---|---|---|---|---|---|
| | Backs | Adjustables | Hit-up fwds | Backs | Adjustables | Hit-up fwds |
| Being tackled | 29.2 (23-36) | 21.5(15-28) | 37.4(29-46) | 17.6 (13-23) | 8.9 (5-13) | 30.4 (23-38) |
| Tackling | 7.1 (4-10) | 12.6 (8-17) | 17.3 (12-23) | 6.4 (3-9) | 12.2 (7-17) | 13.6 (9-18) |
| Running | 7.1 (4-10) | 6.5 (3-10) | 7.5 (4-11) | 4.9 (2-8) | 0.9 (0-2) | 4.7 (2-8) |
| Collision | 6.7 (4-10) | 5.1 (2-8) | 11.2 (7-16) | 4.5 (2-7) | 2.8 (1-5) | 7.0 (3-11) |

**Table 4** Injury rates per 1000 hours (95% CI) for mild, moderate and major injury by positions.

| | Mild | | | Moderate | | | Major | | |
|---|---|---|---|---|---|---|---|---|---|
| | % | /1000hr | 95% CI | % | /1000hr | 95% CI | % | /1000hrs | 95% CI |
| NRL | | | | | | | | | |
| Backs | 56.8 | 35.9 | (28-43) | 28.4 | 18.0 | (13-23) | 14.8 | 9.4 | (6-13) |
| Adjustables | 66.4 | 36.9 | (29-45) | 24.4 | 13.6 | (9-18) | 9.2 | 5.1 | (2-8) |
| Hit-up fwds | 58.9 | 52.4 | (43-62) | 29.5 | 26.2 | (19-33) | 11.6 | 10.3 | (6-15) |
| NYC | | | | | | | | | |
| Backs | 44.8 | 21.0 | (15-26) | 36.8 | 17.2 | (12-22) | 18.4 | 8.6 | (5-12) |
| Adjustables | 54.7 | 22.0 | (16-28) | 29.1 | 11.7 | (7-16) | 16.3 | 6.5 | (3-10) |
| Hit-up fwds | 51.5 | 40.7 | (32-49) | 34.3 | 27.1 | (20-34) | 14.2 | 11.2 | (7-16) |

## 4. CONCLUSION

This paper provides an overview of the incidence rate, site, type and mechanism of injuries sustained across all clubs in the first grade (NRL) and Under 20 years (NYC) rugby league competition. This provides baseline data for individual clubs as well as for monitoring trends in the upcoming years. Professional rugby league is associated with a relatively high injury rate with hit-up forwards recording the highest incidence rate. However, a large percentage of match injuries can be considered as minor, with a relative risk of injury at 5.9% (NYC)–7.3% (NRL). There was no significant difference between playing position and site, type, severity or injury mechanism for either grade.

**Acknowledgements**

This project was funded by the NRL. I would also like to acknowledge the contribution of the NRL clubs and their staff in the reporting of their injury data.

**References**

Alexander, D. *et al.*, 1980, Rugby league football injuries over two competition seasons. *Medical Journal Australia*, **2**, 334–335.

Brooks, J., 2008, Recent trends in rugby union injuries, *Clin Sport Med*, **27**, 51–73.

Gabbett, T., 2003, Incidence of injury in semi professional rugby league players. *Brit J Sports Med*, **37**, 36–44.

Gabbett, T., 2005, Science of rugby league football. *J Sport Sci*, **23**, 961–976.

Gibbs, N., 1993, Injuries in professional rugby league: A three-year prospective study of the South Sydney Professional Rugby League Football Club. *Am J Sports Med*, **21**, 696–700.

Gissane, C. *et al.*, 1997, Differences in the incidence of injuries between rugby league forwards and backs, *Austral J Sci Med Sport*, **29**, 91–94.

Gissane, C. *et al.*, 2001, Physical collisions and injury rates in professional super league rugby. *Cleveland Medical Journal*, **4**, 147–155.

Hodgson Phillips, L. *et al.*, 1998, Effects of seasonal change in rugby league on the incidence of injury. *Brit J Sports Med*, **32**, 144–148.

Hoskins, W. *et al.*, 2006, Injury in rugby league: A review. *J Sci Med Sport*, **9**, 46–56.

King, D. and Gabbett, T., 2009, Injuries in the New Zealand semi-professional rugby league competition. *NZ J Sports Med*, **36**, 6–15.

King, D. *et al.*, 2010, Match and training injuries in rugby league. *Sports Med*, **40**, 163–178.

King, D. *et al.*, 2011, The effect of player positional groups on the nature of tackles that results in tackle-related injuries in professional rugby league matches. *J Sports Med Phys Fit*, **51**, 435–443.

O'Connor, D., 1996, Physiological characteristics of professional rugby league players. *Strength and Conditioning Coach*, **4**, 21–26.

O'Connor D., 2004, Groin injuries in professional rugby league players: A prospective study. *J Sport Sci*, **22**, 629–636.

Orchard J., 2004, Missed time through injury and injury management at an NRL club. *Sport Health*, **22**, 11–19.

Stephenson, S. *et al.*, 1996, Injury in rugby league: A four year prospective survey. *Brit J Sports Med*, **30**, 331–334.

# CHAPTER FIFTY-THREE

# Closed-kinetic chain evaluation of ankle joint proprioception in athletes with functional ankle instability

S. Aminiaghdam and S. Sheikhesmaeili

Department of Physical Education, Islamic Azad University, Saghez Branch, Saghez, Iran

## 1. INTRODUCTION

Ankle injuries are one of the most common injuries occurred in sport activities among athletes, active young and adult peoples (Hale and Hertel, 2005). Eighty-five percent of ankle injuries are sprains, and of these, 85% are sprains of the lateral ligaments due to ankle inversion (Sekir *et al.*, 2007; Yildiz *et al.*, 2008). Ankle sprains not only result in significant time lost from sports participation, they can also cause long-term disability and have a major impact on health care costs (Konradsen, 2002).

After an ankle sprain, 40% of injured athletes report residual disability involving the sensation of giving way or the feeling of instability at the ankle, this disability is referred to as Functional Ankle Instability (FAI) (Sekir *et al.*, 2007). The FAI is defined as the giving-way sensation, weakness, more pain, or loss of function at the ankle than before injury. Individuals with functional ankle instability are more susceptible to new ankle ligament injuries than others (Freeman *et al.*, 1965; Hiller *et al.*, 2006).

Proprioception has three sub-modalities: joint position sense (JPS), kinesthesia (joint motion detection), and sense of tension, and each of these sub-modalities has a specific evaluation method. In studies that have been conducted in context of ankle joint position sense, contradictory results have been observed as any, low or high proprioceptive deficits in the injured ankle.

In studies that have been constructed on subjects with FAI, some authors have used only within-group (compare the injured to the uninjured side) (Halasi *et al.*, 2006) and some have used between-group (compare injured subjects to a healthy group) (Noronha *et al.*, 2007; Nakasa *et al.*, 2008) comparisons and both research designs have their own advantages and disadvantages. Thus conducting both within-group and between-group comparisons simultaneously can detect impairment associated with this type of injury.

The purpose of this study was to investigate proprioceptive deficit in subjects with FAI and compare their ankle proprioception to healthy subjects. Measurement techniques used to evaluate proprioception are different and each of these procedures evaluates proprioception in a different manner.

Considering that balance is maintained in a closed kinetic chain and most of the ankle sprains occurred during physical activities on the weight-bearing foot, therefore, it seems that a closed kinetic chain and weight-bearing proprioception evaluation may detect proprioception deficits in subjects with FAI more accurately.

Previous studies did not have focus on a closed kinetic chain and weight-bearing evaluation of proprioception in four different ankle positions; it seems that tasks and evaluation methods that better mimic circumstances and positions encountered during sport activities and injuries may be more appropriate when assessing athletic individuals. Therefore our purpose is to evaluate proprioception in different positions and angles of the ankle by means of the Halasi *et al.* (2006) method.

## 2. METHODS

Thirty-six male athletes with at least three years of football playing experience voluntarily participated in this study. Eighteen young football players previously diagnosed with a Functional Ankle Instability were matched by age and dominant limb to eighteen non-injured athletes. Functional ankle instability was measured using the Ankle Joint Functional Assessment Tool (AJFAT) (Ross *et al.*, 2008). All participants completed the AJFAT. On the AJFAT, the functionally unstable group scored significantly lower than the healthy group.

**Table 1** Demographic characteristics of subjects.

| Group | Experiment | Control |
|---|---|---|
| Age (yrs) | $23.54 \pm 2.56$ | $24.87 \pm 3.69$ |
| Height (cm) | $176.46 \pm 5.24$ | $176.73 \pm 4.99$ |
| Weight (kg) | $72.00 \pm 8.32$ | $72.86 \pm 10.48$ |
| AJFAT score | $25.2 \pm 1.74$ | $14.13 \pm 3.92$ |

Twelve of the 18 subjects with FAI have experienced symptoms of unilateral ankle instability of their dominant and six on their non-dominant limb. Subjects were excluded if they had bilateral ankle instability, positive result for two orthopedic assessment tests; score higher than 22 points in AJFAT, previous ankle fracture, ankle surgery at past 6 months, visual and vestibular disorders and present injury at spine, hip and knee. Finally, 18 participants with unilateral FAI were matched by height, weight and dominant leg with 18 participants with stable ankles.

The slope-box test was used for assessment of ankle joint position sense. This procedure was conducted in both groups (experiment and control). Before starting the investigation, sequence of slope direction and amplitudes were randomly selected and applied in all the measurements.

Before random selection of the slope, three different slopes (0, 12.5 and 25 degree angles) in each direction were shown to the subjects. The range of angle estimation had to be between 0 (horizontal) and 35 degrees that means subjects should not estimate angles more than 35 degrees. Subjects were asked to tell the direction and the degree of the slope they were putting feet on the adjustable slope-box. The subjects were barefoot, full weight-bearing and their knees in full extension on a single leg. Subjects had no visual information on the horizontal plane and did not see their lower extremity, but could support themselves on a wall in front of them to maintain their balance (Halasi *et al.*, 2006).

Statistical analysis was performed using SPSS version 16.0 software. Statistical differences between the data within the uninjured and injured ankle in the FAI group were investigated using paired sample t-tests, and differences between the FAI and the control groups using independent t-tests. Comparison of proprioceptive deficit for four slope directions on the injured ankle was made using a 1-way analysis of variance (ANOVA) and Tukey honestly significant difference (HSD) follow-up test.

## 3. RESULTS

Since measurements were constructed in four slope directions (anterior, posterior, medial and lateral) and any direction caused one of ankle movements in its range of motion, we used ankle positions in order to easily report results. Slope anterior, posterior, medial and lateral directions are equivalent to plantar-flexion, dorsi-flexion, inversion and eversion respectively.

**Table 2** Difference between JPS of FAI and healthy subjects.

| Ankle positions | Mean Absolute Estimate Error (MAEE) (degree) | | t | sig |
|---|---|---|---|---|
| | Unstable ankle | Matched ankle | | |
| Plantar-flexion | $4.20 \pm 0.80$ | $1.76 \pm 0.39$ | 10.52 | 0.000*** |
| Dorsi-flexion | $3.48 \pm 0.96$ | $1.80 \pm 0.31$ | 6.45 | 0.000*** |
| Inversion | $5.02 \pm 0.81$ | $1.83 \pm 0.48$ | 13.06 | 0.000*** |
| Eversion | $3.83 \pm 1.32$ | $1.80 \pm 0.36$ | 5.718 | 0.000*** |
| $P < 0.001$*** | | | | |

The comparison between injured and uninjured ankles of athletes in FAI group showed a statistically ($p < 0.001$) larger MAEE of injured ankles. The injured ankles of the FAI also had a statistically (p<0.001) larger MAEE than the ipsilateral ankle in the healthy group (Table 2).

The results showed that MAEE (Joint Position Sense) at inversion position was significantly greater than other positions ($F_{(3, 56)}$ = 6.55, p < 0.01). This means that injured ankles have more errors in the inversion position. Post-hoc Tukey comparison indicated that unstable ankle MAEE in inversion was significantly larger than eversion (p < 0.05) and dorsi-flexion positions (p < 0.01).

The side-to-side differences of the mean absolute angle estimation errors in the FAI group were also significantly greater than the control group in four ankle positions (Table 3).

**Table 3** Side-to-side differences of the MAEE in FAI and healthy subjects.

| Ankle positions | Mean Absolute Estimate Error (MAEE) (degree) | | t | sig |
|---|---|---|---|---|
| | Unstable group | Healthy group | | |
| Plantar-flexion | 1.87 ± 0.69 | 0.34 ± 0.30 | 7.76 | 0.000*** |
| Dorsi-flexion | 1.30 ± 1.06 | 0.22 ± 0.12 | 3.92 | 0.001** |
| Inversion | 2.42 ± 0.81 | 0.36 ± 0.27 | 9.35 | 0.000*** |
| Eversion | 1.61 ± 1.39 | 0.13 ± 0.03 | 3.66 | 0.003** |
| P<0.01**   P<0.001*** | | | | |

One-way ANOVA and post-hoc Tukey results showed that side-to-side differences of the MAEE in the inversion position was greater than other positions ($F_{(3,56)}$ = 3.24, p < 0.05) and side-to-side differences of the MAEE in the inversion position was significantly larger than the dorsi-flexion position.

## 4. DISCUSSION

Freeman *et al.* (1965) described that functional instability arose from sensori-motor control deficits. The nerve fibers of the mechanoreceptors are present in the structures of the lateral aspect of the ankle including the lateral ligaments, capsule, and retinaculum, thus damage to that structure by an inversion ankle sprain might result in reduced proprioceptive inputs from the ankle joint and thereafter functional instability.

Sekir *et al.* (2007) investigated the effects of isokinetic exercise on strength, joint position sense and functionality in 24 recreational athletes with FAI. At pre-treatment evaluation, passive reproduction error score of ankle joint position sense at 10° of inversion angle (2.35 ± 1.16°) and 20° of inversion angle (3.10 ± 2.16°) in the injured ankles were significantly higher than the non-injured ankles.

Nakasa *et al.* (2008) evaluated the inversion angle replication errors on a goniometry footplate in 12 patients with FAI and 17 healthy subjects. They concluded that an unstable ankle has a deficit of joint position sense in comparison with a healthy contralateral side in patients with functional instability.

Noronha *et al.* (2007) in a cross-sectional study investigated the relationship between one measure of proprioception and two measures of motor control in 20 people with FAI. They found no relationship between functional ankle instability and loss of proprioception or motor control. They suggested that proprioception should be measured using various methods.

Our within-group comparison finding is in agreement with that of Nakasa *et al.* (2008) and Sekir *et al.* (2007), who demonstrated deficit in proprioception in unstable ankles but in contrary to Noronha *et al.* (2007) results.

Our between-group comparison finding is in agreement with that of Sekir *et al.* (2007) and Halasi *et al.* (2006) who found ankle proprioception deficit in injured subject in comparison to the healthy group but in contrary to Noronha *et al.* (2007) results. In the study conducted by Nakasa *et al.* (2008), the replication error for unstable and stable ankle were $3.4 \pm 1.0°$ and $2.3 \pm 0.8°$, respectively. In the present study the MAEE was $4.14°$. As mentioned earlier, proprioception testing methods according to ankle position and targeting the mechanoreceptors are different.

Thus possible explanations for the difference between our findings and other published data could include applied measurement method, subjects, number of assessed positions for ankle proprioception and sensitivity of this method than other procedures. The previous authors only investigated the proprioception at the inversion and eversion positions; their measurements did not model the real situation of landing well, the subjects did not put their full weight on the tested leg and they were non-athletes.

## 5. CONCLUSIONS

In comparison with intact side and healthy subjects, the inversion position has a higher amount of proprioception impairment than other ankle positions, and side-to-side differences of the MAEE at the inversion position was greater than other positions. Since in the closed kinetic chain, supination consists of dorsi-flexion, inversion, and internal rotation, we can conclude that increased inversion angle replication error may enhance recurrent rolling-over and ankle sprain after an acute initial ankle sprain in sport or activities that include running, jumping, landing or rapid change of direction.

### References

Bahr, R. and Bahr, I.A., 1997, Incidence of acute volleyball injuries: A prospective cohort study of injury mechanisms and risk factors. *Scandinavian J Med Sci Sports*, **7**, 166–171.

Ekstrand, J. and Tropp, H., 1990, The incidence of ankle sprains in soccer. *Foot Ankle*, **11**, 41–44.

Freeman, M.A. *et al.*, 1965, The etiology and prevention of functional instability of the foot. *J Bone Joint Surg*, **47**, 678–685.

Halasi, T. *et al.*, 2006, Changes in joint position sense after conservatively treated chronic lateral ankle instability. *Knee Surgery, Sports Traumatology, Arthroscopy*, **14**, 1299–1306.

Hale, S.A. and Hertel, J., 2005, Reliability and sensitivity of the foot and ankle Disability Index in subjects with chronic ankle instability. *J Athlet Train*, **40**, 35–40.

Hiller, C.E. *et al.*, 2006, The Cumberland Ankle Instability Tool: A report of validity and reliability testing. *Arch Phys Med Rehab*, **87**, 1235–1241.

Hubbard, T.J. and Kaminski, T.W., 2002, Kinesthesia is not affected by functional ankle instability status. *J Athl Train*, **37**, 481–486.

Jerosch, J. and Bischof, M., 1996, Proprioceptive capabilities of the ankle in stable and unstable joints. *Sports Exerc Injury*, **2**, 167–171.

Konradsen, L., 2002, Factors contributing to chronic ankle instability: Kinesthesia and joint position sense. *J Athl Train*, **37**, 381–385.

Nakasa, T. *et al.*, 2008, The deficit of joint position sense in the chronic unstable ankle as measured by inversion angle replication error. *Archives of Orthopedic and Trauma Surgery*, **128**, 445–449.

Noronha, M.D. *et al.*, 2007, Loss of proprioception or motor control is not related to functional ankle instability: An observational study. *Austral J Physiother*, **53**, 193–198.

Riemann, B.L. *et al.*, 2002, Sensorimotor system measurement techniques. *J Athl Train*, **37**, 85–98.

Ross, S.E. *et al.*, 2008, Assessment tools for identifying functional limitations associated with functional ankle instability. *J Athl Train*, **43**, 44–50.

Santos, M.J. and Liu, W., 2008, Possible factors related to functional ankle instability. *J Orthop Sports Physic Ther*, **38**, 150–157.

Sekir, U. *et al.*, 2007, Effect of isokinetic training on strength, functionality and proprioception in athletes with functional ankle instability. *Knee Surgery, Sports Traumatology, Arthroscopy*, **15**, 654–666.

Yildiz, Y. *et al.*, 2008, Reliability of a functional test battery evaluating functionality, proprioception and strength of the ankle joint. *Turk J Med Sci*, **38**, 1–9.

You, S.H. *et al.*, 2004, Effects of circumferential ankle pressure on ankle proprioception, stiffness, and postural stability: A preliminary investigation. *J Orthop Sports Phys Ther*, **34**, 449–460.

# CHAPTER FIFTY-FOUR

# Screening English Premier League football players for exercise-induced bronchoconstriction

J. Dickinson[1], B. Drust[1,2], G. Whyte[1] and P. Brukner[1]

[1]Research Institute for Sport and Exercise Science, Liverpool John Moores University, UK, [2]Liverpool Football Club, Liverpool, UK

## 1. INTRODUCTION

Exercise-induced bronchoconstriction (EIB) is closely related to asthma and is defined as a transient narrowing of the airways, limiting expiration that usually follows a bout of exercise, and is reversible spontaneously or through inhalation of $\beta_2$-Agonists (Anderson, 1997). The prevalence of EIB in elite sport has been reported to range between 10–50% depending on the sport (Dickinson *et al.*, 2005). Athletes are at a higher risk of EIB if they participate in sports that require high minute ventilation (Bougault *et al.*, 2009) or take place in environments which are dry (Evans *et al.*, 2005) or polluted (Rundell *et al.*, 2004). Individual factors such as atopy can also influence EIB prevalence and severity (Helenius *et al.*, 1998).

Symptom-based diagnosis of EIB has been shown to have a low level of sensitivity and specificity. Lund *et al.* (2009) demonstrated that out of 42 symptomatic elite athletes, only 12 could provide objective evidence of asthma. Rundell *et al.* (2001) showed that only 50% of athletes who had genuine EIB reported any symptoms of EIB. This would suggest that many elite athletes fail to associate respiratory symptoms with EIB, perhaps believing their extreme dyspnoea to be a normal part of intense training/competition. Given the poor sensitivity and specificity of symptoms based diagnosis it is recommended all diagnosis of EIB is accompanied by an indirect airway challenge (Carlsen *et al.*, 2005).

The eucapnic voluntary hyperpnoea (EVH) challenge is a surrogate for exercise (Anderson *et al.* 2001). It possesses a high specificity and sensitivity in the diagnosis of EIB in elite athletes (Dickinson *et al.*, 2006). The International Olympic Committee – Medical Commission (IOC-MC) recommends that athletes are tested for EIB using EVH challenges in order to provide evidence of EIB (IOC-MC 2010). Studies that have used objective tests, such as EVH, have identified an alarming sub-group of athletes, who have no previous diagnosis of EIB, but who exhibit a positive response to EVH (Holzer *et al.*, 2002; Parsons *et al.*, 2007;

Dickinson *et al.*, 2010). This has led to the suggestion that elite athletes should be screened periodically for EIB using bronchoprovocation challenges, irrespective of symptoms and previous diagnosis. At present no data exist reporting the use of screening elite level football players for EIB. Thus, the purpose of this study was to screen elite Premier League Football Players for EIB using an EVH challenge.

## 2. MATERIALS AND METHOD

Twenty-one English Premier League football players (mean$\pm$SD; age 21.9$\pm$3.9 years; height 183.0$\pm$6.7 cm; weight 79.0$\pm$6.0 kg) volunteered and provided written informed consent. Each player completed an EVH challenge with maximal flow volume loops measured at baseline and 3, 5, 10 and 15 minutes following the EVH challenge.

The EVH challenge required players to achieve a target minute ventilation ($\dot{V}_E$) of 85% (baseline $FEV_1$ x 30) of their predicted maximal voluntary ventilation rate (MVV) for 6 minutes (Anderson *et al.*, 2001). The air that was inspired during the EVH challenge consisted of 21% $O_2$, 5% $CO_2$ and 74% $N_2$ (inspired air temperature 19°C, humidity <2%). The gas was delivered to each participant via a gas cylinder, reservoir and a two-way valve. $\dot{V}_E$ was recorded by calculating the volume of air passing through a dry gas meter every minute (see Figure 1).

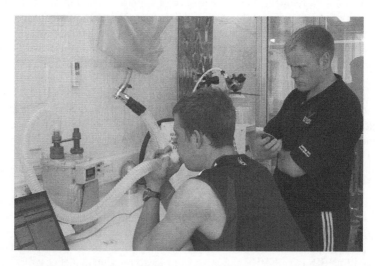

**Figure 1** Athlete undergoing Eucapnic Voluntary Hyperpnoea challenge.

A fall of 10% in forced expiratory volume in one second ($FEV_1$) from baseline at two consecutive time points was deemed positive. One-way ANOVA was conducted to compare the maximal change of $FEV_1$ following EVH between EVH positive (EVH +ve) and EVH negative (EVH –ve) players. Significance was assumed if $p \leq 0.05$.

## 3. RESULTS

Six players (29%) demonstrated EVH +ve. Four out of the six (66%) players who demonstrated EVH +ve did not have a previous diagnosis of EIB. The two EVH +ve players with a previous EIB diagnosis were not currently using any medication to treat EIB. The four EVH +ve players with no previous history had the greatest changes from baseline $FEV_1$. Two players presented with a maximal fall from baseline $FEV_1$ of 10% at one time point but could not demonstrate a second consecutive fall $FEV_1 \geq 10\%$ from baseline. These two players were deemed to have presented EVH –ve (see Figure 2).

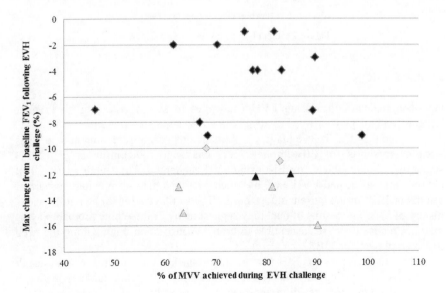

**Figure 2** Individuals maximum $FEV_1$ change from baseline post-EVH challenge.

There was a significant difference between the maximal percent change in $FEV_1$ from baseline following the EVH challenge between EVH +ve and EVH −ve players (-13.3±1.9% vs -5.5±3.5%; p<0.01). At each time point following the EVH challenge the $FEV_1$ fall from baseline was significantly (p<0.05) greater in the EVH +ve players when compared to EVH −ve players (see Figure 3).

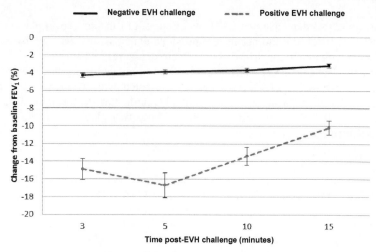

**Figure 3** Fall in $FEV_1$ following EVH challenge.

## 4. DISCUSSION

Our data indicates that using EVH challenges to screen elite English Premier League football players for EIB results in 29% of players presenting EVH +ve. The prevalence of EVH +ve players is similar to reports of screening elite athletes from other sports for EIB through EVH challenges. Dickinson *et al.* (2011) screened 228 elite athletes for EIB using EVH challenges. They reported 78 (34%) elite athletes presented EVH +ve, of which 57 (73%) had no previous history of asthma or EIB. In the current study four EVH +ve players (66%) had no previous history of EIB. The results of our study suggest many of these elite football players may not realise they are susceptible to bronchoconstriction, highlighting the need to screen players for EIB.

Screening players for EIB may be important from a performance and health perspective. Detecting and appropriately treating EIB elite athletes with no previous diagnosis may result in improvements in aerobic performance. Brukner *et al.* (2007) reported that detecting and appropriately treating athletes with previously undiagnosed EIB resulted in a 10% improvement in $VO_2$ peak. This observed improvement can be explained by the inhaled corticosteroid treatment improving airway function, thereby allowing increased alveolar ventilation and improved efficiency of alveolar-to-arterial blood $O_2$ exchange during exercise. From a health perspective it is important to detect and appropriately treat EIB athletes to ensure airway health is not compromised. It is paramount that all athletes with EIB are detected as acute cases of bronchoconstriction can result in significant mortality. Becker *et al.* (2004) reported that in the USA over a seven-year period, 61 asthma-related deaths occurred in close association to physical activity. More than half of these deaths occurred in elite or competitive athletes and nearly 10% of whom had no known history of asthma.

In conclusion the high proportion of previously undiagnosed players who demonstrated EVH +ve suggests that elite football players should be screened routinely for EIB using a suitable bronchoprovocation challenge such as EVH. The practical implications of this study would suggest that players involved with senior elite football squads should be screened for EIB. It may also be appropriate to incorporate EIB screening into the medical of any player signing for a new club.

## References

Anderson, S., 1997, Exercise induced asthma. In *Allergy and Allergic Diseases*, Oxford: Blackwell Scientific, pp. 621–711.

Anderson, S. *et al.*, 2001, Provocation by eucapnic voluntary hyperpnoea to identify exercise induced bronchoconstriction. *Brit J Sports Med*, **35**, 344–347.

Becker, J. *et al.*, 2004, Asthma deaths during sports: Report of a 7 year experience. *J Allergy Clin Immunol*, **113**, 264–267.

Bougault, V. *et al.*, 2009, Asthma, airway inflammation and epithelial damage in swimmers and cold-air athletes. *European Respiratory Journal*, **33**, 740–746.

Brukner, P. *et al.*, 2007, The impact of exercise-induced bronchoconstriction on performance. *Med Sci Sports Exerc*, **39**, S639.

Carlsen, K. *et al.*, 2005, Treatment of exercise-induced asthma, respiratory and allergic disorders in sports and the relationship to doping: Part II of the report from the Joint Task Force of European Respiratory Society (ERS) and European Academy of Allergy and Clinical Immunology (EAACI) in cooperation with GA(2)LEN. *Allergy*, **63**, 492–505.

Dickinson, J. *et al.*, 2005, The impact of the changes in the IOC-MC asthma criteria: A British perspective. *Thorax*, **60**, 629–632.

Dickinson, J. *et al.*, 2006, Screening elite winter athletes for exercise-induced asthma: A comparison of three challenge methods. *Brit J Sports Med*, **40**, 179–183.

Dickinson, J. *et al.*, 2011, Diagnosis of exercise induced bronchoconstriction (EIB): Eucapnic voluntary hyperpnoea challenges identify previously undiagnosed elite athletes with EIB. *Brit J Sports Med*, **45**, 1126–1131.

Evans, T. *et al.*, 2005, Cold air inhalation does not affect the severity of EIB after exercise or eucapnic voluntary hyperventilation. *Med Sci Sports Exerc*, **37**, 544–549.

Helenius, I. *et al.*, 1998, Occurrence of exercise-induced bronchospasm in elite runners: dependence on atopy and exposure to cold air and pollen. *Brit J Sports Med*, **32**,125–129.

Holzer, K. *et al.*, 2002, Exercise in elite summer athletes: Challenges for diagnosis. *J Allergy Clin Immunol*, **110**, 374–380.

International Olympic Committee, Medical Commission, 2010, Beta$_2$ adrenoceptor agonists and the Olympic Games in Beijing 2008. http://multimedi.olympic .org/pdf/en_report_1302.pdf (accessed 28/1/2010).

Lund, T. *et al.*, 2009, Are asthma-like symptoms in elite athletes associated with classical features of asthma? *Brit J Sports Med*, **43**, 1131–1135.

Parsons, J. *et al.*, 2007, Prevalence of exercise induced bronchospasm in a cohort of varsity college athletes. *Med Sci Sports Exerc*, **39**, 1487–1492.

Rundell K. *et al.*, 2001, Self-reported symptoms and exercise-induced asthma in the elite athlete. *Med Sci Sports Exerc*, **33**, 208–213.

Rundell, K. 2004, Pulmonary function decay in women ice hockey players: Is there a relationship to ice rink air quality? *Inhaled Toxicology*, **16**, 117–123.

# CHAPTER FIFTY-FIVE

# A novel method to monitor lower limb muscles flexibility in elite youth soccer players

O. Materne[1,2], F. Fourchet[1,2], T. Hudacek[1,2] and M. Buchheit[1]

[1]ASPIRE, Academy for Sports Excellence, Doha, Qatar
[2] ASPETAR, NSMP, National Sports Medicine Programme, Qatar

## 1. INTRODUCTION

The International Olympic Committee consensus on elite child athlete recognized this population as exclusive in many aspects and requires appropriate supervision to insure a healthy athletic development (Mountjoy *et al.*, 2008). Philippaerts *et al.* (2006) presented the longitudinal change in youth soccer players including the trunk flexibility pattern during the growth period and the rapid modification of this physical factor during this critical phase was emphasized. Witvrouw *et al.* (2003) reported that an increased tightness or length imbalance of the hamstring or quadriceps muscles in professional players may increase the risk of injury. Recently de Lucena *et al.* (2011) stated on Brazilian adolescent a prevalence of 9.8% of Osgood-Schlatter's disease, the factors associated were practising regular sport and the shortness of the rectus femoris muscle (odds ratio, 7.15; 95% CI 2.86, 17.86). Nevertheless, while there is no definitive consensus regarding the possible benefit of stretching on athletic performance or injury prevention (Ben and Harvey, 2010), the development or maintenance of optimal flexibility has become very popular in the past years to prevent injury. An accurate monitoring of the primary lower limb muscle groups performed on a regular basis in youth elite soccer players may, however, help to identify flexibility imbalance of players in order to prescribe specific exercises, to reduce injury risks and football development time loss. The accuracy and the reliability of flexibility measures is of primary interest for clinicians working with elite youth soccer players (i.e., screening, prevention, rehabilitation programmes). Today there is a large body of literature about flexibility assessments. The most common methods rely either on the subject's tolerance to stretch (Law *et al.*, 2009) or on the patient's voluntary activation (Folpp *et al.*, 2006), which likely limits the accuracy of these methods. In an attempt to overcome these weaknesses a new method has recently been developed using a standardized stretch force (Fourchet *et al.*, 2011). This novel procedure is an extension of a previous method using a standardized stretch force on hamstrings (Fredriksen *et al.*, 1997) to the main lower limb muscles groups. The aim of the present study was therefore to, 1) evaluate the reliability of this novel digital video analysis method to assess the flexibility of the lower limb muscles groups in youth elite soccer players, and 2) examine whether changing the operators and/or the video analysers was likely to affect the reliability of the measures.

## 2. METHOD

Ten healthy male adolescents from a sports academy ($15.3 \pm 1.6$ years, $65.4 \pm 26.2$ kg, $171.7 \pm 8.8$ cm and $+1.5 \pm 1.5$ years from peak height velocity (Mirwald *et al.,* 2002) were tested. All participants were without history of musculoskeletal injuries of the lower limbs the previous two months before the study. Prior to testing, informed consent was obtained from all participants and their parents. The study was approved by the local research ethics committee and conformed to the recommendations of the Declaration of Helsinki.

On two occasions, three days apart, the flexibility of eight lower limb muscle groups was examined bilaterally in two phases. Firstly, the angle measurement with video capture of each body part in a stretched position (see Figure 1) was performed by three distinct pairs of operators. A muscle specific standardized force (Table 1) was applied using a hand-held dynamometer (Compact force gauge, Mecmesin, Slinfold, United Kingdom) in order to obtain reliable measurement (Fredriksen *et al.,* 1997, Ben and Harvey 2010, Folpp *et al.,* 2006, Fourchet *et al.,* 2011). Secondly, a computer-aided analysis of the video clips was performed by three different analysers using software (Dartfish Software, TeamPro Classroom 5.5, Fribourg, Switzerland) in order to measure each joint angle in the stretched position.

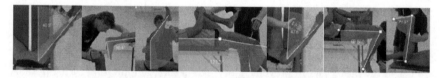

**Figure 1** Angles of measurements of the lower limb muscle groups.
Modified from Fourchet *et al.* (2012), with permission.

The absolute reliability of the overall method was assessed by analysing differences in angles for the two testing sessions. Intraclass correlation coefficient (ICC) and typical error of measurement expressed as a coefficient of variation (CV, %) were calculated. For each of the eight muscle groups, the average of the eight coefficients of variance were compared and the differences in reliability between operators, analysers and all operators/analysers combinations were assessed. The magnitude of these differences were expressed as standardized mean differences (Cohen's d). Additionally, we calculated the chances that the angles or CV values were greater/similar/smaller than, 1) the other day (between-day comparisons of angles measures) or, 2) any analysers and/or operators combinations (between-staff reliability comparisons) (Hopkins *et al.,* 2009).

# 3. RESULTS

Between all muscle groups, CV value ranged from 2.6 to 12.4% (see Table 1). The lowest CV was observed for the hip flexors, while the highest (the worse) was noted for the hip lateral rotators.

**Table 1** Reliability of the flexibility measurements for each lower limb muscle group (data are +/- SD for Endpoint angles and with 90% CL for CV and ICC).

| Muscle Group | n | Force (N) | Endpoint angle (°) | CV (%) | ICC |
|---|---|---|---|---|---|
| **Hip flexors** | 128 | 98.1 | 157 (6) | 2.6 (2.3;2.9) | 0.51 |
| **Hamstring** | 128 | 68.7 | 160 (11) | 3.3 (3.0;3.7) | 0.80 |
| **Quadriceps** | 124 | 78.5 | 48 (11) | 8.3 (7.5;9.3) | 0.86 |
| **Adductors** | 128 | 39.2 | 54 (9) | 7.2 (6.5;8.0) | 0.85 |
| **Hip medial rotators** | 126 | 49.1 | 55 (15) | 9.6 (8.6;10.8) | 0.92 |
| **Hip lateral rotators** | 128 | 49.1 | 44 (14) | 12.4 (12.2;14.0) | 0.91 |
| **Gastrocnemius** | 128 | 147.2 | 74 (7) | 5.7 (5.1;6.3) | 0.66 |
| **Soleus** | 125 | 147.2 | 59 (10) | 4.5 (4.0;5.0) | 0.93 |

The results showed that there was no substantial difference in CV values (see Figure 2), either between the operators or between analysers (all Cohen's d rated as trivial and difference unclear). All combinations of operators and analysers (see Table 2) showed no substantial difference (all Cohen's d rated as trivial and difference as unclear).

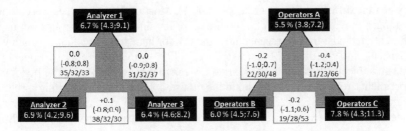

**Figure 2** Measure of reliability for all analysers and operators (Cohen's d (90% CL) and chances for CV values to be greater/similar/smaller). Modified from Fourchet *et al.* (2012), with permission.

**Table 2** Magnitude-based inferences for mean difference in reliability (Cohen's d (90% CL) and chances for CV values to be greater/similar/smaller) between the different analysers and operators.

|  | Operator A | Operator B | Operator C |
|---|---|---|---|
| **Analyser 1** | +0.3 (-0.6;1.1)<br>57/27/16 | +0.1 (-0.7;0.9)<br>42/31/27 | -0.1 (-1.0;0.7)<br>24/31/45 |
| **Analyser 2** | +0.3 (-0.5;1.1)<br>57/27/16 | +0.1 (-0.7;0.9)<br>42/31/27 | -0.2 (-1.0;0.7)<br>23/30/47 |
| **Analyser 3** | -0.2 (-1.0;0.7)<br>22/30/48 | +0.1 (-0.7;0.9)<br>45/31/24 | +0.2 (-0.6;1.1)<br>54/24/18 |

## 4. DISCUSSION

The results of the study presented a moderate to good reliability of the novel method for all involved lower limb muscle groups. There was also no substantial difference between all operators and analysers combinations. To our knowledge, the potential effect of various operators/analysers combinations on the reliability of flexibility measures has not yet been reported with such a method. Most previous reliability studies used the intraclass correlation coefficient (ICC) as a measure of reliability (Berryman, 2002). ICC does not provide an index of the expected trial-to-trial noise in the data, but rather reflects the ability of a test to differentiate between individuals. Moreover, the ICC is sample size dependent and largely affected by the heterogeneity of the between-subject measures. Hopkins (2001) therefore proposed to use the typical error of measurement as the most appropriate measure of reliability. Typical error of measurement represents the noise occurring from trial-to-trial, which might confound the assessment of real changes in repeated measures (i.e., when monitoring changes in players). The ICC obtained with our method was therefore provided for information in Table 1, but will not be discussed in this article. When angle measures were repeated over different days, we observed CV values ranging from 2.6 to 12.4%, with substantial differences between the different muscle groups (Table 1). Most of the CV values were within the ranges previously reported in the literature for similar muscle groups but using different methods. In the present study, the CV for hamstring was 3.3%, which was consistent with the data of Fredriksen *et al.* (1997). Involving only two operators and two subjects, these authors reported CV ranging from 0.8% to 3.2%. In another experiment, reliability of an isokinetic assisted hamstrings stretching protocol yielded a CV of 5.8–6.5% (Magnusson *et al.*, 1997). A recent study (Peeler and Anderson, 2008), exploring the flexibility of the rectus femoris with a modified Thomas test reported a CV value of 13%. In our study, the CV for the quadriceps measure was 8.3%. More recently, a study assessed the reliability of abduction (5.6%) and medial rotation (10.2%) ranges of motion measures using an electromagnetic tracking system (Nussbaumer *et al.*, 2010). We reported similar CV values as these authors for the same movement in our study. As mentioned earlier, it is worth noting that the reliability of the measures was muscle group-dependent: the CVs for the hip rotators were 9.6% and 12.4%, while this latter was only 2.6% for the hip flexors. We postulated that these differences might be related to variability in standardization for some measures. For example, while Berryman (2002) reported that positioning the hip at 0° or at 90° in flexion were equivalent in terms of reliability of measurement, we may consider the 0° position as more accurate (better thigh stability on the bench). The clinical implications of this method could help identify players with specific muscle flexibility imbalances during the pre-season screening, carried out in most football academies. It may help identify players at potential risk of injury due to poor flexibility. Longitudinal and age-specific flexibility measurement/ranges for the main lower limb muscles group could also be derived around the time of peak height velocity. This is a crucial period with regard to growth, the rapid change of intrinsic factors and increased injury risk. The method may provide reference values for players, not only throughout the competitive season but also during the rehabilitation process when a comparison can be made with the pre-injury data. Finally, the opportunity to switch staff without affecting the results is useful in the context of clubs and academies dealing with a large number of players.

## 5. CONCLUSION

The present study investigated the reliability level of a novel method to monitor the flexibility of the main lower limb muscles groups in elite youth soccer players. There were no substantial day-to-day differences in flexibility measures for all muscle groups, with CV ranging for 2.6 to 12.4%, depending on the muscle group considered. The reliability of the method was examiner-independent and there was no substantial difference between all possible operators versus analyser permutations.

## References

Ben, M. and Harvey, L.A., 2010, Regular stretch does not increase muscle extensibility: A randomized controlled trial. *Scand J Med Sci Sports*, **20**, 136–144.

Berryman, R.N., 2002, *Joint Range of Motion and Muscle Length Testing.* Philadelphia, PA: W.B. Saunders Company.

de Lucena, G. *et al.*, 2011, Prevalence and associated factors of Osgood-Schlatter Syndrome in a population-based sample of Brazilian adolescents. *Am J Sports Med*, **39**, 415–420.

Folpp, H. *et al.*, 2006, Can apparent increases in muscle extensibility with regular stretch be explained by changes in tolerance to stretch? *Austr J Physiother*, **52**, 45–50.

Fourchet, F. *et al.*, 2011, Reliability of video-based muscle flexibility measures in adolescent athletes. *Brit J Sports Med*, **45**, 348.

Fourchet, F. *et al.*, 2012, Reliability of a novel procedure to monitor the flexibility of lower limb muscle groups in highly-trained adolescent athletes. *Phys Ther Sport*, **1**, 1–7.

Fredriksen, H. *et al.*, 1997, Passive knee extension test to measure hamstring muscle tightness. *Scan J Med Sci Sports*, **7**, 279–282.

Hopkins, W.G. *et al.*, 2009, Progressive statistics for studies in sports medicine and exercise science. *Med Sci Sports Exerc*, **41**, 3–13.

Hopkins, W.G. *et al.*, 2001, Reliability of power in physical performance tests. *Sports Med*, **31**, 211–234.

Law, R. *et al.*, 2009, Stretch exercises increase tolerance to stretch in patients with chronic musculoskeletal pain: A randomized controlled trial. *Physical Therapy*, **89**, 1016–1026.

Magnusson, S.P. *et al.*, 1997, Determinants of musculoskeletal flexibility: Viscoelastic properties, cross-sectional area, EMG and stretch tolerance, *Scan J Med Sci* Sports, **7**, 195–202.

Mirwald, R.L. *et al.*, 2002, An assessment of maturity from anthropometric measurements. *Med Sci Sports Exerc*, **34**, 689–694.

Mountjoy, M. *et al.*, 2008, IOC consensus statement: Training the elite child athlete, *Brit J Sports Med*, **42**, 163–164.

Nussbaumer, S. *et al.*, 2010, Validity and test-retest reliability of manual goniometers for measuring passive hip range of motion in femoroacetabular impingement patients. *BMC Musculoskeletal Disorders*, **11**, 194–205.

Peeler, J.D. and Anderson, J.E., 2008, Reliability limits of the modified Thomas test for assessing rectus femoris muscle flexibility about the knee joint. *J Athl Train*, **43**, 470–476.

Philippaerts, R. *et al.*, 2006, The relationship between peak height velocity and physical performance in youth soccer players, *J Sports Sci*, **24**, 220–230.

Witvrouw, E. *et al.*, 2003, Muscle flexibility as a risk factor for developing muscle injuries in male professional soccer players: A prospective study. *Am J Sports Med*, **31**, 41–46.

# Part VII

# Training science, coaching and psychology

## CHAPTER FIFTY-SIX

# A case study of coach practices in skill acquisition training

J. F. Barkell and D. O'Connor

University of Sydney, Australia

## 1. INTRODUCTION

In recent years research into skill acquisition has identified a variety of alternate coaching strategies thought to enhance skill learning and overall skill retention. These changes revolve around increasing the amount of contextual interference and the variability of the training session and decreasing the frequency of feedback whilst utilising more implicit forms of instruction within the skill learning process (Ford *et al.*, 2010; Li and Wright, 2000).

Higher levels of contextual interference and variability in practice require the athlete to perform a number of motor skills in a myriad of scenarios so that they cannot generate a series of skill based steps to improve at the one skill. The athletes mind is required to constantly move from one skill to another in no particular order, similar to that of a game. Whilst this form of training increases errors in practice it does develop the cognitive skills of the athlete due to the involvement of decision making, higher levels of concentration, and the ability to refocus on a previously learned task (Porter and Magill, 2010; Robinson, 2010).

Similarly a reduced frequency of feedback has shown no negative effects on retention during practice. Alternatively it has been shown to produce positive retention effects due to athletes developing their own intrinsic feedback systems and less reliance on the coach. Implicit instructions lack the exact answer and require the athlete to discover the processes involved within a skill. This gives the athletes autonomy over their movements requiring less step by step processing throughout the movement (Porter and Magill, 2010; Masters, 2008).

The aim of this case study was to identify and compare coaching practices at the youth developmental level of football with two other team sports and examine how successful coaches at the youth development level give feedback and schedule practice sessions.

## 2. METHOD

### 2.1. Participants

Three premiership winning coaches (Football, Volleyball and Basketball) from Sydney Schoolboy competitions participated in this study. All were accredited coaches in their sport, qualified physical education teachers and former professional players in their chosen sport.

### 2.2. Procedure

Five training sessions from each sport were recorded totalling fifteen sessions. Sessions were video recorded for review and each session was subsequently coded according to five overlapping categories of coaching practice: contextual interference, variability, frequency of feedback, timing of feedback and the nature of feedback instruction.

Contextual interference was coded as blocked (practice that focused repeatedly on a single skill in a grid or drill format); serial (practice that utilised a variety of skills in a regular order); and random (practice that utilised a variety of skills in no specific order). Variability of practice was coded as either constant (practice that was performed repeatedly through grids) or variable (practice performed in a variety of modified game type formats or games).

Feedback was coded into three separate categories. The frequency was recorded by the total number of times feedback was being administered. The timing of feedback was categorised as either concurrent (during the performance) or terminal (after completing a performance or task). The nature of feedback instruction was coded as explicit (giving step by step instructions or corrections) or implicit (the use of analogies, questions or body gestures during feedback).

### 2.3. Data analysis

Data was entered into the Statistics Package for the Social Sciences (SPSS) version 17. For the purpose of exploratory analysis the following descriptive statistics were determined for all measured variables for each group: means (M), standard deviations (SD) and range. One-way analysis of variance with Tukey post-hoc tests at the critical value of $p < .05$ was used for determining statistical significance between the three coaches. One sample t-tests were conducted to determine differences between any variables across the 15 training sessions.

### 3. RESULTS

The mean and standard deviation for the various descriptors are displayed in Table 1. This analysis was the final percentage over the total 15 training sessions. Random practice and variable training were most commonly used in all 15 training sessions (p<0.01). The football coach, however, scheduled significantly more random practice (52.8%, p<0.01) and had greater variability of practice (67.9%, p<0.01) compared to the other coaches. The football coach gave players feedback on less occasions (22 v 53-55 p<0.01). Timing of the football coach's feedback was similar to the other coaches. The football coach used significantly more explicit feedback (91% p<0.01) than implicit feedback.

**Table 1** Mean and standard deviations for various practice descriptors.

| *Descriptor* | *Total* | *Football* | *Volleyball* | *Basketball* |
|---|---|---|---|---|
| Training time | 61.57 ±1.09 | 56.56 ±1.88** | 62.28 ±0.41 | 66.25 ±1.70 |
| Blocked (%) | 23.5 | 24.8 ± 7.71 | 24.01 ± 1.91 | 21.69 ±11.08 |
| Serial (%) | 8.16 | 0 | 3.45 ±3.32 | 21.03 ± 7.61** |
| Random (%) | 32.44 ** | 52.75 ± 3.74** | 25.55 ±2.56 | 18.97 ± 5.72 |
| Constant (%) | 20.4 | 9.7 ± 6.86* * | 29.54 ± 6.16 | 21.97 ± 3.58 |
| Variable (%) | 43.75* | 67.85 ± 4.96** | 23.46 ± 5.04 | 39.93 ± 5.08 |
| Feedback occurrences | 43.9 | 22.2 ± 1.1** | 56.6 ± 1.95 | 53 ± 8.92 |
| Concurrent (%) | 47 | 51.17 ± 12.65 | 52.38 ± 4.36 | 37.56 ± 3.79* |
| Terminal (%) | 53 | 48.83 ± 12.65 | 47.62 ± 4.36 | 62.44 ± 3.79* |
| Explicit (%) | 88* | 91.1 ± 6.2** | 83.99 ± 7.57** | 91.29 ± 4.91** |
| Implicit (%) | 12 | 8.9 ± 6.2 | 16.01 ± 7.57 | 8.71 ± 4.91 |

* P<.05    ** P<.01

# 4. DISCUSSION

## 4.1. Contextual interference

Data analysis of all 15 training sessions indicated that random practice was being used significantly more (p<0.01) than blocked or serial practice, answering the question of whether contextual interference was being applied in the training sessions. However, the football coach applied the principles of contextual interference more effectively by scheduling approximately half of his session as random practice which provides greater opportunities for learning and retention. This may facilitate performance improvement during competitive game situations (Lee and Simon, 2004). Nevertheless, it has been suggested that learning at the youth development level may benefit from an almost totally random environment that closely mirrors the changes in skill usages associated with match play (Williams and Hodges, 2005).

## 4.2. Variability of practice

Findings demonstrated that there was significantly more (p<0.01) time spent in variable practice as opposed to constant practice. This suggests that the youth development coaches are effectively applying skill learning principles to their practice. The football players spent significantly more time (67%, p<0.01) in variable practice utilising small sided games and modified games for much of their time spent on task. In most cases warm ups remained variable using games such as 'piggy in the middle', where players were forced to make decisions with regards to space, defenders and the quality of the pass they were receiving. The football group spent significantly less time (9%, p<0.01) in constant practice which was not consistent with a UK football study that reported football coaches spent a considerable amount of time in constant practice (Training Form) as opposed to variable practice (Playing Form) (Ford *et al.*, 2010). Possible reasons for this difference include the new Football Federation Australia (FFA) Curriculum (FFA, 2008), which highlights the importance of practising skills in modified or small sided game scenarios.

Increasing variability has demonstrated improved decision making skills, the ability to develop numerous skills at a time, develop more intrinsic forms of feedback and enhance skill transfer and retention. Other positives involved are that it involves a larger group of athletes remaining on task as opposed to waiting in turn (Ford *et al.*, 2010; Lawrence and Kingston, 2008).

Ways to increase the amount of variable training include scheduling skill practice into a variety of small sided and modified games. An example of a variable football drill which displayed an emphasis on passing was to pass the ball amongst teammates within a given area, an opposition team needed to try and steal the ball, whilst the emphasis was on passing and ball control, defenders worked on marking players and intercepting skills, whilst attackers needed to identify space, move into space and use communication skills to be effective. Once the attacking team could pass the ball uninterrupted amongst their teammates for eight passes, their team gained a point. This gave players targets and goals to achieve within their skill training.

Due to the amount of time the football group spent in variable practice, these players had the most opportunities to interchange and utilise skill sets whilst on the move due to more practice time being spent in that schema (Butler, 2010). Variable practice tends to be implicit in nature due to the number of skills being used at any one time and it contains fewer opportunities for instruction due to its free flowing nature. This form of practice develops players' cognitive awareness of when to use certain skills more efficiently than constant practice. This gives the players not only the skills needed to apply to the game but also the ability to know when to apply them (Ford *et al.*, 2010; Williams and Hodges, 2005).

### 4.3. Frequency and timing of feedback

The football coach offered feedback on significantly fewer (p<0.05) occasions than the other coaches. Feedback was offered 21% of the time during the football training sessions of which only 16% was terminal, with an average of four episodes of feedback per 10 minutes. Therefore the football players had the greatest opportunity to develop their own intrinsic feedback and develop problem solving skills whilst on the move (Lawrence and Kingston, 2008).

Arguments against high frequency of feedback and reliance on coach feedback refer to the unavailability of feedback whilst in the midst of competition. In numerous team sports (e.g. football) once the game starts players have little contact with the coach and the players must make their own decisions. However, sports such as basketball use time outs and have constant stoppages allowing more access to coach feedback and instruction. This could have some bearing in the way feedback was administered between the three sports.

### 4.4. Instructional feedback

Studies written on the nature of feedback indicate that implicit feedback possesses two quality learning traits. Firstly there is an unconscious learning process that takes place and secondly that it generates an abstract knowledge of a skill rather than step by step instructions (Gebauer and Mackintosh, 2007; Masters and Maxwell, 2004). Within this study very little emphasis was placed on implicit feedback from any of the coaches. Masters (2008) discusses the drawbacks of overusing explicit feedback claiming that athlete reinvestment during pressure situations is one of the major reasons against the use of explicit instructions. Giving athletes the answers takes away the thought process needed to make effective decisions.

The infrequent implicit instructional feedback offered by the football coach was in the form of questioning players, using analogies and non-verbal cues. This form of feedback had the opportunity to be used more frequently, especially during terminal feedback situations. This demonstrates there may be little knowledge of the effects of implicit feedback at this level of coaching.

### 5. CONCLUSIONS

Results of the study suggest there is some awareness into scheduling the various characteristics that enhance skill acquisition into coaching sessions; however, more development into coach education could be carried out within the leading sporting body's coach education system. Interestingly it was the football coach who performed the most random practice, the highest amount of variability and the lowest frequency of feedback. This may be due to the large emphasis placed on training variability and the use of small sided and modified games within the FFA coaching curriculum (FFA, 2008). With regards to coach education it may be hypothesised that other sports place too much emphasis on explicit skill explanations and technical aspects of the sport with little regard to researched coaching principles. This may give coaches the technical knowledge, however, provide little instruction on skill learning principles. This identifies possible practical deficiencies within youth sports coach education programs.

## References

Butler, A.C., 2010, Repeated testing produces superior transfer of learning relative to repeated studying. *J Exp Psychol*, **36**, 1118–1133.

Football Federation Australia, 2008, *FFA National Curriculum.* Australia: FFA.

Ford, P.R. *et al.*, 2010, An analysis of practice activities and instructional behaviours used by youth soccer coaches during practice: Exploring the link between science and application. *J Sports Sci*, **28**, 483–495.

Gebauer, G.F. and Mackintosh, N.J., 2007, Psychometric intelligence dissociates implicit and explicit learning. *J Exp Psychol*, **33**, 34–54.

Lawrence, G. and Kingston, K., 2008, Skill acquisition for coaches. In *An Introduction to Sports Coaching: From Science and Theory to Practice*, London: Routledge, pp.16–27.

Lee, T.D. and Simon, D. A., 2004. Contextual interference. In *Skill Acquisition in Sport: Research, Theory and Practice*, London: Routledge, pp. 29–44.

Li, Y. and Wright, D.L., 2000, An assessment of the attention demands during random and blocked practice schedules. *Quart J Exp Psychol*, **53A**, 591–606.

Masters, R.S.W., 2008, Skill learning the implicit way – say no more! In *Developing Sport Expertise: Researchers and Coaches Put Theory into Practice*, London: Routledge, pp. 89–103.

Masters, R.S.W. and Maxwell, J.P., 2004, Implicit motor learning, reinvestment and movement: What you don't know won't hurt you. In *Skill Acquisition in Sport: Research, Theory and Practice*, London: Routledge, pp. 207–228.

Porter, J.M. and Magill, R.A., 2010, Systematically increasing contextual interference is beneficial for learning sport skills. *J Sports Sci*, **28**, 1277–1285.

Robinson, P.E., 2010, *Foundations of Sports Coaching.* New York: Routledge.

Williams, A.M. and Hodges, N.J., 2005, Practice, instruction and skill acquisition in soccer: Challenging tradition. *J Sports Sci*, **23**, 637–650.

# CHAPTER FIFTY-SEVEN

# The coach–athlete relationship in Australian touch football

A. Bennie[1] and C. Moran[2]

[1]School of Biomedical and Health Sciences, Univ. of Western Sydney, Australia
[2]Human Movement and Health Education, Univ. of Sydney, Australia

## 1. INTRODUCTION

Sporting success is strongly related to the psychological aspects of sport, not merely physical training and natural ability (Iso–Ahola, 1995) and there are many different psychological aspects of sport that influence athletes' experiences. One of the most influential factors is the coach–athlete relationship. This relationship is decisive in competitive sport as it impacts on athlete satisfaction, self-esteem, and performance (Jowett and Cockerill, 2003; Jowett and Meek, 2000; Philippe and Seiler, 2006). For some athletes, the coach–athlete relationship shapes their entire sport experience and has a profound impact on the quality of both practice and athletic performance during competitions (Poczwardowski *et al.*, 2002).

Much of the existing literature on coach–athlete relationships concentrates on either coach *or* athlete perceptions – not both – within *individual* sport settings. This needs to be addressed, because coach–athlete relationships are often didactic and as such, research needs to examine both sides of the coach–athlete relationship to gain a holistic understanding of coach–athlete interactions. Furthermore, team sport environments warrant further investigation, because 'the dynamics involved in individual sports are much different than those in team sports' (Jowett and Meek, 2000). The present research explores the characteristics of coach–athlete relationships within one mixed sex adult touch football team in Australia. The aim is to present a detailed insight into the common experiences of elite team sport coaches and athletes. A further aim is to provide a deeper understanding of the type and nature of coach–athlete relationships that exist within the unique 'mixed' team sport setting of touch football in Australia.

## 2. METHODS

The adult mixed touch football team recruited for this study compete in Australian representative competitions at local (Sydney based competition known as *Vawdon Cup*), state (New South Wales [NSW] *State Cup*) and national (*National Touch League, NTL*) level in Australia. In 2010, the team finished second in the *NTL* and in 2008-2009, they finished third in the *Vawdon Cup*, *NSW State Cup* and *NTL*.

One male coach and 11 athletes (male=7; female=4) participated in semi-structured individual or focus-group interviews.

The interpersonal constructs of Closeness, Co-orientation and Complementarity (3Cs; Jowett and Cockerill, 2003) guided both the interview questions and data analysis process as recommended by previous studies investigating the coach–athlete relationship (Philippe and Seiler, 2006; Jowett and Meek, 2000). The 3Cs refer to *Closeness* (emotional bond that exists between an athlete and a coach), *Co-orientation* (both the coach and athlete have shared goals, beliefs, values and expectations) and *Complementarity* (interactions between a coach and an athlete which promote teamwork, common goals and collaboration; Jowett and Cockerill, 2003). These three constructs provide a reliable and valid framework for researching the characteristics and qualities of positive and negative coach–athlete relationships (Philippe and Seiler, 2006). The interview schedule was adapted from Jowett and Cockerill's (2003) standardised open ended interview schedule by using the same questions but adapting terminology to suit touch football participants (Moran, 2010). Following verbatim transcription of the interviews, qualitative content analysis was undertaken (Philippe and Seiler, 2006; Weber, 1990). The researcher examined the responses, highlighting key words and sentences containing these words. These key words/sentences represented a single first order. For example, the following statements represented the initial code termed 'Respect': 'The respect I have for him mainly, knowing what he knows and how good a player he is' (MP11). Similar terms or quotes containing these themes were collated and allocated to second order themes, which were then placed into the pre-defined constructs of the 3Cs (see Table 1).

To maintain anonymity, participants were allocated terms such as FP1, meaning Female Player 1. To ensure trustworthiness in the research process, member checking occurred where the data was sent back to the participants to confirm the credibility of the information derived from the data analysis (Creswell and Miller, 2000). No changes were required after this procedure. The use of focus groups also helped to increase the trustworthiness of the data, as other team members were present and able to identify any discrepancies in the information provided (Flick, 2005).

## 3. RESULTS AND DISCUSSION

The discussion has been structured according to the three constructs of Closeness, Co-orientation and Complementarity and their underlying themes (see Table 1). It was impossible to include quotes from the participants throughout this section given the enormity of data generated and paper length. Please refer to Moran (2010) for detailed participant accounts.

Two key themes emerged under the construct of Closeness—Personal Feelings and Essential Coach–Athlete Requirements. Personal Feelings such as trust and friendship have an important influence on establishing the relationship, as researchers have identified the significance of an emotional connection between the coach and the athlete (Philippe and Seiler, 2006). Essential Coach–Athlete Requirements referred to critical factors that help establish and maintain the relationship such as mutual respect, belief and admiration. In the current study, many of the participants' responses referred to the respect and admiration they have for the coach due to his knowledge, previous success and ability (playing and coaching). For example, Male Player 2 stated that 'I have a high level of respect for my coach. The amount of technical knowledge ... and time that goes into his coaching ... is much more than any other coach I have had in the past.' The high value placed on mutual respect, belief and admiration and the essential role they play in the nature of coach–athlete relationships has also been identified in preceding studies with athletes from individual and team sports at recreational to international level (Olympiou *et al.*, 2008). The nature of the coach–athlete relationship in this unique mixed team sport environment, where multiple additional variables to do with gender and ability may influence the development and ongoing nature of the coach–athlete relationship, is similar to that of individual and other team sports contexts. Hence, these findings confirm that Personal Feelings and Essential Coach–Athlete Requirements form key elements of Closeness that are the basis for positive coach–athlete relationships in team and individual sport settings.

**Table 1** Constructs and themes from data analysis.

| Construct | 2nd Order Themes | 1st Order Themes | | |
|---|---|---|---|---|
| **Closeness** | **Personal Feelings** | Like | Trust | Friendship |
| | **Essential Coach–Athlete Requirements** | Respect | Belief | Admiration |
| **Co-orientation** | **Communication and Sharing Knowledge** | Technical communication/ instruction | Individualised communication | |
| | **Goals and Shared Understanding** | Common goals | Respecting the goals set | |
| **Complementarity** | **Helping Transactions** | Seeing the positives | Selflessness | |
| | **Respecting the Roles** | Roles and tasks | | |

Co-orientation was underpinned by the themes of Communication and Sharing Knowledge, and Goals and Shared Understanding. The theme Communication and Sharing Knowledge reflected the coach's technical communication and how the transfer of technical information helped provide a shared understanding of the game, a crucial outcome of Co-orientation. Other coaching research has also shown that a high level of technical knowledge is considered vital for effective coaching (Côté and Gilbert, 2009) and greatly contributes to the overall nature of the coach–athlete relationship (Stirling and Kerr, 2009). At times however, the immense level of knowledge the coach possessed had a negative impact on the coach–athlete relationship. The coach also highlighted how poor communication inevitably caused problems developing player performances:

... sometimes people say 'Yes I understand' but really they mean 'No, I do not understand but I do not want to say anything'. This makes our training ineffective as we spend time working on ... our defensive policy ... Then we start running and they let in tries ... This wastes time as we then have to go over the policy again.

As in previous research, this comment shows that professional knowledge alone is insufficient for developing positive coach–athlete relationships (Côté and Gilbert, 2009). The present study also highlighted the value of understanding how different athletes learn and react to various forms of communication. For example, Female Player 7 stated that:

The only area where I think the relationship could be improved is an increase in positive feedback. I know he is highlighting things we need to improve but our team can get down if we are not playing well and it is hard to turn that around ... when there is no positive feedback.

Alternatively, Male Player 10 identified the coach's use of critical feedback as an important part of their relationship: 'His constant communication about areas of improvement. He will talk to me after a game and after training about things I might need to work on.' This supports previous research where female athletes were more likely to respond to and desire positive feedback, whereas male athletes were more likely to respond to critical feedback (Sherman *et al.*, 2000). As athletes react and learn in different ways, it is important for coaches to continuously develop their interpersonal knowledge base so that they can communicate appropriately and effectively with their particular athletes (Côté and Gilbert, 2009). Hence, coaches need to establish good communication skills in order to develop successful relationships with their athletes. In the construct of Co-orientation, the second theme of Goals and Shared Understanding represented explanations about common goals and respecting the goals set. These features were crucial to the athlete-coach relationship, as shown by Male Player 5:

... as long as my interest is similar he is happy to work with me as much as I want. He also has a sincere interest in making me a better player. He doesn't want our team to win based on one person's skills, he would rather us win because we all played a part.

This supports previous research which found that an athlete's knowledge of, contribution to, and agreement with, team goals play an important part in the coach–athlete relationship (Poczwardowski *et al.*, 2002). The entire team must share the respect for the goals, as goals will only be achieved if enough of the team are motivated and desire the same outcome (Widmeyer and Ducharme, 1997). The findings highlight the high value placed on the coach's communication and goal setting skills. These factors were linked to the construct of Co-orientation and were crucial to developing strong coach–athlete relationships.

The themes that emerged under the construct of Complementarity were Helping Transactions and Respecting the Roles. Helping Transactions included times when the coach was selfless in developing player potential and saw the positives in challenging situations. Being selfless was something that this coach made a clear priority with his players and the players acknowledged this as positive attribute about the coach. For example, Male Player 3 indicates:

> He is happy to do extra hours with you [and that] has helped heaps of us. It also frees up time at training if he has already done some one-on-one stuff with someone so we can focus on team stuff at training instead.

Selflessness is important for both the coach and athletes within a team environment as it enhances their relationship through complimentary feelings. This notion supports Jackson and Delehanty's beliefs that 'selflessness is the soul of teamwork' (1995, p.6). The coach needs to be selfless in offering their support, knowledge and time to develop athlete performance. In return, athletes also need to be selfless by being prepared to train, work hard and execute their own role in the team.

Respecting the Roles was characterised by having respect for each member's roles and tasks in relation to how they contribute to the team. Players considered the coach–athlete relationship to be positive when there was a mutual respect of the roles and expectations required within the team. The coach shared this perspective and previous research found that mutual respect for each other's roles increases persistence, effort and interest in achieving team goals (Gill, 2000). These findings and previous research show that clear delegation of individual roles and respect for these roles are increasingly vital for the development of positive coach–athlete relationships in team sports (Potrac *et al.*, 2007). They also indicate that the nature of the coach–athlete relationship in mixed team sport settings is comparable to that in individual sport contexts.

## 4. CONCLUSION

The findings show how the coach–athlete relationship was characterised by personal feelings, such as trust, respect, belief and admiration. Instruction offered by the coach, and the way in which this was communicated to the individual, were integral characteristics of the relationship. Seeing the positives in one another, selflessness and respecting the roles and tasks assigned by the coach were also important characteristics of the relationship. As such, the findings support the three interpersonal constructs of Closeness, Co-orientation and Complementarity. One major finding from this study was that the nature of the coach–athlete relationship in a team sport setting remained similar to that in an individual sporting context. This conclusion was surprising given the unique mixed environment of the elite team in the present study where a male coach worked with male and female athletes. It would therefore be prudent for future research to compare team and individual sport perspectives to clarify where key similarities and differences exist across each setting. A comparative study with junior athletes would also be useful, as few studies thus far have considered the nature of the coach–athlete relationship in the youth context. Overall, this research builds on existing beliefs about coach–athlete relationships and demonstrates how positive coach–athlete relationships act as a major contributor to the satisfaction, self-esteem and performance of an athlete in various sport settings.

## References

Côté, J. and Gilbert, W., 2009, An integrative definition of coaching effectiveness and expertise. *Int J Sports Sci Coaching*, **4**, 307–323.

Creswell, J. and Miller, D., 2000, Determining validity in qualitative inquiry. *Theory into Practice*, **39**, 124–130.

Flick, U., 2005, *An Introduction to Qualitative Research*. London: Sage Pubs.

Gill, D., 2000, *Psychological Dynamics of Sport and Exercise*, 2nd ed., Champaign: Human Kinetics.

Iso-Ahola, S.E., 1995, Intrapersonal and interpersonal factors in athletic performance. *Scand J Med Sci Sports*, **5**, 191–199.

Jackson, P. and Delehanty, H., 1995, *Sacred Hoops: Spiritual Lessons of a Hardwood Warrior*, New York: Hyperion.

Jowett, S. and Cockerill, I.M., 2003, Olympic medallists' perspective of the athlete–coach relationship. *Psych Sport Exerc*, **4**, 313–331.

Jowett, S. and Meek, G.A., 2000, The coach–athlete relationship in married couples: An exploratory content analysis. *The Sport Psychologist*, **14**, 157–175.

Moran, C., 2010, The coach–athlete relationship in touch football: A qualitative investigation of coach and athlete perceptions. Honours Thesis, Univ. Sydney.

Olympiou, A. *et al.*, 2008, The psychological interface between the coach-created motivational climate and the coach–athlete relationship in team sports. *The Sport Psychologist*, **3**, 423–438.

Philippe, R.A. and Seiler, R., 2006, Closeness, co-orientation and complementarity in coach–athlete relationships. *Psych Spor Exerc*, **7**, 159–171.

Poczwardowski, A. *et al.*, 2002, The athlete and coach: Their relationship and its meaning. Results of an interpretive study. *Int J Sport Psych*, **33**, 116–140.

Potrac, P. *et al.*, 2007, Understanding power and the coach's role in professional English soccer. *Soccer and Society*, **8**, 33–49.

Sherman, C. *et al.*, 2000, Gender comparisons of preferred coaching behaviours in Australian sports. *J Sport Behav*, **23**, 389–406.

Stirling, A. and Kerr, G., 2009, Abused athletes' perceptions of the coach–athlete relationship. *Sport in Society*, **12**, 227–239.

Weber, R.P., 1990, *Basic Content Analysis*, 2nd ed., London: Sage Publications.

Widmeyer, N. and Ducharme, K., 1997, Team building through team goal setting. *J Appl Sport Psych*, **9**, 97–113.

# CHAPTER FIFTY-EIGHT

# Perceptions of effective coaching in Australian professional team sports

A. Bennie[1] and D. O'Connor[2]

[1]School of Biomedical and Health Sciences, Univ. of Western Sydney, Australia
[2]Human Movement, Health and Coach Education, Univ. of Sydney, Australia

## 1. INTRODUCTION

Effective coaching is a multifarious term described in many ways over time. While research into effective coaching was conducted intermittently throughout the 1960s, it was not until the late 1970s that research in this area began to flourish (see Chelladurai and Carron, 1978; Smith *et al.*, 1977). The topic of effective coaching has featured in leadership research (Chelladurai, 1984), systematic observation of coach behaviour (Smith *et al.*, 1983) and more recently qualitative research with expert coaches (see Côté *et al.*, 1995; Côté and Sedgwick, 2003). Despite the broad strategies employed by previous researchers to investigate effective coaching, the term 'effective coaching' remains problematic.

## 2. METHOD

This study examined the concept of effective coaching based on the perceptions (through interviews) and behaviours (via observations) of four, male, professional coaches and 17 athletes from Australia. The aim was to explore what professional coaches do, and what makes coaches effective in their day-to-day roles. The participants were from two teams; one from the *National Rugby League* (highest level of club rugby league in the world) and one from the *Super Rugby* (highest level of provincial rugby union in the southern hemisphere). Interviews enabled participants to discuss their interpretations of their unique professional contexts from their own point of view while the observational data identified various coaching strategies and interactions with players during training and competition contexts. The analysis of data involved Grounded Theory (GT) analytic procedures (Côté *et al.*, 1993). This involves constant comparative analytic procedures where the researcher compares, contrasts, and re-analyses the data to make sure that what is reported accurately details the information from the interviews and observations. The constant comparison method was used to create (a) tags, (b) properties, and (c) categories (Côté *et al.*, 1993).

## 3. RESULTS AND DISCUSSION

The analysis of observation and interview data revealed a total of 636 raw data units that included statements and quotations from a few words to entire paragraphs. There were a similar number of meaning units per sport with rugby league at 317 and rugby union 319. Further inductive analysis produced 70 tags, 22 properties and 8 major categories. The 8 major categories include: (1) Personal Coach Characteristics and Knowledge; (2) Coach Philosophy; (3) Leadership; (4) Communication; (5) People Management; (6) Planning; (7) Developing a Positive Team Environment; and (8) Team Culture. It was impossible to include quotes from the participants throughout this section given the enormity of data generated and paper length. Please refer to Bennie (2009) for detailed participant accounts.

### 3.1. Personal coach characteristics and knowledge

The coaches and players in the current study outlined that effective coaching involves the possession of various personal qualities (e.g. empathy, approachable), knowledge (e.g. technical and tactical understanding of the game), characteristics (e.g. calm, honest) and skills (e.g. organisation skills). The present research identified many qualities and skills of effective coaching that were widely recognised in previous studies with individual and team sport participants, across geographic localities and with coaches and athletes from youth to Olympic sport arenas (Durand-Bush and Salmela, 2002; Gilbert and Trudel, 2000). The findings also support Côté and Gilbert's (2009) recent contention that the coach's knowledge of sport related information as well as inter and intrapersonal skills forms a core part of coaching effectiveness. The qualities, knowledge and skills outlined by these Australian participants suggest that there are specific characteristics valued by both coaches and players from different professional team sport contexts.

### 3.2. Coach philosophy

When describing their own philosophies, which they inherently believe to underpin effective coaching, the coaches suggested their ultimate goal was to educate players so that they developed both on and off the field as people and players. This concurs with previous research across a variety of team (Kellett, 1999) and individual sport contexts (Côté *et al.*, 1995) where the ultimate goal of coaching was to develop the athlete and improve performance. More recently, however, coaches have acknowledged the vital role they play in developing the total person (Bennie and O'Connor, 2010; Vallée and Bloom, 2005) rather than merely developing player performance. This is significant because in many professional sport environments, the coach's win-loss record generally supersedes these more holistic aims.

## 3.3. Leadership

The findings show that coaches possess their own personal approach to leadership and that various leadership strategies are considered effective. Importantly, the coach's leadership approach must align with the players' preferred leadership style for the coach to be considered effective. This shows support for previous research (Chelladurai 1984; Côté and Gilbert, 2009), which suggested that the coach's leadership behaviour is dependent on the situation, the coach and the group members. Therefore, various leadership approaches can be employed for a coach to be considered effective and experience success. Effective coaching also involves the head coach being able to adequately delegate clear roles and responsibilities and their ability to make significant decisions based on the team's on- and off-field requirements. Empowerment is a formative concept that also evolved from research with college basketball and volleyball (Vallée and Bloom, 2005) as well as professional AFL coaches (Kellett, 1999) where the head coach's role involved overseeing the entire coaching process and facilitating player development. This type of approach has become increasingly prominent with the advent of professionalism in Australian sport, and the rising number of assistant coaches and support staff associated with the coaching process.

## 3.4. Communication

When analysing the data, it became apparent that effective communication surfaced as one of the most crucial concepts outlined by both the players and coaches. This concurs with previous research that identified good communication as a key interactive, negotiation and teaching skill in coaching (Côté and Sedgwick, 2003). Effective coaching involves honest and open communication to develop and maintain trust and respect between players and coaching staff. Coaches in the present study provided tactical instructions and feedback to players during meetings and training sessions more frequently than any other form of communication. Further to this, a steady, transparent approach in day-to-day coaching was effective as it instils confidence in the players during the highs and lows of their sporting experiences. These findings support Dorfman (2003) who suggested that predictability in communication provides confidence and security for the players while also allowing them to focus on what they are doing instead of what the coach may do. Participants in the current study also mentioned that effective coaching occurs when coaches understand how their players learn and tailor their communication strategy to suit their needs. This is important as each individual responds differently to feedback or instructions provided in a public or private environment.

## 3.5. People management

The current research revealed that effective coaching requires people management skills that reflect the coachs' ability to develop and then manage relationships with and between players, and create a team environment where everyone works cohesively towards common outcomes. Interestingly, players and coaches in the current study provided different opinions about the extent to which the relationship should exist beyond the nature of the training environment. Some professional coaches and players feel socialisation is significant for the development of coach-player relationships while other participants believe that effective coaching involves knowing when to talk 'work' and when to generate other conversations with players. This highlights the unique social and contextual nature of the coaching process, whereby different types of relationships exist between sport contexts yet are considered equally effective by various players and coaches. Identifying individual needs emerged as a significant category in the current research and in previous studies on expert coaching (Côté and Sedgwick, 2003). Under the auspice of people management, effective coaching also includes the ability to identify and cater for the individual needs of each player in the team. This is crucial for managing the team dynamic and building player confidence.

## 3.6. Planning

Crucial to the development and ongoing maintenance of player confidence and a positive environment are the coaches' planning skills. Effective coaching requires coaches to plan sessions that are enjoyable and challenging to develop player competency levels on a consistent basis. Effective coaches plan training sessions so that players can practice game specific skills. They also provide for players to adequately recover, review their own performance, and contribute to the development of strategies for the team, prior to competition. In these professional settings, effective coaching involved the careful construction of an appropriate framework for training sessions to accommodate both team and individual training needs that are relevant to their sport (Côté and Sedgwick, 2003).

## 3.7. Developing a positive team environment

To achieve the ultimate goal of player development on and off the field, effective coaches create an environment that makes players feel supported, confident and comfortable. In these professional contexts, coaches developed a safe learning environment by allowing athletes to take risks, make mistakes and by guiding them in the right direction rather than punishing them for errors made. The above findings are similar to previous qualitative research that claims it is essential for coaches to provide a supportive (Kellett, 1999) or positive (Côté and Sedgwick, 2003) environment for players to learn and develop. Furthermore, research with professional coaches (Jones et al., 2004) presented empirical support for the notion that a positive learning environment enhances athlete performance and that athlete satisfaction is a pre-requisite for success at the highest level (Riemer and Chelladurai, 1998).

## 3.8. Team culture

Effective coaching involves the development of a common direction for the team where everyone involved with the team works together to achieve the team's goals. These features were often symbolised in a team 'trademark' or 'vision statement' which previous studies of team sport participants have described as a key organisational task of the head coach (Vallée and Bloom, 2005). The present research also supports the recent notion that developing 'connection' amongst the team is integral to coaching effectiveness (Côté and Gilbert, 2009). Effective coaching encourages a player-driven culture based on a strong work ethic which inspires players to train hard and work together to improve their individual and team performances. Kidman (2001) claims that an athlete-centred approach – where athletes gain and take ownership of knowledge, development and decision-making – helps maximise athlete performance by promoting a sense of belonging and a shared approach to learning. This demonstrates that coaches and players recognise the benefits of promoting a player-driven team culture and that one of the coach's most important roles is to influence the psyche of the players and build an appropriate framework for the players to achieve success.

## 4. CONCLUSION

Participants from rugby union and rugby league suggested that effective coaches placed less focus on the technical and tactical elements of coaching in comparison to the emphasis placed on the need for professional coaches to be good at working with people. It is plausible that one centrally agreed upon definition or model of 'effective coaching' may never exist, however, the current investigation offered an additional perspective on effective coaching – one that includes the perspectives of professional coaches and players from an Australian sports context. Acquiring the characteristics, qualities and skills outlined in this research involves a long-term process that draws on personal experiences in sport as a player, coach and member of society.

## References

Bennie, A., 2009, Effective coaching in cricket, rugby league and rugby union: A qualitative investigation involving professional coaches and players from Australia. PhD Thesis, University of Sydney.

Bennie, A. and O'Connor, D., 2010, Coaching philosophies: Perceptions from professional cricket, rugby league and rugby union players and coaches in Australia. *Int J Sports Sci Coach*, **5**, 309–320.

Chelladurai, P., 1984, Discrepancy between preferences and perceptions of leadership behavior and satisfaction of athletes in varying sports. *J Sport Psych*, **6**, 27–41.

Chelladurai, P. and Carron, A.V., 1978, *Leadership*. Vanier City: Canadian Association for Health, Physical Education and Recreation.

Côté, J. and Gilbert, W., 2009, An integrative definition of coaching effectiveness and expertise. *Int J Sports Sci Coach*, **4**, 307–323.

Côté, J. and Sedgwick, W.A., 2003, Effective behaviors of expert rowing coaches: A qualitative investigation of Canadian athletes and coaches. *International Sports Journal*, **7**, 62–78.

Côté, J. *et al.*, 1993, Organizing and interpreting unstructured qualitative data. *The Sport Psychologist*, **7**, 127–137.

Côté, J. *et al.*, 1995, The coaching model: A grounded assessment of expert gymnastic coaches' knowledge. *J Sport Exerc Psych*, **17**, 1–17.

Dorfman, H.A., 2003, *Coaching the Mental Game: Leadership Philosophies and Strategies for Peak Performance in Sports, and Everyday Life*. Lanham: Taylor Trade Publishing.

Durand-Bush, N. and Salmela, J.H., 2002, The development and maintenance of expert athletic performance: Perceptions of World and Olympic champions. *J Appl Sport Psych*, **14**, 154–171.

Gilbert, W.D. and Trudel, P., 2000, Validation of the coaching model (CM) in a team sport context. *International Sports Journal*, **4**, 120–128.

Jones, R. *et al.*, 2004, *Sports Coaching Cultures*. London: Routledge.

Kellett, P., 1999, Organisational leadership lessons from professional coaches. *Sport Management Review*, **2**, 150–171.

Kidman, L., 2001, *Developing Decision Makers: An Empowerment Approach to Coaching*, Christchurch: Innovative Print Communications Ltd.

Riemer, H.A. and Chelladurai, P., 1998, Development of the Athlete Satisfaction Questionnaire (ASQ). *J Sport Exerc Psych*, **20**, 127–156.

Smith, R.E. *et al.*., 1977, A system for the behavioral assessment of athletic coaches. *Research Quarterly*, **48**, 401–407.

Smith, R.E. *et al.*, 1983, Behavioral assessment in youth sports: Coaching behaviors and children's attitudes. *Med Sci Sports Exerc*, **15**, 208–214.

Vallée, C.N. and Bloom, G.A., 2005, Building a successful university program: Key and common elements of expert coaches. *J Appl Sport Psych*, **17**, 179–196.

# CHAPTER FIFTY-NINE

# Monitoring exercise load and recovery during the 2010 FIFA Soccer World Cup

M. Tschopp[1,2] and Z. Komes[2]

[1] Swiss Federal Institute of Sports Magglingen, Switzerland
[2] Swiss Football Association, Muri b. Bern, Switzerland

## 1. INTRODUCTION

When preparing soccer players for competition, it is crucial to apply a balanced load and recovery routine during the training process. Too heavy a load or insufficient recovery can result in decreased performance (Kenttä and Hassmén, 1998) and possible injuries (Gabbett and Jenkins, 2011). In contrast, too light a load will not lead to the desired training adaptations. Importantly, the physical preparation for a tournament such as the FIFA World Cup differs from that of regular season preparation for a variety of reasons (Bangsbo, 1998). This tournament with games at the highest competitive level occurs at the end of the regular season when players may be physically and mentally fatigued. For national teams, the players play in different clubs or leagues with seasons ending at different times. Therefore, players may be in different condition at the beginning of the preparation. In addition, the tournament may take place in specific environmental conditions, such as altitude at the FIFA 2010 World Cup in South Africa, that has an effect on the relative intensity of playing soccer (Levine et al., 2008) and as a consequence on training load. A tournament including preparation lasting for several weeks may also have a psychological stress for the players living separated from their usual social environment over a long period.

Considering these factors, a well-balanced dosage of exercise load and recovery is essential for optimal preparation. For appropriate planning and control of training process, many methods exist to quantify and monitor training load (Lambert and Borresen, 2010). The session Rating of Perceived Exertion method (RPE-method) (Foster et al., 1996) has become popular in recent years and was validated for soccer (Impellizzeri et al., 2004). Compared to methods based on heart rate, the session RPE-method includes training stress from a variety of training types (e.g., high-intensity exercise, plyometric or sprint training) (Foster et al., 2001), as well as non-physiological factors such as psychological stress. Therefore, it may be more appropriate for tournament preparation.

Interestingly, less attention has been paid to monitoring daily recovery in soccer to date. However, it is known that high training load normally leads to reduced recovery (Fry *et al.*, 1991). This reduction may differ between players because it depends on a number of factors including the quantity of the previous load, fitness level and recovery strategies (Borresen and Lambert, 2009). In this regard, it seems important to know the recovery state of the team and the players to plan the next training load properly. Kenttä and Hassmén (1998) described a method for monitoring recovery, which is similar to the session RPE-method. It involves a self-evaluation of the overall psychophysiological recovery of the athlete once a day for the previous 24 hours using a scale (6–20 point Total Quality Recovery (TQR) Scale). However, in the existent literature, only a few studies have explored monitoring training process in elite soccer players.

Taken together, the specific situation of a tournament such as the FIFA World Cup 2010 may have a particular exercise load and recovery interaction in soccer players. The aim of this study was therefore to quantify exercise load during both the preparation and tournament phases of the 2010 FIFA World Cup ($WC_{2010}$), and to evaluate its effects on the ability of players to recover.

## 2. METHOD

The exercise load of 23 Swiss national team soccer players (age: $27.1 \pm 3.9$ years, height: $183.3 \pm 6.9$cm, weight: $80.9 \pm 5.8$kg) was recorded during 33 days of the 2010 FIFA soccer World Cup ($WC_{2010}$). This included 25 training sessions (TS) and five games (two preparation games and three final-round games). Of these, 15 training sessions and 1 final-round game were carried out at a low altitude level (1350–1600m above sea level). Training sessions included specific conditioning exercises (e.g. plyometrics, sprints), small sided games and technical as well as tactical exercises. Individual training, training in small groups, and training beside the pitch were not included in the analysis. The global exercise load was obtained using the session-RPE method ($L_{RPE}$), as described by Foster *et al.* (1996). Players were asked to rate their perceived exertion 15–25 minutes after each TS. For games, the duration of the warm up was added to the official game playing time and only players who played the entire game were included. Heart rate (HR) was measured in 23 training sessions with radio technology data transmission from players' chest belts to a central receiver unit (Acentas, Hörgertshausen, Germany). HR-based training load ($L_{HRI}$) was calculated using a method similar to that of Edwards (Impellizzeri *et al.*, 2004). This involved multiplying the accumulated training time (in minutes) of 4 HR zones by a coefficient relative to each zone according to a formula provided by the manufacturer (60-80% of $HR_{max} = 1$, 80–90% of $HR_{max} = 2$, 90–95% of $HR_{max} = 4$, 95–100% of $HR_{max} = 8$). Every morning before breakfast, the players were asked to record their recovery score (RS) on a scale from 1 (no recovery at all) to 10 (maximal recovery) (adapted from the TQR Scale, Kenttä and Hassmén, 1998). The rational for adapting the 6–20 point TQR Scale was to use an analogous 1–10 point range as for the RPE scale. All players were accustomed to using session-RPE and the adapted TQR. For data analysis, the mean training load per day (per training, respectively) was calculated by dividing the mean of the individual total training load by the number of days (number of TS for calculating the mean load per TS, respectively) in the corresponding training phase (building phase: 13 days/14 TS, tapering phase: 10 days/6 TS and tournament phase: 10 days/5 TS, respectively). Standard deviation (SD) refers to between players and not to between TS or games differences. A repeated-measures ANOVA was used for the analysis of differences in training load and RS, respectively. Training phase was the independent variable as within-subject factor with three levels (building, tapering and tournament). Pearson's correlation coefficient was used to calculate the relationship between $L_{RPE}$, $L_{HRI}$ and RS respectively. The level of statistical significance was set at $p \leq 0.05$.

## 3. RESULTS

The mean $L_{RPE}$ per player in the different tournament phases are presented in Table 1. $L_{RPE}$/day in the tapering phase and tournament phase was only 56% and 75% of the $L_{RPE}$/day in the building phase, respectively. $L_{RPE}$/TS was significantly lower during the tournament phase compared to the building and tapering phase. The mean $L_{RPE}$/game was significantly higher in the tournament phase compared to the building phase and almost 3 times higer than for a training session.

**Table 1.** Mean and standard deviation of the exercise load ($L_{RPE}$) per player per day, training session (TS) and game respectively during the 3 phases in arbitrary units (AU). [a] Only players who played the entire game included. * Statistically different to building phase, [#] statistically different to tapering phase.

|  | $L_{RPE}$/day Mean±SD | $L_{RPE}$/TS Mean±SD | $L_{RPE}$/game[a] Mean±SD |
|---|---|---|---|
| Building phase (13 days) | 347±53 AU | 290±45 AU | 678±121 AU |
| Tapering phase (10 days) | 196±23 AU* | 269±49 AU |  |
| Tournament phase (10 days) | 261±73 AU*[#] | 243±70 AU * | 796±143* AU |

Mean RS for the building phase (4.9±1.0) was significantly lower than for the tapering (5.5±0.8) and tournament phases (5.5±1.1), respectively. The highest RS was found on the day of a game (6.8±1.1), and the lowest RS was found on the day after a game day (3.6±0.8) (only players who played the entire game were included).

The variance of the $L_{RPE}$ the day before explained 52% of the RS variance (see Figure 1). RS was significantly and more tightly correlated with $L_{RPE}$/day than with $L_{HR}$/day (r: 0.92 vs. 0.76) in training days. There was a significant correlation between $L_{RPE}$ and $L_{HR}$ (r: 0.76) in TS (see Figure 2).

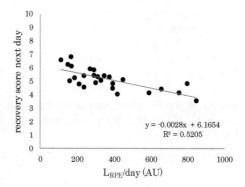

**Figure 1** Correlation between the mean daily exercise load (arbitrary units: AU) using the RPE-method and the mean recovery score the following day using the Adapted TQR-Scale.

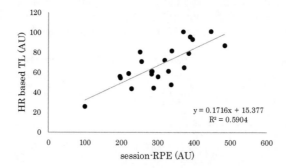

**Figure 2** Correlation between the mean training load using the RPE-method (session-RPE) and the mean training load based on heart rate measurement (HR based TL) (Arbitrary units: AU).

## 4. DISCUSSION

This is the first study monitoring training load and recovery during high-level tournament preparation and competition in elite soccer athletes. There are significant differences in mean daily training load between the different phases. The highest daily training load was measured during the 13-day building phase that ended 10 days prior to the first final round game. The recovery score was lowest during this phase, indicating a slight functional overreaching (Meeusen *et al.*, 2006). It can be assumed that the higher training load leads to a reduced recovery as we found a significant correlation between training load and the recovery score the next morning. It must be considered that during the building phase, players lived at altitude (1500m above sea level), which may have contributed to reduced recovery (Levine *et al.*, 2008). The reduction in training load (training volume) during the tapering phase was lower than recommended for optimal tapering (60–90%) (Muijka and Padilla, 2003). This may be because when approaching the start of the tournament, the focus was on technical and tactical aspects of the game, which required time for perfection, especially for national team players that rarely played together during the regular season. Nevertheless, recovery increased during this phase and was highest the day of the final-round games. The load of the games was much higher than for the training sessions, and for the competitive games significantly higher than for the friendly games. As a consequence, the recovery score was lowest the day after the final round games. Therefore, it seems to be important to implement recovery strategies after demanding games or training sessions (Bishop *et al.*, 2008). Interestingly, recovery level during the whole tournament phase was similar to the tapering phase. Players at this level may be habituated to high game load and emphasising recovery strategies may have reduced fatigue. However, cumulative fatigue might be expected with longer duration of the tournament phase. Training load using the RPE-method correlated significantly with the HR-based method, as shown earlier in soccer (Impellizzeri *et al.*, 2004). It must be added that the method for calculating TL from HR was specific to the HR system used and not exactly the same as described by Impellizzeri and colleagues. However, the correlation between the recovery score of the next day and the training load based on the RPE-method was higher than between recovery score and training load based on HR. This may be because both the RPE-method and the adapted TQR include psychophysiological aspects such as mental and social, as well as different physiological stress and recovery factors respectively (Foster *et al.*, 1996; Kenttä and Hassmén, 1998).

The training process during a tournament and its preparation phase is influenced not only by external training load, but also by multiple factors such as players' fitness level, differences in game load between players, length of the preparation period, as well as travelling and environmental circumstances. Therefore, it is crucial to monitor players' perception of training load and recovery to adapt the training plan if necessary. The session RPE-method and the adapted form of the TQR may be good instruments for optimising training for elite soccer players, as both methods can be administered daily in an applied setting such as tournament football. The session RPE-method is already well established, in contrast the adapted form of the TQR should be further validated.

## References

Bangsbo, J., 1998, Optimal preparation for the World Cup in soccer. *Clin Sports Med*, **17**, 697–709.

Bishop, P. *et al.*, 2008, Recovery from training: A brief review. *J Strength Cond Res*, **22**, 1015–1024.

Borresen, J. and Lambert, M.I., 2009, The quantification of training load, the training response and the effect on performance. *Sports Medicine*, **39**, 779–795.

Foster, C. *et al.*, 1996, Athletic performance in relation to training load. *Wisconsin Medical Journal*, **95**, 370–374.

Foster, C. *et al.*, 2001, A new method to monitoring exercise training. *J Strength Cond Res*, **15**, 109–115.

Fry, R.W. *et al.*, 1991, Overtraining in athletes: An update. *Sports Medicine*, **12**, 32–65.

Gabbett, T.J. and Jenkins, D.G., 2011, Relationship between training load and injury in professional rugby league players. *J Sci Med Sport*, **14**, 204–209.

Impellizzeri, F.M. *et al.*, 2004, Use of RPE-based training load in soccer. *Med Sci Sports Exerc*, **36**, 1042–1047.

Kenttä, G. and Hassmén, P., 1998, Overtraining and recovery: A conceptual model. *Sports Medicine*, **26**, 1–16.

Lambert, M.I. and Borresen, J., 2010. Measuring training load in sports. *Int J Sports Physiol Perf*, **5**, 406–411.

Levine, B.D. *et al.*, 2008, Effect of altitude on football performance. *Scan J Med Sci Sports*, **18**, 76–84.

Meeusen, R. *et al.*, 2006, Prevention, diagnosis and treatment of the overtraining syndrome: ECSS position statement task force. *Eur J Sport Sci*, **6**, 1–14.

Muijka, I. and Padilla, S., 2003, Scientific bases for precompetition tapering strategies. *Med Sci Sports Exerc*, **35**, 1182–1187.

CHAPTER SIXTY

# Small-sided games present an effective training stimulus in Gaelic football

K. Collins[1], D. Doran[2] and T. Reilly[2]

[1]Institute of Technology Tallaght, Dublin, Ireland, [2]Research Institute for Sport and Exercise Sciences, Liverpool John Moores University, Liverpool, UK

## 1. INTRODUCTION

Gaelic football teams with sports science support systems may benefit by gaining advantage over their opponents by being better trained and prepared. Current sport science knowledge of Gaelic football has been garnered from other field games, with limited research existing into the sport itself (Reilly and Collins, 2008). Gaelic football is an intermittent high intensity team game with higher work-rates than that observed for FA Premier League soccer players. In Gaelic football the players are required to perform longer higher intensity bursts with shorter recovery than their professional counterparts (O'Donoghue and King, 2004). The physiological demands of the game mean that players must be competent in several aspects of fitness which include: aerobic and anaerobic power, muscle strength, flexibility and agility (Reilly and Doran, 2001).

The amateur status and the consequential time demands of players requires an appreciation of training strategies which best serves the development of technical skill as well as the attainment of desired fitness levels. The most obvious means of inducing appropriate exercise stress that is compatible with Gaelic football match play is by replication of game play in the training setting. In soccer, small-sided games (SSGs) provide an equal physiological training stimuli compared to classic interval training (Reilly and White, 2005). It is believed SSGs replicate the movement patterns, physiological intensity and technical requirements of competitive match-play (Gabbett and Mulvey, 2008). However, the efficacy of SSGs for Gaelic football preparation and conditioning remains unknown. The purpose of this current study then was to assess the effects of eight weeks of SSGs training on the anthropometric and physiological performance of sub-elite Gaelic footballers.

## 2. METHODS

Seventeen sub-elite (club) Gaelic football players (Mean ± SD: age: 26 ± 4 yrs; stature: 180 ± 6.8 cm) participated in the study. Anthropometric measurements were taken prior to fitness testing and made in accordance with the standards of the

International Society for the Advancement of Kinanthropometry (ISAK). Whole-body fat mass was estimated by measuring the thickness of subcutaneous fat tissue in millimetres at four sites (biceps, triceps, subscapular and suprailiac) using Harpenden skin-fold calipers (Harpenden Instruments Ltd, England). The percentage body fat was calculated from the sum of the four skinfolds using the equation of Durnin and Womersley (1974).

A counter-movement jump (CMJ) was measured using a jump mat (Powertimer, Newtest Oy, Finland). Peak power was calculated using the equation of Sayers *et al.* (1999) and the relative peak power was identified. The sprint times of a participant was measured over 20 m, timing gates being located at 5, 10, and 20 m (Newtest Oy, Finland). Repeated sprint ability (RSA) was assessed using 12 x 20 m sprints with 20 sec recovery between each sprint. Overall time, mean time and sprint decrement was calculated using the equation of Fitzsimmons *et al.*, (1993). Cardio-respiratory fitness was assessed using the multi-stage fitness test (MSFT), which gives an estimation of maximal oxygen uptake ($\dot{V}O_{2max}$) (Ramsbottom, Brewer and Williams, 1988). Heart rate (HR) was measured every 5 s during the MSFT via short-range telemetry using the Polar Team System (Polar Electro, Finland). Heart rate was also classified into five intensity zones: these were recovery (<60% of $HR_{max}$), light intensity (60–75%), medium intensity (75–85%), high intensity (85–95%) and maximal (95–100%).

The intensity of exercise was monitored by means of HR response (Polar Team System, Polar Electro, Finland). The training involved small-sided games (4 vs 4) of 6 x 4 min (performed at >90% $HR_{max}$), with 3 min active recovery (performed at <60% $HR_{max}$) performed over an eight-week period (a total of 20 SSG sessions undertaken) (Reilly and White, 2005). The playing area was 80 x 20 m. The sessions were incorporated into the normal weekly programme of the players. Descriptive statistics (means and standard deviations) were calculated. A univariate analysis of variance (ANOVA) was performed using the Statistical Package for Social Sciences software (SPSS Version 16 program for MacOSX, Chicago, IL). Statistical significance was set at p<0.05.

## 3. RESULTS

Measurements were categorized into anthropometric (body mass, sum of four skinfolds and percentage body fat) and physiological characteristics (CMJ, peak power, relative peak power, 5-, 10-, 20-m sprint times, RSA (overall time, mean time and sprint decrement and estimated $\dot{V}O_{2max}$). Specific details of the variables measured are summarized in Table 1. The results from the experimental period show there was no significant change ($F_{1,32}$=.000; p=.989) in body mass. A non-significant reduction in the sum of four skinfolds ($F_{1,32}$=2.634; p=.114) and body fat ($F_{1,32}$=2.666; p=.112) was observed. The CMJ height ($F_{1,32}$=.866; p=.359), peak power ($F_{1,32}$=.357; p=.554) and relative peak power ($F_{1,32}$=.977; p=.330) improved, however, the change was not significant. Sprint speed over 5 m ($F_{1,32}$=6.237;

p=.018) improved significantly over the course of the intervention whilst sprint speed over 10 m ($F_{1,32}$=3.003; p=.093) and 20 m ($F_{1,32}$=1.881; p=.180), improved but not significantly. The RSA total time ($F_{1,32}$=15.074; p=.000), mean time ($F_{1,32}$=14.966; p=.001) and sprint decrement ($F_{1,32}$=4.396; p=.044) improved significantly. The estimated $\dot{V}O_{2max}$ ($F_{1,32}$=12.631; p=.001) significantly increased. The heart rate response during the SSGs averaged 91.8% of $HR_{max}$ and is within the target intensity thought to be effective in enhancing aerobic fitness (Helgerud *et al.*, 2001).

**Table 1** The anthropometric and physiological characteristics (mean ± sd) pre- and post-SSG training intervention.

| Variable | Pre intervention | Post intervention |
|---|---|---|
| **Anthropomteric** | | |
| Body mass (kg) | 79.3 ± 9 | 79.3 ± 8.7 |
| $\sum$4 Skinfolds (mm) | 28.9 ± 5.3 | 26.4 ± 3.7 |
| Bodyfat (%) | 12.1 ± 2.1 | 11.6 ± 1.6 |
| **Physiological** | | |
| CMJ (cm) | 43.1 ± 6.5 | 45.4 ± 7.8 |
| Peak power (W) | 4148 ± 651 | 4289 ± 723 |
| Relative peak power (W/kg) | 52.3 ± 4.7 | 53.98 ± 5.5 |
| 5 m (s) | 1.14 ± .08 | 1.08 ± .05* |
| 10 m (s) | 1.91 ± .09 | 1.86 ± .08 |
| 20 m (s) | 3.19 ± .12 | 3.13 ± .11 |
| RSA – Overall time (s) | 41.94 ± 1.21 | 40.63 ± .71* |
| RSA – Mean time (s) | 3.49 ± .09 | 3.39 ± .06* |
| RSA – Sprint decrement (%) | 7.4 ± 2.6 | 5.7 ± 1.9* |
| Estimated $\dot{V}O_{2max}$ ($mL^{-1}.kg.min^{-1}$) | 56.9 ± 1.9 | 59.4 ± 2.2* |

*Significant difference (p<0.05).

## 4. DISCUSSION

The current study is the first to describe the utilization of SSGs as a training methodology for Gaelic football conditioning. Despite its widespread application in other codes (Hill-Haas *et al.*, 2011) its use particularly in Gaelic football is limited. The major finding of study was that SSGs significantly improved in sub-elite Gaelic footballers aspects of high-intensity sprint repeatability and aerobic performance. The efficacy of SSG rests in their ability to stimulate both the skill-based, and the physiological stimulus representative of, or exceeding match-play (Hill-Hass *et al.*, 2011). In the present work SSG intensity exceeded the 85% $HR_{max}$ normally reported for Gaelic games (Reilly and Doran, 2001). The use of a 4 x 4 player ratio and larger pitch (80 m x 20 m) acts to increase the relative pitch area; in this context providing an efficient physiological stimulus similar to that observed with interval training (Sassi *et al.*, 2004; Reilly and White, 2005).

The SSG training programme proved an effective training stimulus in improving sprint repeatability. The current findings are in contrast to Hill-Haas *et al.* (2009) who utilizing the same assessment protocol observed no change in RSA in elite youth soccer players. Resultant from the SSG intervention protocol estimated maximal aerobic power increased by ~4.4 per cent, although lower than that reported for SSG training interventions in soccer players (Impellizzeri *et al.*, 2006) it exceeds that reported by others (Hill-Haas *et al.*, 2009). The lower values observed in the present study perhaps reflecting a shorter duration of training; 8 vs 12 weeks, and the amateur vs professional nature of the populations. Despite such variations across codes, the increase noted in aerobic capacity represents an important adaptation to SSG training given the critical role of high aerobic capacities in supporting recovery during the acyclical intermittent exercise observed during Gaelic football match-play.

In addition to the improvements in RSA and aerobic capacity, the power and high intensity performance were noted to improve, with CMJ and sprint speed over 5-, 10- and 20-m sprints enhanced, but attaining significance in only the 5-m split time. These improvements may reflect the increased training volume and intensity of the SSGs training intervention encouraging more explosive movements that results in a better 5-m split time. Such performance improvements may be reflected by an increase in the frequency of aerial fielding of the ball (jumping) required during an SSG and the requirement to apply short bursts of power to sprint over very short distances. Additionally, the influence of breaking contact from the man to man marking strategy commonly applied in Gaelic football (in order to make space to receive or distribute the ball) should also be considered as a training effect for these explosive capacities. As such the observed physical adaptations over the 8-week training period reflect the nature of the SSG stimulus applied. The lack of significant alterations in the longer duration sprints (20 m) is reflective of that noted by others in soccer specific SSGs (Hill-Hass *et al.*, 2009).

It should be noted as no control group was used it is unclear if the SSG is better than a traditional training methodology. However, it can be concluded that SSGs training presents an appropriate physiological training stimulus and therefore an effective training mode to enhance performance in sub-elite Gaelic football players. The evidence in the current study demonstrated that an 8-week SSG training intervention improved Gaelic football 5-m sprint speed, RSA and endurance performance. Careful selection of SSG format is required to optimize technical and tactical demands of the game. Future research should identify if SSG protocols would benefit elite Gaelic footballers who possess higher fitness levels than the sub-elite participants of the current study.

# References

Durnin, J.V. and Womersley, J., 1974, Body fat assessed from total body density and its estimation from skinfold thickness: Measurements on 481 men and women aged from 16 to 72 years. *Brit J Nutr*, **32**, 77–97.

Fitzsimons, M. *et al.*, 1993, Cycling and running tests of repeated sprint ability. *Austr J Sci Med Sport*, **25**, 82–87.

Gabbett, T. and Mulvey, M., 2008, Time-motion analysis of small-sided training games and competition in elite women soccer players. *J Strength Cond Res*, **22**, 543–552.

Helgerud, J. *et al.*, 2001, Aerobic endurance training improves soccer performance. *Med Sci Sports Exerc*, **33**, 1925–1931.

Hill-Haas, S.V. *et al.*, 2009, Generic versus small-sided game training in soccer. *Int J Sports Med*, **30**, 636–642.

Hill-Haas, S.V. *et al.*, 2011, Physiology of small-sided games training in football. *Sports Med*, **41**, 199–220.

Impellizzeri, F.M. *et al.*, 2006, Physiological and performance effects of generic versus specific aerobic training in soccer players. *Int J Sports Med*, **27**, 483–492.

Meckel, Y. *et al.*, 2009, Relationship among repeated sprint tests, aerobic fitness, and anaerobic fitness in elite adolescent soccer players. *J Strength Cond Res*, **23**, 163–169.

O' Donoghue, P.G. and King, S.M., 2005, Activity profile of men's Gaelic football, In *Science and Football V*, London: Routledge, pp. 205–210.

Ramsbottom, R. *et al.*, 1988, A progressive shuttle run test to estimate maximal oxygen uptake. *Brit J Sports Med*, **22**, 141–144.

Reilly, T. and Collins, K., 2008, Science of Gaelic sports: Gaelic football and hurling. *Eur J Sports Sci*, **1**, 84–94.

Reilly, T. and Doran, D., 2001, Science and Gaelic football: A review. *J Sports Sci*, **19**, 181–193.

Reilly, T. and White, C., 2005, Small-sided games as an alternative to interval training. In: *Science and Football V*, London: Routledge, pp. 344–347.

Sayers, S.P. *et al.*, 1999, Cross-validation of three jump power equations. *Med Sci Sport Exerc*, **31**, 572–577.

# CHAPTER SIXTY-ONE

# The effect of a training evaluation tool on youth coaches

W. Cotton and D. O'Connor

University of Sydney, Sydney, Australia

## 1. INTRODUCTION

According to the New South Wales (NSW) Department of Education and Training (2000) the time needed for an adolescent to develop a proficient level in a fundamental movement skill such as catching ranges from 240 to 600 minutes. However, recent research (Booth *et al.*, 2006) suggests that only 15–20 % of boys achieve mastery of a skill like a catch by Year 10. This evidence highlights the importance and place of a coach in the development of players' fundamental movement skills.

The NSW Department of Sport and Recreation recognised also this connection and in 2009 they commissioned O'Connor and Cotton to undertake a large scale study investigating, in part, skill development during youth coaching sessions (O'Connor and Cotton, 2009). Their research involved directly observing 70 coaching sessions involving 407 under 10 Rugby League (RL) and Rugby Union (RU) players, as well as 37 of their coaches. The results of their study revealed that 44% or 24.2 minutes of a training session were spent specifically on skill development, with catching and passing being the most prevalent skill practiced. However, simply having specific skill development time, does not necessary mean quality skill development time, as Siegel (2008, p. 9) suggests that 'the manner in which they [the skill sessions] are run by the coaches ... is also critical' (pg.9). O'Connor and Cotton (2009) identified that junior coaches spend large amounts of time instructing (48%) and managing (13%) players during training sessions, often at the expense of activity time, with players being inactive for 36% of a training session. O'Connor and Cotton (2009) also revealed youth coaches consistently overestimate the amount of time they spend during a coaching session on skill development and giving instructions.

Following on from these findings a paper based Training Evaluation Tool (TET) was developed to assist youth coaches by enabling the coaches to easily and accurately gather information about the skill development opportunities and physical activity levels of players during their training sessions. It was hypothesised that by using the TET, coaches could more accurately review their training sessions and potentially increase the activity levels and skill development opportunities of their players.

## 2. METHOD

The research methodology for the study was guided by the principles of controlled experimental design. The systematic observation of 64 under 10 coaching sessions included 480 Rugby League and Rugby Union players and 32 coaches.

The primary outcome of the study was to test if a six-week intervention targeting coaching behaviour could increase player activity levels and skill development opportunities. The intervention involved the use of the developed (TET).

### 2.1. The Training Evaluation Tool

The NSW Department of Sport and Recreation initially developed the TET to assist coaches to more accurately review their training sessions. The purpose was to cut down 'dead time' (inactivity) during a training session, and to improve skill development opportunities. The TET contained three sections. Section one focused on pre-activity instruction and group management analysis. This section provided a way, with the help of an assistant using a stopwatch, for a coach to determine the total time in which the players were not active in their training session. Section two was designed to help a coach review the number of times a player performed a particular skill during a specific activity in a training session (i.e. number of times a player tackles during a tackling drill). Again this involved the use of an assistant. The final section gave space for the coach to review what they have learnt about their coaching session and what they plan to do in the future to improve their coaching.

After the initial development, the TET was viewed by coaching experts both within and external to the NSW Department of Sport and Recreation, including coaches from the NSW Rugby League, Australian Rugby Union, Australian Sports Commission and the University of Sydney. Any suggested changes to the initial TET were considered by the NSW Department of Sport and Recreation and made where required.

The TET was tested for content validity and test-retest reliability. To examine content validity a panel of three experts in the field of coaching were asked to see if TET measures what it purports to measure. Several minor refinements were suggested and subsequently implemented before the panel of experts were satisfied that the criteria for content validity were met. The final version of the TET was then trialled with a group of youth coaches (n=5) to establish test-retest reliability. The retest was held two weeks after the original test. Data pertaining to the reliability was recorded and analysed and test-retest reliability was calculated using interclass correlation coefficients (ICC). The ICC for the first and second parts of the TET was 0.76 and 0.79 respectively. As these are above Nunnally's (1978) recommended minimum value of 0.70 the TET can be seen as a reliable instrument. The final version of the TET can be seen in *Community Junior Sport Coaching: Part 2 Final Report* (O'Conner and Cotton, 2010).

## 2.2. Measures

Data were collected within individual team settings. Baseline data were collected by trained research assistances from April and May 2010. After this period the intervention coaches (n=15) were trained in how to use the Training Evaluation Tool (TET) and were asked to use the TET, while the control coaches (n=17) continued with their regular coaching sessions. Subsequent follow-up data collection took place six weeks later in July and August 2010. Coach behaviour, player activity types and physical activity levels were measured using the following instruments:

- A modified version of McKenzie, Sallis and Nader's (1991) System for Observing Fitness Instruction Time (SOFIT). A momentary time sampling and an interval recording instrument.
- Pre- and post-session semi-structured coach interviews.
- An observational instrument adapted from the Coach Behavioural Assessment System (Smith, Smoll and Hunt, 1977) combined with the Arizona State University observation instrument (Lacy and Darst, 1984).

Each team (including coach and players) were observed twice and at baseline and twice at follow up. In-depth semi-structured interviews were also conducted after the intervention period with coaches who utilised the TET to obtain a deeper understanding of the coaches use of the TET.

## 2.3. Data analysis

Data collected during this research project was analysed in three different ways depending on the nature of the data gathered. First, the digital video recordings of each training session were captured on computer and uploaded into a web-based computer system called EVA (Educational Video Annotation). Each time a specified coach behaviour was observed, a trained research assistant coded the occurrence and the duration. This coding of the training session allowed for the coach behaviour to be quantified.

The second analytic procedure involved the data from the modified SOFIT instrument which indicated how physically active athletes were, how the coaches spent their time during training, and in the case of this study, what skills were performed during the training session. These data were again quantified and entered with the data from the video recording into the Statistical Package for the Social Sciences (SPSS ver. 17). A series of one-way Analysis of Variances

(ANOVAs), Chi-Square tests and correlations were performed on the data to determine if there were any significant differences between, or relationships within specific data fields.The third process involved analysing the qualitative data collected from the semi-structured interviews. Here, data analysis followed the techniques as recommended by Miles and Huberman (1994) and McCracken (1988). The analysis involved transcribing the data before coding pertinent comments into similar categories.

## 3. RESULTS

Results from the study revealed that no significant differences ($p<0.05$) between the intervention and control groups were found on any of the variables at the baseline collection point. Nor were any significant differences ($p<0.05$) found after the intervention period in session length, physical activity levels or with the time spent on fitness activities, practicing skills, or playing games. An overview of these and other outcome variables can be seen below in Table 1.

**Table 1** Post-test outcome measures of the control and intervention participants.

|  | *Control Group* | *Intervention Group* |
|---|---|---|
| **Coaching Session Length** (mins) | 52.4±12.5 | 53.5±17.0 |
| **Physical Activity Levels of Players** | | |
| Percentage time in sedentary intensity | 32.9±14.7 | 41.0±9.2 |
| Percentage time in moderate-to-vigorous activity | 65.1±10.1 | 59.0±4.8 |
| **Context of the Training Session** | | |
| Percentage time spent on fitness | 7.0±7.8 | 3.8±5.3 |
| Percentage time spent on skills practice | 46.9±19.1 | 48.8±21.4 |
| Percentage time spent in game play | 18.3±16.1 | 20.7±21.4 |
| **Skills Performed During Training Session** | | |
| Percentage time allocated to passing/catching | 11.9±12.7 | 3.5±3.8 |
| Percentage time allocated to ball carrying | 4.2±5.0 | 2.8±2.4 |
| Percentage time allocated to tackling | 12.2±11.6 | 4.7±8.3 |
| Percentage time allocated to kicking | 0.6±1.9 | 0.1±0.2 |
| **Coach Behaviour** | | |
| Percentage time giving instructions | 38.8± 8.2 | 33.5±6.3* |
| Percentage time on management/organisation | 16.8±9.7 | 18.6±8.7 |
| Percentage time spent on observations | 22.4±6.9 | 28.7±12.6 |
| Percentage time not on task | 7.9±6.1 | 6.4±5.9 |
| Percentage time affective behaviour | 10.1±4.2 | 8.9±6.0 |

* $p<.05$

A more detailed breakdown of the coach behaviour variables revealed that coaches who used the TET were found to give significantly shorter pre-activity instructions and significantly shorter concurrent instructions.

The qualitative results from the semi-structured interviews indicated that the majority of coaches who used the TET were surprised that the physical activity levels of their players during their training sessions had not increased as the coaches indicated that they had specifically focused on maximising player participation. However, the majority of coaches did report that they believe the TET assisted them to make positive changes to their coaching.

## 4. DISCUSSION

Results reveal that the TET is effective in providing accurate information regarding the amount of time players are not involved in physical activity, the number of stoppages during a training session, and the number of repetitions a skill is performed by a player. The interviews revealed that coaches generally liked the TET and that coaches using the TET perceived that they 'improved their sessions' (Coach D) by increasing the player activity level and by decreasing stoppages and 'talking too much' (Coach A). Interestingly, their perceptions were not supported by quantitative data as there were no significant differences ($p<0.05$) between the control group of coaches ($n=17$) and coaches using the TET ($n=15$) in the following areas: physical activity levels; amount and type of skills practice; and coach behaviour (organisation, instruction etc.). However, coaches who used the TET gave shorter pre-activity and concurrent instructions. This type of instruction can be consider more effective (Fisher *et al.*, 1982).

Coaches who used the TET generally only used it on one or two occasions. Most literature on changing behaviour would suggest it needs to be used over a longer period of time and at least five times to be effective.

## 5. CONCLUSIONS

The results of this study indicate that the use of the Training Evaluation Tool (TET) as an intervention to enable coaches to increase the physical activity levels and skill development opportunities for their players is limited. However, it is believed that the TET is perhaps the first step in improving community coaching practice, by increasing the coach's awareness of what actually happens during their coaching session. Further research still needs to be undertaken to investigate the best use of the additional knowledge produced by the TET.

## Acknowledgements

This project was funded by the Australian Sports Commission and the NSW Department of Education and Communities (Sport and Recreation). Credit for the initial development of the Training Evaluation Tool goes to Simon Woinarski from the NSW Department of Sport and Recreation.

## References

Booth, M. *et al.*, 2006, *NSW Schools Physical Activity and Nutrition Survey (SPANS) 2004: Full Report.* Sydney: NSW Department of Health.

Fisher, C. *et al.*, 1982, Coach–athlete interactions and team climate. *J Sport Psychol*, **4**, 388–404.

Lacy, A. and Goldston, P., 1990, Behaviour analysis of male and female coaches in female basketball. *J Sport Behav*, **13**, 29–30.

McCracken, G., 1988, *The Long Interview*. Newbury Park, CA: Sage Publications.

McKenzie, T.L. *et al.*, 1991, SOFIT: System for observing fitness instruction time. *J Teach Phys Educ*, **11**,195–205.

Miles, M.B. and Huberman, A.M., 1994, *Qualitative Data Analysis: An Expanded Sourcebook* (2nd ed.), Newbury Park, CA: Sage Publications.

NSW Department of Education and Training, 2000, *Get Skilled: Get Active. A K-6 Resource to Support the Teaching of Fundamental Movement Skills*, NSW Department of Education and Training.

Nunnally, J.C., 1978, *Psychometric Theory* (2nd ed.). New York: McGraw-Hill.

O'Connor, D and Cotton, W., 2009, *Community Junior Sport Coaching: Final Report.* Commissioned by the NSW Department of Sport and Recreation and the Australian Sports Commission.

O'Connor, D. and Cotton, W., 2010, *Community Junior Sport Coaching: Part 2 Final Report.* Commissioned by the NSW Department of Sport and Recreation and the Australian Sports Commission.

Siegel, D., 2008, How do youth sports affect a child's daily activity level? *J Phys Educ Recreation Dance*, **79**, 9.

Smith, R. *et al.*, 1977, A system for the behavioural assessment of athletic coaches. *Res Q*, **48**, 401–407.

# CHAPTER SIXTY-TWO

# The relevance of sports science information to coaches of football and rugby league

C. Nash and R. Martindale

Edinburgh Napier University, Edinburgh, Scotland, UK

## 1. INTRODUCTION

Sport science research into various areas, e.g. strength and conditioning, psychology, motor skill acquisition, has generated vast quantities of information for sport coaches (Bishop, 2008; Reid *et al.*, 2004; Williams and Kendall, 2007a). Sports scientists claim to make a significant contribution to the body of knowledge that influences athletic practice and performance (Bishop, 2008).

Recent studies have shown that coaches tend not to value information that cannot be readily translated into practical activities for use in their coaching (Nash and Sproule, in press; Williams and Kendall, 2007a; Quinlan, 2002). Spinks (1997) drew attention to differences between the focus of sports science research projects and coaches perceptions of the knowledge necessary to enhance their coaching.

Canadian University coaches (CIS) reportedly believe that sport science makes an important contribution to high-performance sport but gaps exist between what coaches are looking for and the research that is being conducted (Reade *et al.*, 2008). The Australian model favours multidisciplinary support teams, comprising assistant coaches, physiologists, psychologists, performance analysts and physiotherapists, managed by the coach (Reid *et al.*, 2004). Much of the sport science research carried out in Australia is quantitative in nature, and tends to focus on the sports of cycling, rowing, athletics and swimming (Williams and Kendall, 2007b).

The aim of this study was to determine how helpful sport coaches within football and rugby league found sports science support within their specific sports and coaching environments within a UK context. Given that research highlights that coaches feel there is a lack of practical application and direct relevance to their needs, a qualitative methodology, focus groups, was considered to be most suitable.

## 2. METHODS

Six groups of coaches were interviewed in focus groups, three each from football and rugby league. Each group consisted of 5-7 coaches, of novice, developmental or elite level in their respective sport and at the respective level. The semi-structured interviews lasted between 60 and 80 minutes, were digitally recorded and transcribed verbatim. Questions were asked around coaches' experience of sport science support, their understanding of the term sports science and the impact of sports science on their coaching. The data was inductively analyzed to interpret the meaning of the phrases used by coaches in response to questions as well as the discussion arising from the group interviews (Côté *et al.*, 1995).

## 3. RESULTS AND DISCUSSION

The analysis revealed 206 raw data themes that were developed into three distinct themes (with numbers of raw data themes in parenthesis):

- language (81)
- practical application (69)
- ease of access (56).

There were key differences between both sport and level of coaching. These findings are discussed using the coaches own words to highlight the depth and richness of their responses. The coaches have been named for clarity as follows: RL=Rugby League; F=Football; N=Novice; D=Developmental and E=Elite.

### 3.1. Language

There was much discussion of the language in which sports science research for academic publication was written. A National Coach (FE1) from the Football Association (FA) said:

> I'm a big believer that there shouldn't be a barrier to information and if the language used is of an academic nature, then that's a barrier too and it's not decrying grass roots culture, because sometimes it's a barrier to me. If that's a barrier, then it needs to be removed.

This view was backed by an elite rugby league coach (RLE1), who thought: Rugby league coaches have rugby league jargon and researchers have researcher jargon. However this was followed by his own personal reflection that: 'I believe we have a duty to educate coaches coming through as much as we can. Some of the jargon, if you like, has still got to stay there.'

The language being used appeared to these coaches to be unnecessarily difficult to understand in the minds of these coaches, which has been found in similar studies (Nash and Sproule, in press: Williams and Kendall, 2007a and 2007b). A developmental rugby league coach (RLD1) felt that he would not attempt to read them as: 'You get pages of tables of statistics and you look at N equals de de de de' although a football development coach (FD1) offered the following suggestion, thinking:

> I'm not saying get people to read it for you but if someone has read it and there's a clear message coming from a journal, can it be summarised and put on one page, these are the eight points that come out of this journal, fact, you know, they've done the research, it's backed by X, Y and Z as well in whatever it is, there you go. So you get the messages. That sounds a bit lazy but...

A national football coach (FE2) also stated: 'The idea of sitting down with a 30 page journal, you know, with a cuppa tea does not turn me on at all.' Some coaches have identified a need for more dissemination of research findings via coaching clinics and sports-specific magazines, and the use of more appropriate 'lay' language in information dissemination (Bishop, 2007).

### 3.2. Practical application

The elite rugby league coaches and developmental football coaches agreed emphatically that unless sports scientists could demonstrate how research findings could be applied to benefit players and coaches there was little point to their studies. An elite rugby league coach (RLE2) stated:

> I've come across a lot of theoretically very sound sport scientists who perhaps haven't been practical and that's really what you need from sport science is not only the knowledge but the ability to practically apply it.

And another (RLE3) backed this up saying: 'You don't improve players, you don't win trophies through theory. You do it practically.' A football development coach (FD2) reflected:

> I think coaches, in general terms, they like to see things applied. So for me I'd like to see that research applied to what I'm doing and even maybe be involved in the research itself, so that I can see how it's all gone about and what the outcome was at the end of it. So if there's a follow up to a piece of research going on and I can be involved in it, it'll be fantastic because then I would be more inclined to use it.

Another football development coach (FD1) took the aspect of practical application of sports science one step further:

> So if it's the science, it's not just the how you do it, it's what you're actually doing it for – the why. But why are we actually doing that and what are we

improving in the kids? Is it not just their physical literacy or is it the whole rounded person?

The influence of sports science on physical literacy was debunked by an elite football coach (FE3) who was of the opinion that: 'It's the most natural thing in the world. There's nothing scientific about me growing up being able to run and jump and play, it's just nature.' The aspect of practical application led to a heated discussion amongst these coaches about the strong influence that they perceived sport science and sports scientists to have within their sports. An elite rugby league coach (RLE3) indicated: 'I think that in sport in general, sports science is leading too many sports rather than the sports leading the sport science.' A football national coach (FE1) was of a similar opinion, saying:

> I think we're the sport definitely in danger of letting the sport science go off in this direction and drag the game with it when actually the game's the game, sport science should enhance the game. The pendulum's gone too far in the other direction in my opinion and it needs to come back a little bit.

The protectiveness of these coaches was apparent when discussing their perceptions of both the control given to sports scientists rather than the coaches as well as the difficulties associated with applications to coaching practice. The multidisciplinary research mentioned earlier found that most conflict between coaches and support teams arose when athlete issues were involved (Reid *et al.*, 2004). It also suggested that clear delineation of roles be established initially to allow harmonious development of a coaching programme, a concept the coaches in this study have not accepted.

### 3.3. Ease of access

Many coaches admitted that they did not work with sport scientists, or indeed any support, on a regular basis. The elite coaches, from both rugby league and football, had different experiences, with the football coaches utilising them extensively within the competitive environment but FE4 also thought:

> I think too often certainly in the club environment from my experience where they're left in isolation and I think that's what the negative is they're just seen as someone who warms the players up.

A professional rugby league coach (RLE4) was of the opinion that:

> as a sport, we're one of the leading lights in terms of embracing sport science, aren't we? In terms of new ideas and thoughts and things and we're forever

looking for those extra edges. But when you get to my level, you're a jack of all trades really, so as you coach, you tend to use a bit of everything.

He continued on to say:

It's the relationship between coaches and sport scientists that's the interesting bit, isn't it? How much is the coach also a sport scientist? You need to be able to ask the right questions, don't you?

This relationship he referred to takes time to develop and can only be reached when coaches and sports scientists interact on a regular basis, building a good working relationship. This was explained by a coach of a top English football team (FE5), stating that sports scientists needed to:

Be a part of the team, not apart from the team. So I've had experiences where there's been some terrific sport science working within the structure of the club guided and managed by the head coach or whoever, particularly for pre-season and rehab. I think that's a vital commodity.

A novice rugby league coach (RLN1) said: 'I don't see any sports scientists in my coaching, they're not really necessary and I don't know if I would use them even if they were available.' Another elite level football coach (FE3) agreed that sports science was not a high priority, thinking:

You don't need it that often. It's like one of those ones where you get a first aid certificate, you pray you never have to use it. So I mean, you don't lose it but, you know, if you're asked, you know, a test on the spot, so it's been refreshed I would suggest, once a year on various CPD things first aid, for injury, training and stuff like that.

So far, there has been little evidence to suggest that coaches rely on sport scientists for their information, which would indicate minimal interaction between sport scientists and coaches (Reade *et al.*, 2008). Over the years, sport science has mainly been viewed by coaches as inaccessible, too technical, or in many cases, non-applicable to the actual sport setting. There is a widening gap between scientific knowledge and practice and that, in general, the utilisation of research in practice is poor (Bishop, 2008).

There was also considerable debate within all of the groups as to what sports science actually was, some individuals favouring inclusive definitions whereas others stuck to very rigid criteria, for example, one football coach (FN1) seemed to consider sports science as physiology, saying: 'most academies will have dedicated sport science but very few have dedicated psychologists.' The British Association of Sport and Exercise Science (BASES) encourages accreditation in the disciplines of physiology, psychology and biomechanics as well as in interdisciplinary focus. Other coaches seemed to favour a more holistic definition, an example being FD4, thinking that:

> the way you structure practices and also consider the needs of the players – the age and the stage of their development and whether they are enjoying the sport – is all sports science to me.

Perhaps the national governing bodies of sport, in this case rugby league and football, need to introduce sports science and perhaps more importantly, sports scientists to coaches earlier in their development. One novice rugby league coach (RLN2) confirmed this by saying: 'I've only heard of sport science – never seen any at the club. This may allow a meaningful relationship to develop, enabling coaches and sports scientists to develop their own communication methods and meaningful applications to not just the sport but the players and the coaches. At present the situation was summed up by one football coach (FE5), who said:

> I mean, there were two great quotes on it. One was Winston Churchill who said, 'scientists should be on tap, not on top'. And Gerard Houllier said, 'football is too important to leave in the hands of sport scientists.'

## References

Bishop, D., 2008, An applied research model for the sport sciences, *Sports Med*, **38**, 253–263.

Côté, J. *et al.*, 1995, The coaching model: A grounded assessment of expert gymnastic coaches' knowledge, *J Sport Exerc Psychol*, **2**, 1–17.

Nash, C. and Sproule, J., (in press) Coaches' perceptions of their coach education experiences. *Int J Sport Psychol.*

Quinlan, D., 2002, More art than science: Top coach Dennis Quinlan joins the ongoing distance running debate. *Athletics Weekly*, **56**, 26–27.

Reade, I. *et al.*, 2008, New ideas for high performance coaches: A case study of knowledge transfer in sport science. *Int J Sports Sci Coach*, **3**, 335–364.

Reid, C. *et al.*, 2004, Multidisciplinary sport science teams in elite sport: Comprehensive servicing or conflict and confusion? *The Sport Psychologist*, **18**, 204–217.

Spinks, W.L., 1997, Sports research and the coach. *Sports Coach*, **19**, 18–19.

Williams, S.J. and Kendall, L., 2007a, Perceptions of elite coaches and sports scientists of the research needs for elite coaching practice. *J Sports Sci*, **25**, 1577–1586.

Williams, S.J. and Kendall, L., 2007b, A profile of sports science research (1983–2003). *J Sci Med Sport*, **10**, 193–200.

# CHAPTER SIXTY-THREE

# Coaching practice: turning the camera on yourself

D. O'Connor

The University of Sydney, Australia

## 1. INTRODUCTION

Coaches strive to create an effective learning environment for their athletes and have embraced video technology to provide objective information regarding the performance of their athletes and their opponents. Video analysis has been used to assist with the planning of future practice sessions, provide feedback to players and enhance learning and performance. However, video analysis is rarely used to improve coach learning and performance.

The first section of this paper provides an overview of the current literature on coaching effectiveness and expertise. Although a lack of consensus exists regarding what defines an expert coach we now have a better understanding of the coaching behaviours displayed by coaches. Systematic observation instruments have been used in previous research to identify the behaviours that coaches demonstrate in their coaching practice. This has enabled us to gain a better understanding of 'what' expert coaches do as well as identify how closely coaching practice reflects the research related to skill acquisition and athlete learning. More recently research is examining 'why' coaches exhibit these behaviours or utilise practice activities and the impact it has on athlete learning, performance and enjoyment. Finally, the use of a web-based video analysis system used to assist coach development is examined. This system provides access for coaches to analyse and annotate videos of expert coaches conducting practice sessions. Video analysis of themselves during practice sessions and competition is another method to assist with self-monitoring and highlight a coach's strengths and areas for improvement.

## 2. COACHING EFFECTIVENESS AND EXPERTISE

Coaching effectiveness or expertise is difficult to identify and has often been defined by one or more of the following:

- an athlete's level of achievement, e.g. win-loss record; developing national players; winning premierships or world championships
- athlete's personal attributes, e.g. athlete satisfaction and enjoyment

- a coach's years of experience, e.g. 10 years coaching and playing experience (Côté and Gilbert, 2009; Horton and Deakin, 2008)

Whilst at the elite level winning is of primary importance, other factors may better demonstrate a coach's performance. Similarly, the athletic result is not solely dependent on the coach's performance – player talent can be restricted due to salary cap and draft pressures, and injuries sustained by senior players are all influencing variables. In proposing a new definition of coaching effectiveness Côté and Gilbert (2009) question whether any research exists on expert coaches as the inclusion criteria has relied on experience or performance records. Their definition states coaching effectiveness is 'The consistent application of integrated professional, interpersonal, and intrapersonal knowledge to improve athletes' competence, confidence, connection, and character in specific coaching contexts' (p. 316).

Nevertheless, what do we currently know about expert coaches? In line with the above definition expert coaches have extensive knowledge in a number of areas and have developed this knowledge through a range of formal (e.g. university courses, certification programs), non-formal (e.g. coaching clinics, workshops and conferences) and informal learning situations (e.g. reading, coaching experience, interactions with other coaches) (Cushion *et al.*, 2010; Nelson *et al.*, 2006). Expert coaches invest in detailed planning and have contingency plans covering potential scenarios. Their knowledge and experience allows them to intuitively make decisions – with coaches often saying they go with their 'gut feelings' (Ericsson *et al.*, 2006; Schempp *et al.*, 2006) – and they can provide better solutions to problems (Chi *et al.*, 1981 cited in Schempp and McCullick, 2010). Expert coaches strive to continually learn and develop. They have strong self-reflection skills. They closely monitor the things they do well and they identify specific things that can be improved (DeMarco and McCullick, 1997; Schempp *et al.*, 2007).

Expert coaches are great teachers. They 'know what to say and when to say it' (Schempp and McCullick, 2010, p. 224). Expert coaches appear to 'see' more and offer better feedback to their players; they are able to distinguish between the important and unimportant (Ericsson *et al.*, 2006; Schempp and McCullick, 2010). They place a high priority on communication skills, are able to adapt to the learning preferences of their players and understand the players' perspective (Webster, 2009). They continually use key words or cues (e.g. John Wooden often used 5–8 words – 'hard, driving, quick steps' Coyle, 2009, p. 168) rather than lengthy instructions and frequently use purposeful questions (Schempp *et al.*, 2004).

Expert coaches achieve a consistent and superior performance. Any coach can become a 'more-expert' coach and as Schempp and McCullick (2010) note this can be achieved by 'identifying clear goals, undertaking the practice of important coaching skills, and learning all that can be learned from one's experiences and from others' (p. 230).

## 3. SYSTEMATIC OBSERVATION OF COACHING BEHAVIOURS

Case study research on coaches at various levels confirms that the behaviours of effective coaches consist of a high percentage of instructional strategies such as explanations, demonstrations, questioning and feedback (Becker and Wrisberg, 2008; Cushion and Jones, 2001; Lacy and Darst, 1985; Potrac *et al.*, 2007). The majority of these studies used either the Arizona State University Observation Instrument or the Coaching Behaviour Assessment Scheme to code coaching behaviours. Table 1 indicates that elite coaches spend 32–63% of a training session 'instructing' their players.

**Table 1** Amount of practice time spent on instruction.

| Sport | % practice spent on 'instruction' | Reference |
|---|---|---|
| Professional Soccer | 59.8 | Potrac *et al.* (2007) |
| Elite Soccer | 50.3 | Vangucci *et al.* (1997) |
| Youth Soccer | 58.2 | Cushion & Jones (2001) |
| College Basketball (John Wooden) | 62.7 | Tharp & Gallimore (1976) |
| College Basketball (Pat Summit) | 48.1 | Becker & Wrisberg (2008) |
| National team (soccer and basketball) | 32.0 | Horton *et al.* (2005) |

Interestingly, the most frequent type of instruction given by the legendary college basketball coaches was concurrent instruction which allows players to continue practicing while receiving brief, concise feedback often using 'cue' words (Becker and Wrisberg, 2008; Cushion and Jones, 2001). National coaches often only have access to their players in camp situations prior to major championships. In this context Horton *et al.* (2005) reported that coaches spend the majority of practice observing players (silence) with the emphasis when instructing players on tactics rather than technique. Observing players is now seen as a deliberate coaching strategy to enhance player learning while allowing the coach to observe and analyse player performance (Cushion, 2010).

Systematic observation research allows the comparison of coaching behaviours under different sporting contexts (e.g. youth v elite). This research revealed that a large number of team sport practices often suffer from under-utilisation of time. For example, during elite volleyball practices players are generally only inactive for 7% of the total training session compared to 36% during junior rugby league and rugby union training sessions (O'Connor and Cotton, 2010) and 48% of junior ice hockey practices (Horton and Deakin, 2008). Expert coaches have smooth transitions from one activity to another, use cues or give feedback on the 'run' and minimise the stoppages during practice for instruction. Not surprising, the amount of time the coach spends 'managing' or organising players also varies depending on the context. Coaches of youth teams spend approximately 13–15% managing players (O'Connor and Cotton, 2009) compared to 5–6.4% at the college or elite level (Potrac *et al.*, 2007; Vangucci *et al.*, 1997).

## 4. WEB-BASED VIDEO ANALYSIS

Video analysis of coaching practice can play an integral role in coach development. In the postgraduate coaching degree at the University of Sydney a web-based video analysis system (EVA) is employed. This system allows coaches to observe, analyse and annotate videos of national coaches conducting practice sessions that they often wouldn't otherwise get access to. Videotaping expert coaches highlights the emphasis placed on pressure, intensity and simulated game conditions during their practice sessions. Coaches observing these sessions can critically focus on areas such as communication (use of questions, cues and feedback), and the scheduling and type of practice activities compared to what they may do. This also assists the coaches to bridge the theory-practice gap in their development.

Coaches can also upload video of their own coaching or team meetings. Videotaping coaches in action so they can view their behaviours contributes to raising their awareness of what they actually do. This is beneficial as coaches' perceptions of their own behaviour are limited (Cushion, 2010; O'Connor and Cotton, 2009). Using the EVA system coaches can log-in from anywhere in the world and insert their observations and self-analysis into the comment box. Coaches can also respond to time-coded annotations made by other coaches.

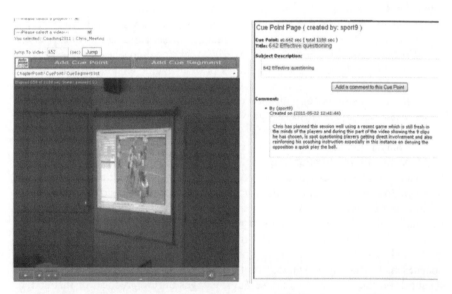

**Figure 1** Screen shot of web-based video analysis system allowing annotations.

This assists in creating a student centred learning environment that encourages exploration, lifelong learning and the fulfilment of one's potential. Knowles *et al.*

(2006) recommends the inclusion of 'reflection practices' to enhance learning. The EVA system allows reflecting-in and reflecting-on practice dilemmas (Schön, 1983) as part of coach development. For change to take place the coach must be aware of the issue or behaviour, actually want to change and then be supported and guided if new behaviour patterns are to be adopted (Stratford, 2001). In a number of instances, the coach identified specific aspects of their coaching behaviour to be evaluated indicating their acceptance and commitment to the learning process. Receiving valid feedback from colleagues or observing themselves coaching often provided the necessary evidence to stimulate the commitment to change. Coach action plans often involved identifying what to keep doing, start doing and stop doing. Below are comments from two coaches:

> After watching numerous coaches' tapes and video clips one of the specific items I'm going to implement this weekend in our games is the use of the assistant coach and myself to provide individual feedback to each player at half-time of our game.

> This type of team meeting is a regular occurrence for me and I felt comfortable in doing it. The video analysis system allowed me to look at the areas I need to improve. I really enjoyed the feedback from my peers – I wasn't aware that I failed to give players enough time to respond to my questions.

## 4. CONCLUSION

It has been reported that expert coaches are not only knowledgeable in the techniques and tactics of their sport but they also know how to interact with their athletes, plan effectively, have good teaching skills and self-monitor their own performance. The coaches reported that using the web-based video analysis system allowed them to receive honest feedback in a safe environment; become more accurate in their self reflections; assisted them in identifying their strengths and areas to improve and ultimately enhanced their confidence. Therefore, the application of this technology has many benefits and supports the reflective practitioner approach.

### References

Becker, A. and Wrisberg, C., 2008, Effective coaching in action: Observations of legendary collegiate basketball coach Pat Summit, *Sport Psychol*, **22**, 197–211.
Côté, J. and Gilbert, W., 2009, An integrative definition of coaching effectiveness and expertise. *Int J Sports Sci Coach*, **4**, 307–323.
Cushion, C, 2010, Coach behaviour, In *Sports Coaching: Professionalisation and Practice*, London: Churchill Livingstone, pp. 42–61.

Cushion, C. and Jones, R., 2001, A systematic observation of professional top-level youth soccer coaches. *J Sport Behav*, **24**, 354–375.

Cushion, C. *et al.*, 2010, *Coach Learning and Development: A Review of the Literature*, Leeds, UK: Sports Coach UK.

DeMarco, G. and McCullick, B., 1997, Developing expertise in coaching: Learning from the legends, *J Phys Educ Recr Dance*, **8**, 37–41.

Ericsson, K. *et al.*, 2006, *The Cambridge Handbook of Expertise and Expert Performance*. Cambridge UK: Cambridge University Press.

Horton, S. *et al.*, 2005, Experts in action: A systematic observation of 5 national team coaches, *Int J Sport Psychol*, **36**, 299–319.

Horton, S. and Deakin, J., 2008, Expert coaches in action. In *Developing Sport Expertise: Researchers and Coaches Put Theory into Practice*, London: Routledge, pp. 75–88.

Knowles, Z. *et al.*, 2006, Reflecting on reflection: Exploring the practice of sports coaching graduates. *Reflect Prac*, **7**, 163–179.

Lacy, A and Darst, P., 1985, Systematic observation of behaviours of winning high school football coaches. *J Teach Phys Educ*, **4**, 256–270.

Nelson, L. *et al.*, 2006, Formal, nonformal and informal coach learning: A holistic conceptualisation. *Int J Sports Sci Coach*, **1**, 247–259.

O'Connor, D and Cotton, W., 2009, *Community Junior Sport Coaching: Final Report.* Commissioned by the NSW Department of Sport and Recreation and the Australian Sports Commission.

Potrac, P. *et al.*, 2007, Understanding power and the coach's role in professional English soccer. *Soccer and Society*, **8**, 33–49.

Schempp, P. and McCullick, B., 2010, Coaches' expertise. In *Sports Coaching: Professionalisation and Practice*, London: Churchill Livingstone, pp. 221–231.

Schempp, P. *et al.*, 2004, Expert golf instructors' student-teacher interaction patterns. *Res Quart Exerc Sport*, **75**, 60–70.

Schempp, P. *et al.*, 2007, How the best get better: An analysis of the self-monitoring strategies used by expert golf instructors. *Sport Educ Soc*, **12**, 175–192.

Schempp, P. *et al.*, 2006, The development of expert coaching. In *The Sports Coach as Educator: Re-conceptualising Sports Coaching*, London: Routledge, pp. 145–161.

Schön D., 1983, *The Reflective Practitioner*. San-Francisco: Harper Collins.

Stratford, D., 2001, *Executive Coaching: The Key for Performance Improvement Through Personal Growth.* Melbourne: Information Australia.

Tharp, R. and Gallimore, R., 1976, What a coach can teach a teacher, *Psychology Today*, **9**, 75–78.

Vangucci, M. *et al.*, 1997, A systematic observation of elite women's soccer coaches. *J Interdiscip Res Phys Educ*, **1**, 1–17.

Webster, C., 2009, Expert teachers' instructional communication in golf. *Int J Sport Comm*, **2**, 205–222.

# CHAPTER SIXTY-FOUR

# Offensive sequences in youth soccer: experience and small-sided games effects

C. H. Almeida, A. P. Ferreira, A. Volossovitch and R. Duarte

Sport Expertise Laboratory, Technical University of Lisbon, Portugal

## 1. INTRODUCTION

The interactional effects of deliberate practice and its task constraints are not sufficiently explained in the skill acquisition and developmental programs of young soccer players. Some studies argued that capacities and knowledge of skilled players are essentially related to the time spent and quality of sport-specific practice, rather than to the maturation process (e.g., Williams, 2000; Vaeyens *et al.*, 2007; Ford and Williams, 2012). In a recent review, Ericsson (2006) suggested that the effects of mere experience differ greatly from those of deliberate practice (i.e., activities specifically designed to improve performance). We can assume that the time spent in these types of activities, which can be defined as deliberate practice experience, can be an important particularity in youth soccer developmental programs.

On the other hand, the use of small-sided games (SSGs) in these processes is a current circumstance that has triggered the attention of some researchers. Previous studies have pointed out that SSGs are an efficient strategy to increase players' specific practice time, eliciting simultaneously physical and technical aspects within a major tactical involvement (e.g., Duarte *et al.*, 2009; Hill-Haas *et al.*, 2009; Katis and Kellis, 2009). Thus, the acquisition of technical and tactical skills can be thought according to a net of interacting constraints such as the individual, task and the environmental constraints (Handford *et al.*, 1997; Williams and Hodges, 2005). In the scope of a constraints-led approach, the game format presented to players constraints them to solve specific game problems with implications on the individual and collective actions that are performed (Handford *et al.*, 1997). Nevertheless, it is not clear how players with different levels of experience respond to similar practice tasks.

Given the world-wide popularity of soccer compared to other team sports, the lack of scientific interest in the relationship between the deliberate practice experience and the manipulation of task constraints in the development of game performance is surprising (for an exception see Ford and Williams, 2012). Therefore, to better understand the attacking playing patterns emerging during SSGs performance, this study aimed to analyze the combined effects of both deliberate practice experience and SSG format on performance indicators that characterize the offensive sequences produced by teams of youth soccer players.

## 2. METHODS

Twenty-eight U-15 males were selected as participants. Parental written consent was received prior to the study. Participants were separated in two groups according to their deliberate practice experience in soccer. The Non-Experienced group (N-Exp) was constituted by 14 participants (age: 12.84 ± 0.63 years) selected from physical education classes with no deliberate practice experience in soccer. The Experienced group (Exp) was formed by 14 participants (age: 12.91 ± 0.59 years) selected from a U-15 team competing at the Portuguese regional level and with 3.93 ± 1.00 years of deliberate practice experience in soccer. Each group was divided into two balanced teams in the 7-a-side games: 1 goalkeeper, 2 defenders, 3 midfielders and 1 forward; and in the 4-a-side games, the same goalkeeper, one of the defenders, one of the midfielders and the forward took part in the experiment. Matches were always contested by teams with the same experience level.

Both groups of participants completed three independent sessions separated by one-week intervals. In each session, both groups performed the two SSGs – 4-a-side (3vs.3+GKs) and 7-a-side (6vs.6+GKs) games – during periods of 10 minutes interspersed with 5 minutes of passive recovery. The total number of SSGs performed was 12 (i.e., three of 4-a-side and three of 7-a-side games per group), and they were presented in a random order in each session. Whereas the 4-a-side game is frequently employed in training practices in youth soccer, the 7-a-side game is an official competitive game format used in younger age categories, across several countries. In the present study, these SSGs were played in pitches of size 46 x 31m and 62 x 40.4m (length x width), respectively. The relative space available for each player (ratio of pitch area per player), and the dimensions of goalkeeper areas (9 x 24m; length x width) were similar in both game situations. Prior to SSGs, participants performed a 10-min standardized warm-up. All the official rules of soccer have been implemented apart from the offside rule.

The units of analysis were the offensive sequences, which were understood as the execution of one or more individual and/or collective tactical-technical actions, defined according to criteria of beginning and end of ball possession. The characterization of each offensive sequence was carried out through a hand notational analysis system specifically designed for this purpose – Offensive Sequences Characterization System – and includes performance indicators previously applied in other investigations. Thus, the offensive sequences were characterized in terms of Duration of ball possession (Hughes and Churchill, 2005), number of Players involved (Garganta *et al.*, 2002), number of Ball Touches (Garganta *et al.*, 2002), number of Passes (e.g., Hughes and Franks, 2005), and number of Shots (e.g., Hughes and Franks, 2005). Since these performance indicators directly derived from the behaviors observed through the system, they will be designated as simple indicators. Moreover, some composite indicators were also analyzed to assist data interpretation. The composite indicators were defined as 'ratios' obtained by dividing two simple indicators (Hughes and Bartlett, 2002): Players involved/Duration of ball possession, Ball Touches/Duration of ball possession, Passes/Duration of ball possession, Ball Touches/Players involved, Passes/Players involved, Passes/Ball Touches, and Goal/Shots. Additionally, the simple and composite indicators were grouped in one of the two levels configured to characterize the offensive sequences: development and finalization.

The statistical analyses were held by applying non-parametric MANOVAs to assess the effects of 'experience level' and 'SSG format' on simple and composite indicators. Afterwards, multiple non-parametric Mann-Whitney tests were applied to discriminate pair wise differences. For all statistical procedures alpha ($\alpha$) was set at 0.05.

## 3. RESULTS

In the 12 matches played, an overall of 398 offensive sequences were identified. Table 1 presents the descriptive statistics (mean ± standard deviations) of performance indicators that characterize the offensive sequences revealed by players in each SSG.

**Table 1** Characterization of the offensive sequences: performance indicators values (mean ± s).

| | 4-a-side | | 7-a-side | |
| --- | --- | --- | --- | --- |
| Performance Indicators | N-Exp $\bar{x} \pm s$ | Exp $\bar{x} \pm s$ | N-Exp $\bar{x} \pm s$ | Exp $\bar{x} \pm s$ |
| **DEVELOPMENT** | | | | |
| Duration of ball possession (s) | 10.67 ± 6.53 | 12.39 ± 7.94# | 12.28 ± 9.04* | 15.17±10.10*# |
| Players involved | 2.28 ± 0.83*# | 2.64 ± 0.85*# | 2.80 ± 1.26*# | 3.40 ± 1.47*# |
| Ball Touches | 7.31 ± 4.67 | 8.47 ± 5.77 | 7.42 ± 5.45* | 9.64 ± 6.00* |
| Passes | 1.61 ± 1.48* | 2.58 ± 2.04* | 1.83 ± 1.68* | 3.03 ± 2.50* |
| Players involved/Duration | 0.28 ± 0.18 | 0.27 ± 0.14 | 0.29 ± 0.15 | 0.27 ± 0.11 |
| Ball Touches/Duration | 0.72 ± 0.25# | 0.69 ± 0.22 | 0.64 ± 0.23# | 0.66 ± 0.20 |
| Passes/Duration | 0.16 ± 0.13* | 0.2 ± 0.11* | 0.16 ± 0.11* | 0.19 ± 0.11* |
| Ball Touches/Players involved | 3.22 ± 2.04# | 3.04 ± 1.48 | 2.55 ± 1.22# | 2.83 ± 1.31 |
| Passes/Players involved | 0.59 ± 0.48* | 0.87 ± 0.56* | 0.55 ± 0.36* | 0.77 ± 0.50* |
| Passes/Ball Touches | 0.21 ± 0.16* | 0.29 ± 0.15* | 0.24 ± 0.15* | 0.29 ± 0.15* |
| **FINALIZATION** | | | | |
| Shots | 0.39 ± 0.56# | 0.5 ± 0.64# | 0.24 ± 0.53# | 0.28 ± 0.52# |
| Goals/Shots | 0.38 ± 0.48 | 0.17 ± 0.36 | 0.29 ± 0.44 | 0.26 ± 0.44 |
| **OFFENSIVE SEQUENCES** | **103** | **102** | **107** | **86** |

\* Significant difference ($P < 0.05$) between experience levels in each SSG format.
\# Significant difference ($P < 0.05$) between SSG formats in each experience level.

In 4-a-side games, the non-parametric MANOVAs demonstrated that the factor 'experience level' had a significant effect on simple and composite indicators that characterize the offensive sequences ($P = 0.001$ and $P = 0.001$, respectively). Concerning the development of offensive sequences, Mann-Whitney tests exhibit significant differences between groups (N-Exp vs. Exp) in number of: Players involved ($P = 0.003$), Passes ($P = 0.001$), Passes/Duration ($P = 0.005$), Passes/Players ($P = 0.001$), and Passes/Ball Touches ($P = 0.001$). No differences between experience levels were observed in performance indicators associated to the finalization of offensive sequences.

The application of non-parametric MANOVAs testified that the deliberate practice experience showed a significant effect on simple and composite performance indicators in 7-a-side games ($P = 0.012$ and $P = 0.024$, respectively). The Mann-Whitney test revealed that the offensive sequences differed significantly between both groups in the performance indicators: Duration of ball possession ($P = 0.016$), Players involved ($P = 0.004$), Ball Touches ($P = 0.003$), Passes ($P = 0.001$), Passes/Duration ($P = 0.009$), Passes/Players involved ($P = 0.001$), and Passes/Ball Touches ($P = 0.008$). No significant differences were observed at finalization level in any of the performance indicators analyzed.

The factor 'SSG format' evidenced a significant influence on simple and composite indicators of the offensive sequences produced by the 'N-Exp' group ($P = 0.001$ and $P = 0.001$, respectively). Significant differences were discriminated between SSGs in the following performance indicators: Players involved ($P = 0.003$), Ball Touches/Duration ($P = 0.003$), Ball Touches/Players involved ($P = 0.005$), and Shots ($P = 0.02$). Regarding the 'Exp' group, the non-parametric MANOVA reported a significant effect of the factor 'SSG format' only on simple indicators ($P = 0.001$). Hence, the differences between game formats in the 'Exp' group were only significant for the Duration of ball possession ($P = 0.033$), Players involved ($P = 0.001$), and Shots ($P = 0.011$).

## 4. DISCUSSION

Results from our investigation indicate that deliberate practice experience in soccer significantly influenced the characteristics of the offensive sequences produced by young footballers during SGGs. Differences between groups were identified in the performance indicators characterizing the development of offensive sequences, with a larger distinction in 7-a-side games. Overall, experienced participants adopted a 'possession playing' style, since they performed significantly longer offensive sequences, with a greater number of players involved, who, in turn, executed more touches on the ball and more passing actions. The non-experienced participants showed a tendency to build offensive sequences through individual actions, possibly trying to quickly explore the defensive disorganization that is common in lower skill levels. In this group, offensive sequences were, on average, shorter and involved fewer players, which is associated with the execution of a low number of passing actions.

The configuration of the SSG format (i.e., pitch size and number of players) manifested a significant effect on performance indicators. Evidence confirms that manipulating task constraints may induce modifications in specific behaviors of practitioners and, thereby, foster the development and improvement of technical, tactical, and strategic skills in team sports (Williams and Hodges, 2005). Data from the N-Exp group confirmed findings from other investigations (e.g., Duarte *et al.*, 2009; Katis and Kellis, 2009; Casamichana and Castellano, 2010), in which each player revealed a more effective relationship with the ball in smaller game formats. The Exp group exhibited greater stability in collective performance profiles between both game formats. The duration of ball possession and the number of players involved presented significantly higher values in 7-a-side games, which underscore the ability of the experienced teams to keep the ball in larger pitch sizes and involving more players.

Furthermore, decreasing the pitch size and player numbers provided an increase in the number of shots and goals. Such findings are consistent with previous research (e.g., Katis and Kellis, 2009; Casamichana and Castellano, 2010), which revealed that players had more opportunities for shooting and scored more goals in smaller game formats. Our data suggested that the game format clearly affects the quantity and quality of performed tactical-technical actions and, consequently, the offensive sequences' characteristics. Katis and Kellis (2009) argued also that SSGs can serve several purposes as specific means of training. Smaller game situations seem to be more appropriate for developing individual skills, particularly for those on the ball. In larger game formats, the number of actions that each player performs on the ball (i.e., Ball Touches/Players involved and Passes/Players involved) tends to decrease, increasing the number of 'off-the-ball' movements and the need to form an effective unit of cooperation with teammates. Such game formats may be useful to practice the specific movement requirements of competitive situations (Hill-Haas *et al.*, 2009).

## 5. CONCLUSIONS

Deliberate practice experience in soccer influenced the characteristics of the offensive sequences, which confirms the importance of an accurate diagnosis of the players' skill level in the design of specific skills acquisition and talent developmental programs for young soccer players. Besides, the manipulation of the pitch size and the number of players also affected the characteristics of the offensive sequences. Regardless of experience level, the results authenticate the propensity of participants to perform more shots and achieve more goals in smaller game formats. Therefore, we conclude that the smaller game formats are especially suitable for children/youngsters with no deliberate practice experience or a lower skill level in soccer, since they constrain the development of sport-specific skills based on a major involvement with the ball. On the other hand, larger SSG formats are useful in order to replicate specific requirements of a competitive situation and should be carefully considered as young soccer players improve game understanding and specific motor skills.

## References

Casamichana, D. and Castellano, J., 2010, Time-motion, heart rate, perceptual and motor behaviour demands in small-sided soccer games: Effects of pitch size. *J Sports Sci*, **28**, 1615–1623.

Duarte, R. *et al.*, 2009, Effects of duration and number of players in heart rate responses and technical skills during futsal small-sided games. *Open Sports Sci J*, **2**, 37–41.

Ericsson, K.A., 2006, The influence of experience and deliberate practice on the development of superior expert performance. In *The Cambridge Handbook of Expertise and Expert Performance*, New York: Cambridge University Press, pp. 685–705.

Ford, P.R. and Williams, A.M., 2012, The development activities engaged in by elite youth soccer players who progressed to professional status compared to those who did not. *Psychol Sport Exerc*, **13**, 349–352.

Garganta, J. *et al.*, 2002, Modelação táctica do jogo de futebol. Estudo da organização da fase ofensiva em equipas de alto rendimento. In *A investigação em futebol: Estudos ibéricos*, Porto: FCDEF-UP, pp. 51–66.

Handford, C. *et al.*, 1997, Skill acquisition in sport: Some applications of an evolving practice ecology. *J Sports Sci*, **15**, 621–640.

Hill-Haas, S.V. *et al.*, 2009, Physiological responses and time-motion characteristics of various small-sided soccer games in youth players. *J Sports Sci*, **27**, 1–8.

Hughes, M.D. and Bartlett, R.M., 2002, The use of performance indicators in performance analysis. *J Sports Sc*, **20**, 739–754.

Hughes, M. and Churchill, S., 2005, Attacking profiles of successful and unsuccessful teams in Copa America 2001. In *Science and Football V*, London: Routledge, pp. 222–228.

Hughes, M. and Franks, I., 2005, Analysis of passing sequences, shots and goals in soccer. *J Sports Sci*, **23**, 509–514.

Katis, A. and Kellis, E., 2009, Effects of small-sided games on physical conditioning and performance in youth soccer players. *J Sports Sci Med*, **8**, 374–380.

Vaeyens, R. *et al.*, 2007, The effects of task constraints on visual search behavior and decision-making skill in youth soccer players. *J Sport Exerc Psychol*, **29**, 147–169.

Williams, A.M., 2000, Perceptual skill in soccer: Implications for the talent identification and development. *J Sport Sci*, **18**, 737–750.

Williams, A.M. and Hodges, N.J., 2005, Practice, instruction and skill acquisition in soccer: Challenging tradition. *J Sport Sci*, **23**, 637–650.

# CHAPTER SIXTY-FIVE

# The use of accelerometers to quantify the training load in soccer

D. Casamichana, J. Castellano, J. Calleja-González and J. San Román

University of the Basque Country (UPV-EHU), Spain

## 1. INTRODUCTION

Traditionally, the ability of coaches to prescribe training load so as to optimize performance was the product of many years of experience (Borresen and Lambert, 2008). However, due to recent advances in the field of sport science the use of new technologies can now provide more specific information about workload, thereby facilitating the attainment of optimum performance (Barris and Button, 2008). The quantification of training load is therefore a key aspect when it comes to assessing the extent to which the objectives set prior to training have been met, and also enables this load to be modulated according to the period or phase of activity.

Actually a range of indicators have been employed to quantify workload in team sports, and they have been shown to be highly correlated with one another (Alexiou and Coutts, 2008; Borresen and Lambert, 2008; Foster *et al.*, 2001; Manzi *et al.*, 2010; Impellizzeri *et al.*, 2004). The main indicators in this regard are those based on heart rate: 1) the TRIMP method, proposed by Bannister (1991) and based on the duration of training, the maximum heart rate, the resting heart rate and the mean heart rate during exercise, and 2) the Edwards method (Edwards, 1993), which sums the values obtained in each heart rate zone.

In an attempt to simplify the quantification of training, and as an alternative to methods based on heart rate, Foster *et al.* (1996) developed what is known as the session rating of perceived exertion (session-RPE). The session-RPE is calculated using a 10-point scale (Borg scale) as a measure of intensity and then multiplying the value obtained by the duration of the training session (in minutes, which represents the volume of training).

Moving on to indicators of external training load, several techniques and instruments have been developed to measure this, with varying degrees of reliability (Barris and Button, 2008). In soccer, where intermittent activity is commonplace, the incorporation of new technology such as GPS devices is enabling new aspects of external load to be monitored among players. Furthermore, they can also be fitted with accelerometers, which are useful in any acyclic sport because the analysis of accelerations has certain advantages over traditional measures such as the distance covered or heart rate, since it takes into account actions other than just running (jumps, tackles, etc.). More specifically, accelerometry can be used to calculate *player load*, a measure of effort that has recently been employed to monitor the training of elite athletes in certain sports (Cunniffe *et al.*, 2009; Montgomery *et al.*, 2010). Consequently, the aim of the present study was to determine the validity of the *player-load* as an indicator of training load in soccer, based on correlations with other methods of quantification used in team sports.

## 2. METHODS

Participants were 28 semiprofessional soccer players (mean (±SD) age 22.9 (±4.2) years, height 177 (±5) cm, body mass 73.6 (±4.4) kg) who all played for the same team in the Spanish Third Division. All the players were notified of the research design and its requirements, as well as the potential benefits and risks, and they each gave their informed consent prior to the start. The Ethics Committee of the University of the Basque Country (CEISH) also gave its institutional approval of the study.

The players' external load was monitored and quantified by means of portable GPS devices (MinimaxX, v.4.0, Catapult Innovations) operating at a sampling frequency of 10 Hz and incorporating a 100 Hz triaxial accelerometer. The reliability and validity of the devices used in this study can produce better results (Castellano *et al.*, 2011) than those obtained in previous studies (Duffield *et al.*, 2010; Jennings *et al.*, 2010), which used a sampling frequency of 1 and 5 Hz. After recording, the data were downloaded to a PC and analysed using the software *Logan Plus v.4.4* (Catapult Innovations, 2010).

In order to monitor and quantify internal load, players wore a chest-strap monitor (Polar Oy, Finland) to record heart rate continuously during the training sessions. The RPE was obtained using the 10-point Borg scale as modified by Foster (1998), this being individually completed 30 min after training ended, thereby ensuring that players rated their physical exertion for the session as a whole. The details of the procedure followed has been described elsewhere (Alexiou and Coutts, 2008; Foster *et al.*, 2001; Manzi *et al.*, 2010; Impellizzeri *et al.*, 2004).

During the weeks prior to the study the players were familiarized with the equipment to be used. Then, before commencing the study, the maximum heart rate ($HR_{max}$) of each player was assessed by means of a specific resistance test, the Yo-Yo Intermittent Recovery Test Level 1 (YYIRT1). This provided a measure of both their $HR_{max}$ and the individual heart rate zones (Krustrup *et al.*, 2003).

A total of 44 training sessions were then monitored between January and April of the 2009–10 competitive season. Two to three sessions were monitored each week, with a mean duration of 90.4 (±23.0) min per session. In all 44 training sessions we monitored external load using the GPS devices, heart rate by means of the chest-strap monitors, and RPE with the Borg scale. All the sessions observed had been designed by the team's main coach and fitness trainer, who were present throughout.

The indicators of internal load were the Edwards method (Edwards, 1993) and the session-RPE. The former is based on heart rate and is calculated by multiplying the accumulated time in each heart rate zone (in min) by the weighting assigned to each zone of $HR_{max}$ (50–60% = 1; 60–70% = 2; 70–80% = 3; 80–90% = 4; and 90–100% = 5) and then summing the results obtained. The second indicator, the session-RPE, is obtained by multiplying the duration of each training session (in min) by the intensity assigned to that session on the RPE scale (Foster *et al.*, 1996). All sessions were recorded in their entirety, including recovery periods. The indicators of external load was *player load*, obtained via accelerometry (Cunniffe *et al.*, 2009; Montgomery *et al.*, 2010), combining the accelerations produced in three planes of body movement by means of a 100 Hz triaxial accelerometer. *Player load* is a new indicator which seems to be highly correlated with both heart rate and blood lactate levels (Montgomery *et al.*, 2010). The instantaneous value (1/100-s) is calculated using the following formula:

$$Player\ load_{(i)} = \sqrt{((aca_i - aca_{i-1})^2 + (act_i - act_{i-1})^2 + (acv_i - acv_{i-1})^2)}$$

where *aca* is the acceleration in the anteroposterior or horizontal axis, *act* is the acceleration in the transverse or lateral axis, *acv* is the acceleration in the vertical axis, *i* is the current time. These values are then accumulated over the sessions. The data are presented as means and standard deviations (±SD). The homogeneity of variances was examined by means of Levene's test, while the Pearson coefficient was used to assess the correlations between the different indicators of workload. All the statistical analyses were performed using *SPSS 16.0 for Windows*, with significance being set at $p < 0.05$ and $p < 0.01$.

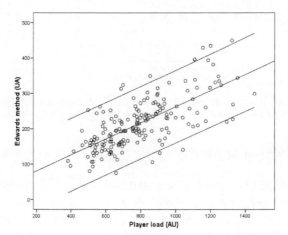

**Figure 1** Relationship between *player load* (determined by accelerometry) and the training load indicator obtained via the Edwards method for the 210 recordings made ($r = 0.70$; $p < 0.01$).

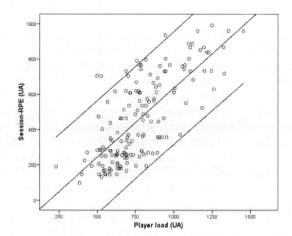

**Figure 2** Relationship between *player load* (determined by accelerometry) and the session-RPE indicator for the 210 recordings made ($r = 0.74$; $p < 0.01$).

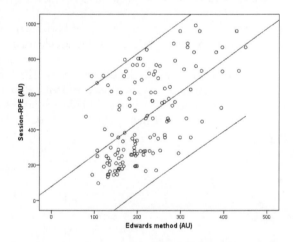

**Figure 3** Relationship between the session-RPE indicator and the training load indicator obtained via the Edwards method for the 210 recordings made ($r = 0.57$; $p < 0.01$).

## 3. RESULTS AND DISCUSSION

The average value of *player load* was 789.2 ±224.9 AU, while the *session-RPE* average was 462.4±237.9 AU and *Edwards' TL* was 216.3±72.6 AU. Figure 1 plots the correlation between *player load* (determined by accelerometry) and the training load indicator obtained via the Edwards method ($r = 0.70$; $p < 0.01$). Analysis of the correlation between *player load* (determined by accelerometry) and the session-

RPE indicator gave r = 0.74 ($p$ < 0.01; Figure 2). Analysis of the correlation between the session-RPE indicator and the training load indicator obtained via the Edwards method gave r = 0.57 ($p$ < 0.01; Figure 3).

The purpose of this study was to examine the relationship between workload indicators used to quantify full training sessions in soccer, with both internal and external load indicators being considered. The analysis revealed significant correlations between *player load* and the session-RPE indicator, as well as with the training load indicator obtained via the Edwards method (based on heart rate). It can therefore be concluded that player load is a valid indicator for quantifying workload during full training sessions in soccer.

Although the session-RPE indicator has been related to various indicators of physiological load (Alexiou and Coutts, 2008; Borresen and Lambert, 2008; Foster *et al.*, 2001; Impellizzeri *et al.*, 2004; Manzi *et al.*, 2010) we are unaware of any study that has examined its relationship with external training load, it therefore being unclear whether session-RPE is a valid indicator for determining physical load during training. The present analysis revealed that the session-RPE indicator was significantly correlated ($p$ < 0.01) with *player-load* based on accelerometry (Figure 2). In team sports, which involve rapid and nonlinear accelerations and decelerations, it is highly useful to have a parameter that quantifies the efforts made in this regard.

The present analysis of the relationship between *player load* and the two indicators of internal load (session-RPE and the Edwards method) revealed a higher correlation with session-RPE (r = 0.74; Figure 2) than with the indicator obtained via the Edwards method (r = 0.70; Figure 1). Future studies should examine the validity and reliability of this indicator in different training contexts and at different points during the season so as to determine its sensitivity when it comes to quantifying training load. In this regard, one of the main limitations of the present study is that it did not examine the correlation between training load indicators at different points in the season or across different training sessions (with different content, different workload levels or on different days of the week), these being factors which could influence training load and alter the relationships between indicators (Manzi *et al.*, 2010, Impellizzeri *et al.*, 2004).

## 4. CONCLUSION

On the basis of the results obtained for the external load of training sessions, monitored by means of GPS devices, and the internal load, estimated according to the session-RPE and the Edwards method, it can be concluded that in the context of team sports, which are characterized by intermittent activity and where high-intensity and sometimes nonlinear efforts alternate with periods of incomplete recovery, both these methods of quantification are highly correlated with the *player load*. This indicator, termed *player load*, is obtained via accelerometry and takes into account the accelerations made in intermittent and acyclic activities, in other words, maximum and brief efforts made in three planes of movement. Despite being a new indicator it has already been applied to different training contexts (Cunniffe *et al.*, 2009; Montgomery *et al.*, 2010), and the present results confirm that *player load* is a valid indicator for quantifying workload in full training sessions in soccer.

## Acknowledgements

We gratefully acknowledge the support of the Spanish government project Innovaciones en la evaluación de contextos naturales: Aplicaciones al ámbito del deporte [Grant number BSO2001-3368] and to the University of Basque Country (UPV-EHU).

## References

Alexiou, H. and Coutts, A., 2008, A comparison of methods used for quantifying internal training load in women soccer players. *Int J Sport Physiol Perf*, **3**, 320–330.

Bannister, E.W., 1991, Modelling elite athletic performance. In *Physiological Testing of the High-Performance Athlete*, 2nd ed., Champaign, IL: Human Kinetics Books, pp. 403–425.

Barris, S. and Button, C., 2008, A review of vision-based motion analysis in sport. *Sports Medicine*, **38**, 1025–1043.

Borresen, J. and Lambert, M., 2008, Quantifying training load: A comparison of subjective and objective methods. *Int J Sports Perf*, **3**, 16–30.

Castellano, J. *et al.*, 2011, Reliability and accuracy of 10 *Hz* GPS devices for short-distance exercise. *J Science Med Sport*, **10**, 233–234.

Cunniffe, B. *et al.*, 2009, An evaluation of the physiological demands of elite rugby union using global positioning system tracking software. *J Strength Cond Res*, **23**, 1195–1203.

Edwards, S., 1993, *The Heart Rate Monitor Book*. Sacramento, CA: Fleet Feet Press.

Foster, C. *et al.*, 1996, Athletic performance in relation to training load. *Wisconsin Medical Journal*, **95**, 370–374.

Foster C., 1998, Monitoring training in athletes with reference to overtraining syndrome. *Med Sci Sports Exerc*, **30**, 1164–1168.

Foster, C. *et al.*, 2001, A new approach to monitoring exercise training. *J Strength Cond Res*, **15**, 109–115.

Impellizzeri, F. *et al.*, 2004, Use of RPE-based training load in soccer. *Med Sci Sports Exerc*, **36**, 1042–1047.

Jennings, D. *et al.*, 2010, The validity and reliability of GPS units for measuring distance in team sport specific running patterns. *Int J Sports Physiol Perf*, **5**, 328–341.

Krustrup, P. *et al.*, 2003, The Yo-Yo Intermittent Recovery Test: Physiological response, reliability and validity. *Med Sci Sports Exerc*, **35**, 697–705.

Manzi, V. *et al.*, 2010, Profile of weekly training load in elite male professional basketball players. *J Strength Cond Res*, **24**, 1399–1406.

Montgomery, P.G. *et al.*, 2010, The physical and physiological demands of basketball training and competition. *Int J Sports Physiol Perf*, **5**, 75–86.

# CHAPTER SIXTY-SIX

# What is the work-load during training sessions in Rugby Union?

G. Da Lozzo and S. Pogliaghi

Faculty of Human Movement Sciences, University of Verona, Italy

## 1. INTRODUCTION

The determination of the work-load related to specific activities is essential to design training programs with adequate volume and intensity and to plan the optimal sequence of load and recovery. This allows reaching the highest levels of performance while minimizing the risk of injuries and overtraining. Furthermore, the monitoring of the individual effort allows the evaluation of the players' performance and commitment and can be used to reinforce motivation. Finally, this information is essential to quantify the athletes' energy requirements and the prevalent energy substrate involved in the training activity and to customize the dietary regime.

Three main components determine the training load: *frequency*, which is the number of sessions that take place in a given time; *volume*, which is the total length of training sessions; and *intensity*, which is the degree of effort that the athletes exert in each session. This last component is the most elusive in team sports (Duthie *et al.*, 2003). In rugby, the quantification of exercise intensity is further complicated by the variability of tasks, in the whole team and in positional groups, and by the high variability in players' somatotype. Differences in playing ability, age and gender pose additional challenges to the determination of exercise intensity at the team and individual level.

Possible approaches to the characterization of the physical demands of rugby are the quantification of frequency and/or duration of specific tasks by video movement analysis (Duthie *et al.*, 2005; Deutsch *et al.*, 2007) and the determination of the accelerations/decelerations using GPS tracking devices or accelerometers (Cunniffe *et al.*, 2009). Along with the high costs, a number of validity issues may limit the usefulness of the above approaches: i) estimation of exercise intensity based on absolute load (also called external load); ii) simplification of movement patterns into categories (while the actual play involves a dynamic combination of tasks, skills and tactics); iii) limitations of accuracy and reliability, especially for high intensity activities (Coutts and Duffield, 2010; Duthie *et al.*, 2003).

An alternative approach to the quantification of exercise intensity is based on the well known linear relationship between heart rate (HR) and oxygen uptake

(VO$_2$). The advantages of this approach are: simplicity of use; relatively low cost; easy and transparent data handling; measurement of both absolute and relative loads. Within some limitations (i.e. potential perturbation of HR by ambient and internal confounders; overestimation of HR during high-intensity isometric activities; inability of HR to account for the anaerobic component of exercise intensity; relatively slow adaptation of HR at the onset and offset of changes in work rate), the HR method provides satisfactory average estimates of exercise intensity for a group (Achten and Jeukendrup, 2003) and it has been widely used in individual and team sports (Foster *et al.*, 2001; Impellizzeri *et al.*, 2004).

Based on the determination of individual HR/VO$_2$ relationship, a number of indexes of absolute (VO$_2$, caloric expenditure) and relative exercise intensity (%HR$_{max}$, %VO$_{2max}$) can be determined. Furthermore, based on the knowledge of the athlete's ventilatory thresholds, the individual work-load can be quantified (Lucia *et al.*, 2003). HR-based quantification of exercise intensity has seldom been applied in rugby (Deutsch *et al.*, 1998; Duthie *et al.*, 2003) due to the difficulty in obtaining reliable HR measures during highly vigorous contacts (Duthie *et al.*, 2003). The availability of new, dependable HR monitors may allow the application of this approach on a large scale.

The few previous studies focused their attention on the determination of work-load in competitive matches (Deutsch *et al.*, 1998; Duthie *et al.,* 2005; Deutsch *et al.*, 2007). Regarding training sessions, the influence of duration and frequency on injuries was evaluated (Brooks *et al.*, 2008), but the component of intensity wasn't investigated. The lack of knowledge on specific training sessions' loads surely limits the accuracy of the training process' design and control. The aim of this study was to investigate the exercise intensity and work-load of two types of training sessions (Team Session and Unit Training) typically used in rugby union, based on the session HR, the individual HR/VO$_2$ relationship and the knowledge of individual ventilatory thresholds.

## 2. METHODS

**Subjects:** Fifteen rugby players (8 forwards (FW) and 7 backs (BK)) from the same Italian 1st Division rugby team were involved in the study (Table 1).

**Laboratory Tests:** Body mass (digital scale, Seca 877, Seca, Leicester, UK), stature (vertical stadiometer, Seca, Leicester, UK) and % body fat (plicometry, Holtain T/W skinfold caliper, Holtain limited, UK) were measured. Thereafter, athletes performed an incremental treadmill test to exhaustion (RunRace Technogym, Italy): after one minute standing still, subjects started running at 6.0 Km·h$^{-1}$ at an inclination of 1%. After three minutes, the treadmill speed was increased to 8.0 Km·h$^{-1}$ and then by 0.5 Km·h$^{-1}$ every minute until exhaustion. Throughout the test, respiratory variables and HR were measured breath-by-breath (Quark b$^2$ Cosmed, Italy).

**Field tests:** Twelve afternoon training sessions (6 Team Sessions (TS) and 6 Unit Trainings (UT)) were monitored within a 4-week period, during the mid-season competition break (January-February). During TS all the players were involved in similar activities: attack and defence movements on narrow or wide spaces, breakdown plays, pattern plays. During UT, forwards were trained mainly on scrums and lineouts; backs performed 3vs2 and 4vs2 attack and defence patterns, kicking game and counterattack movements. Throughout the sessions HR was measured every 10 seconds (Memory Belt, Suunto, Finland).

**Calculations:** Based on the laboratory test, the sub-maximal and maximal values of HR and $VO_2$ were calculated as the average of the last 10s of each work-load and of the last 10s before exhaustion, respectively. Furthermore the ventilatory thresholds were detected with standard technique (Wasserman *et al.*, 1973) and the individual HR/$VO_2$ relationship was determined by linear regression. Based on the ventilatory thresholds, three intensity zones were defined: a) Light Intensity Zone (LI zone): below the first ventilatory threshold ($VT_1$); b) Moderate Intensity Zone (MI zone): between $VT_1$ and the second ventilatory threshold ($VT_2$ or respiratory compensation point); c) High Intensity Zone (HI zone): over $VT_2$ (Lucia *et al.*, 2003).

Regarding the field tests, the training duration and the HR data were evaluated after the removal of the initial, standardized warm-up phase (~15min). HR data were expressed as percentage of maximum heart rate (%$HR_{max}$) and the energy expenditure ($Kcal \cdot Kg^{-1} \cdot min^{-1}$) was calculated, after conversion of individual HR into $VO_2$ data, based on a caloric equivalent of oxygen of 5 $kcal \cdot l^{-1}$. Furthermore, the training impulse (TRIMP), a cumulative indicator of work-load, was calculated as the sum of the minutes spent in the three different intensity zones, each multiplied by a specific coefficient equal to 1 for LI zone, 2 for MI zone and 3 for HI zone (Lucia *et al.*, 2003).

**Statistics:** Mean and standard deviation were calculated for all parameters and data were compared by t test.

## 3. RESULTS

Players had 12±3 years playing experience and their anthropometric and functional characteristics (Table 1) are representative of the Italian 1st Division championship. As expected, FW were taller, heavier and had a larger fat free mass compared to BK, yet the aerobic fitness was not different between groups.

**Table 1** Average ± standard deviation of the anthropometric and functional characteristics of forwards (FW) and backs (BK). * indicates a significant (p<0.05) difference from FW.

|    | Age (yrs) | Mass (kg) | Height (cm) | Fat mass (%) | Lean body mass (kg) | $VO_{2max}$ $(ml \cdot kg^{-1} \cdot min^{-1})$ |
|----|-----------|-----------|-------------|--------------|---------------------|--------------------|
| FW | 25±4 | 106±10 | 188±9 | 18±6 | 87±4 | 47±5 |
| BK | 24±3 | 92±12* | 181±11* | 14±6 | 79±6* | 47±3 |

Regarding the monitoring of training sessions, a minimal data loss was experienced (11 measures out of the initially programmed 180 were lost, 8 due to athlete's absence, 3 due to malfunction of the heart rate monitor). The characteristics of the training sessions are summarized in Table 2. TS and UT had similar overall duration. TS were conducted at a higher relative intensity and caused a higher energy expenditure compared to UT in both FW and BK. Accordingly, TS had a higher training-load (i.e. TRIMP) compared to UT.

**Table 2** Average ± standard deviation of the duration (min), intensity (% of maximal heart rate - $\%HR_{max}$- and energy expenditure - $Kcal \cdot kg^{-1} \cdot min^{-1}$) and work-load (training impulse or TRIMP and % of time spent in each intensity zone during training sessions) of team (TS) and in unit (UT) training sessions, in positional groups: forwards (FW) and backs (BK). * and § indicate, respectively, a significant (p<0.05) difference *vs* FW and *vs* TS.

|  | Team session training (TS) | | Unit training (UT) | |
|---|---|---|---|---|
|  | FW | BK | FW | BK |
| Duration (min) | 59±12 | 59±12 | 56±17 | 51±17§ |
| HR ($\%HR_{max}$) | 72±8 | 74±6 | 63±7§ | 70±5*§ |
| Energy Expenditure ($Kcal \cdot kg^{-1} \cdot min^{-1}$) | 0.13±0.03 | 0.14±0.02 | 0.11±0.03§ | 0.12±0.03*§ |
| TRIMP (min·training session$^{-1}$) | 69.4±16.0 | 67.4±21.2 | 58.5±23.5§ | 55.5±23.6§ |
| Time in zone 1 (%) | 88±14 | 89±15 | 91±8 | 89±10 |
| Time in zone 2 (%) | 8±9 | 6±8 | 6±5 | 8±7 |
| Time in zone 3 (%) | 4±8 | 5±8 | 3±5 | 3±5 |

## 4. DISCUSSION

The present study was the first to determine exercise intensity and work-load of two types of training sessions (Team Session and Unit Training) typically performed in rugby union, based on the session HR, the individual $HR/VO_2$ relationship and the knowledge of individual ventilatory thresholds. In this team of senior, semi-professional players, the absolute and relative intensity and the work-load of training sessions were successfully determined.

TS, during which all the players were involved in similar, mostly dynamic, activities (attack and defence movements on narrow or wide spaces, breakdown plays, pattern plays), were performed in the moderate intensity domain and produced a relatively low energy expenditure. During UT forwards performed high-intensity activities with a large isometric component (i.e. scrums and lineouts), interspersed by complete recovery periods while backs performed dynamic activities (3vs2 and 4vs2 attack and defence patterns, kicking game and counterattack movements). Surprisingly, UT were characterized by a lower absolute and relative exercise intensity and by a lower work-load compared to TS for both FW and BK.

During both types of activity, yet specially so for UT, the ability of HR to accurately track exercise intensity may be reduced due to the following: a) an overestimation of HR of about $10 \cdot bmin^{-1}$ has been documented in mixed, static-dynamic activities compared to only dynamic activities (Patterson *et al.*, 1985). In the present study, this would have caused a 10% overestimation of energy expenditure; b) HR does not account for the anaerobic component of exercise, therefore potentially causing an underestimation of caloric expenditure of highly intense, intermittent activities. In the present study, average intensity was relatively low (~70% $HR_{max}$) and homogeneous (average within session coefficient of variation <10%), suggesting a rather small contribution of the anaerobic metabolism to the overall energy production; c) at exercise onset and offset, both HR and $VO_2$ adapt to the changes in work rate with a 30s to 1 min delay in trained individuals. Particularly so for highly intermittent exercise, this may cause an underestimation of exercise intensity in the on-transient that is mirrored by (and therefore can be dampened by) an overestimation during the off-transient.

Notwithstanding the above potential limitations the HR method provides satisfactory average estimates of exercise intensity for a group of athletes (Achten and Jeukendrup, 2003) that has been widely used in individual and team sports (Foster *et al.*, 2001; Impellizzeri *et al.*, 2004) in which a direct $VO_2$ determination cannot be performed.

In accordance with the literature (Duthie *et al.*, 2003; Scott *et al.*, 2003; Duthie *et al.*, 2006), our data document significant role differences in anthropometric parameters between FW and BK. This confirms the specificity in the physical requirements of rugby union in individual playing positions. Our players appear shorter, lighter, with a lower fat free mass and a larger fat mass compared to elite Italian and international players. Such differences may reflect the lower playing ability, selection and training work-load that is typical of our semi-professional national championship.

Functional evaluation of aerobic performance was also performed in our study. $VO_{2max}$ values in both FW and BK appear lower than indicated in previous studies (Duthie *et al.*, 2003). The importance of $VO_{2max}$ is controversial in rugby union. Although, as in many other team sports, a high $VO_{2max}$ facilitates the repetition of high intensity anaerobic efforts, it is not usually considered a fundamental component of the rugby player's fitness profile. Therefore the low $VO_{2max}$ observed in our study could be ascribed to both a low work-load and to the fact that training is normally not addressed at improving this functional parameter.

In summary, this is the first study to evaluate the absolute and relative intensity and the work-load during specific training sessions in rugby union. These parameters can be useful to establish the physical requirements of both training and match-play, to identify role differences and to support training decisions. Only by increasing the number of published data in the scientific literature, can we have reliable reference data on this small and poorly understood subject. Furthermore, periodic monitoring of a variety of playing populations is necessary to quantify and compare the evolving demands of rugby union.

## References

Achten, J. and Jeukendrup, A.E., 2003, Heart rate monitoring: Applications and limitations. *Sports Med*, **33**, 517–538.

Åstrand P.O. *et al.*, 2003, *Textbook of Work Physiology.* 4th edition, Champaign, IL: Human Kinetics.

Brooks, J.H. *et al.*, 2008, An assessment of training volume in professional rugby union and its impact on the incidence, severity, and nature of match and training injuries. *J Sports Sci*, **26**, 863–873.

Coutts, A.J. and Duffield, R., 2010, Validity and reliability of GPS devices for measuring movement demands of team sports. *J Sci Med Sport*, **13**, 133–135.

Cunniffe, B. *et al.*, 2009, An evaluation of the physiological demands of elite rugby union using Global Positioning System tracking software. *J Strength Cond Res*, **23**, 1195–1203.

Deutsch, M.U. *et al.*, 2007, Time-motion analysis of professional rugby union players during match-play. *J Sports Sci*, **25**, 461–472.

Deutsch, M.U. *et al.*, 1998, Heart rate, blood lactate and kinematic data of elite colts (under-19) rugby union players during competition. *J Sports Sci*, **16**, 561–570.

Duthie, G. *et al.*, 2003, Applied physiology and game analysis of rugby union. *Sports Med*, **33**, 973–991.

Duthie, G. *et al.*, 2005, Time motion analysis of 2001 and 2002 Super 12 rugby. *J Sports Sci*, **23**, 523–530.

Duthie, G.M. *et al.*, 2006, Anthropometry profiles of elite rugby players: Quantifying changes in lean mass. *Brit J Sports Med*, **40**, 202–207.

Foster, C. *et al.*, 2001, A new approach to monitoring exercise training. *J Strength Cond Res*, **15**, 109–115.

Impellizzeri, F.M. *et al.*, 2004, Use of RPE-based training load in soccer. *Med Sci Sports Exerc*, **36**, 1042–1047.

Lucia, A. *et al.*, 2003, Tour de France versus Vuelta a Espana: Which is harder? *Med Sci Sports Exerc*, **35**, 872–878.

Patterson, R.P. *et al.*, 1985, Work-rest periods: Their effects on normal physiologic response to isometric and dynamic work. *Arch Phys Med Rehabil*, **66**, 348–352.

Scott, A. C. *et al.*, 2003, Aerobic exercise physiology in a professional rugby union team. *Int J Cardiol*, **87**, 173–177.

Wasserman, K. *et al.*, 1973, Anaerobic threshold and respiratory gas exchange during exercise. *J Appl Physiol*, **35**, 236–243.

# CHAPTER SIXTY-SEVEN

# Influence of age and fitness on match and training activity profiles in junior Australian football

P. B. Gastin[1,3], G. Bennett[1] and J. Cook [2,3]

[1]Centre for Exercise and Sport Science, Deakin University, Australia
[2] Department of Physiotherapy, Monash University, Australia
[3]Australian Centre for Research into Sports Injury and its Prevention, Monash University, Australia

## 1. INTRODUCTION

The physical attributes that increase during childhood and adolescence are well established (Nevill *et al.* 1998; Van Praagh and Dore, 2002). Increased height and weight have an impact on aerobic and anaerobic capacities, muscular strength, power and running speeds, leading to an increased sporting performance throughout pubertal growth (Malina *et al.*, 2004). This gives a distinct advantage in sporting performance to older individuals or those more biologically mature within an age group (Armstrong and Welsman, 2005). Selection bias and the relative age effect (Barnsley *et al.*, 1992), where a predominance of selected players are from the first quarter or half of the year, have previously been observed in the football codes at both junior and senior levels (Cobley *et al.*, 2009), suggesting that players born earlier in the selection year have an advantage in the sport.

While age-related differences in measures of fitness have been documented in soccer (Mendez-Villanueva *et al.*, 2010, 2011), little data is available to evaluate whether these underlying age-related fitness parameters translate into improvements in on-field measures of performance. It has recently been observed that match running performance increased with age in highly trained youth soccer players (Buchheit *et al.*, 2010) while in elite under eighteen Australian football (AF) shorter and lighter players who possessed high levels of speed and endurance were more likely to acquire possessions and be awarded votes in competition (Young and Pryor, 2007). However time-motion analysis and the relationships between running performance and fitness have not been documented in junior recreational AF. The purpose of this study therefore was to assess baseline fitness characteristics and their relationships with activity profiles in training and competition in junior AF. A secondary aim was to describe the time-motion demands of AF beyond those reported for elite senior football.

## 2. METHODS

Forty-seven healthy male junior AF players from four age groups ranging from under elevens (U11) to under seventeens (U17) were recruited for this study from a local junior AF club in Melbourne, Australia. The study protocol was approved by the Deakin University Human Research Ethics Committee and informed consent obtained from participants and their parents/guardians.

This study used an observational cross sectional design, and was conducted over an eight week period (June-July) during the second half of the AF season. Pre-testing measures included age, standing height, weight, 20 m multi-stage shuttle run and 20 m sprint. Data relating to running movements during training and competition were collected using GPS technology.

Height and weight were measured (shoes off in training uniform) to the nearest 0.1 cm and 0.1 kg, respectively. Running speed was measured during a 20 m sprint using infra-red timing gates (Smartspeed, FusionSport Pty Ltd, Australia),with the best of three trials being recorded. Aerobic fitness level was determined using an incremental 20 m shuttle run test (Multi-stage Fitness Test, Australian Coaching Council, Australian Sports Commission, 1999). Both speed and aerobic fitness were assessed following a warm-up and prior to football training and were conducted on grass with players wearing football boots.

Participants from each age group were fitted with a GPS device (SPI Pro, 5 Hz, GPSports Pty Ltd, Australia) in one to four regular training sessions (mean = 3.0) and one to two matches (mean = 1.7) for a total of 197 individual samples. Each participant wore the same GPS unit for each training session and match. GPS data from the SPI Pro unit was downloaded to a personal computer for analysis using the Team AMS proprietary software provided by the manufacturer (version 2.1.05 P2, GPSports Pty Ltd, Australia).

GPS data analysis included measures of total distance, peak speed, high-speed running (HSR) distance, high-speed efforts (HSE) and number of sprints. Any running recorded above 14.4 km/h was considered HSR/HSE, whereas any effort in excess of 23 km/h was considered a sprint. These speed zones were selected as they reflected the zones previously reported in recent time-motion analysis literature in field-based team sports (Coutts *et al.*, 2010; Mohr *et al.*, 2003; Rampinini *et al.*, 2007, 2009).

Training data was split using Team AMS software from the recorded start time to the end time of each session. Match data was split into four quarters to eliminate the warm up and quarter time breaks from data analysis. All training and match data was expressed relative to time (i.e. per minute) to compensate for different training and match times observed across the age groups. For each player a paired sample of mean training and match data was used in the analysis.

Data are presented as means and standard deviations. All statistical analyses were conducted using Statistical Package for the Social Sciences software (SPSS 17.0.0, SPSS Inc., USA). Statistical significance was set at $p < 0.05$. One-way ANOVA for independent measures with Tukey post-hoc comparison were used to test differences between age groups. Pearson's correlation coefficients (r) were calculated to examine the relationships between age, running fitness and activity profiles during training and competition. Correlation coefficients are discussed as very strong ($r \geq \pm 0.7$), strong ($r \geq \pm 0.5$), moderate ($\pm 0.5 > r \geq \pm 0.3$) and weak ($\pm 0.3 > r \geq \pm 0.1$).

## 3. RESULTS

Descriptive statistics of participant physical characteristics and aerobic fitness and speed test results are summarised in Table 1. Significant differences were evident between the younger (U11, U13) and older (U15, U17) age groups for weight, height, aerobic fitness and 20 m sprint. Figure 1 shows a very strong positive correlation between age in years and 20 m shuttle run score ($r = 0.825$) and a very strong negative correlation between age and 20 m sprint time ($r = -0.807$). This confirms that aerobic and anaerobic fitness improves with age in junior AF players, although inspection of individual data points within each age group suggests that considerable variability exists in individuals of similar age.

The activity demands of AF during both training and competition increase with age as is evident by significant correlations for all distance and high-speed running variables (Table 2). Relationships are, however, stronger in training compared to match conditions.

**Table 1** Descriptive statistics of participants (mean ± SD).

| Age Group | U11 (n = 10) | U13 (n = 16) | U15 (n = 14) | U17 (n = 7) |
|---|---|---|---|---|
| Age (yrs) | 11.0 ± 0.3 | 12.9 ± 0.4[a] | 15.0 ± 0.3[ab] | 16.2 ± 0.5[abc] |
| Height (cm) | 149.5 ± 5.9 | 158.8 ± 8.3 | 172.5 ± 8.9[ab] | 173.4 ± 5.1[ab] |
| Weight (kg) | 40.3 ± 6.0 | 48.6 ± 9.1 | 63.7 ± 10.1[ab] | 67.0 ± 4.2[ab] |
| 20 m shuttle (level) | 6.3 ± 1.6 | 7.5 ± 1.6 | 11.8 ± 1.1[ab] | 11.8 ± 1.9[ab] |
| 20 m sprint (s) | 3.99 ± 0.31 | 3.75 ± 0.22 | 3.26 ± 0.15[ab] | 3.27 ± 0.24[ab] |

Post-hoc comparisons with groups to the left:
[a] significantly different (p<0.05) from U11; [b] from U13; [c] from U15

Similar relationships between measures of aerobic fitness and speed and AF training and match activity profiles were also observed (Table 3), with relationships again being stronger for the training data. Interestingly aerobic fitness correlated most highly with HSR and peak speed in training.

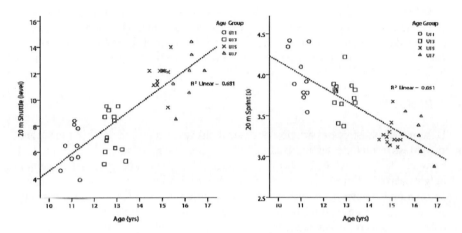

**Figure 1** Relationships between age and 20 m shuttle run and 20 m sprint.

**Table 2** Relationships between age and Australian football activity profiles.

|            | Training Data* | Match Data* |
|------------|----------------|-------------|
| Distance   | 0.899          | 0.408       |
| HSR        | 0.870          | 0.612       |
| HSE        | 0.827          | 0.585       |
| Sprints    | 0.616          | 0.599       |
| Peak Speed | 0.464          | 0.582       |

HSR = high-speed running distance, HSE = high-speed efforts
*All correlations (Pearson's r) significant at the 0.01 level (2-tailed)

**Table 3** Relationships between indices of fitness and Australian football activity profiles.

|                   | Distance* | HSR*   | HSE*   | Peak Speed* |
|-------------------|-----------|--------|--------|-------------|
| Training Data     |           |        |        |             |
| 20 m shuttle run  | 0.801     | 0.923  | 0.578  | 0.930       |
| 20 m sprint       | -0.752    | -0.825 | -0.626 | -0.833      |
| Match Data        |           |        |        |             |
| 20 m shuttle run  | 0.649     | 0.746  | 0.720  | 0.675       |
| 20 m sprint       | -0.637    | -0.785 | -0.782 | -0.740      |

*All correlations (Pearson's r) significant at the 0.01 level (2-tailed)

Training and competition match data (Table 4) show incremental increases across the age groups for most GPS derived running variables, with significant differences being evident between the younger and older age groups, but not typically between the U11 and U13 or the U15 and U17. The match activity profile was significantly greater than that achieved during training for all age groups except in the U17 group or for peak speed and number of sprints.

**Table 4** Measures of training and match activity profiles for each age group.

| Age Group | U11 (n = 10) | U13 (n = 16) | U15 (n = 14) | U17 (n = 7) |
|---|---|---|---|---|
| Training Data | | | | |
| Duration (min) | 70.0 ± 5.5 | 72.3 ± 6.2 | 84.8 ± 2.7[ab] | 59.6 ± 1.7[abc] |
| Distance (m/min) | 48.4 ± 4.5 | 66.3 ± 5.4[a] | 74.3 ± 5.8[ab] | 89.7 ± 4.4[abc] |
| HSR (m/min) | 3.4 ± 2.1 | 7.4 ± 2.2[a] | 14.8 ± 3.7[ab] | 18.6 ± 5.2[ab] |
| HSE (number/min) | 0.2 ± 0.1 | 0.4 ± 0.1[a] | 0.8 ± 0.1[ab] | 0.8 ± 0.2[ab] |
| Sprints (number) | 0.0 ± 0.1 | 0.2 ± 0.1 | 2.0 ± 1.8[ab] | 4.2 ± 3.2[abc] |
| Peak Speed (km/h) | 23.4 ± 5.0 | 23.5 ± 3.1 | 26.7 ± 3.1 | 27.7 ± 3.4 |
| Match Data | | | | |
| Duration (min) | 60.0 ± 0.0* | 60.0 ± 0.0[a]* | 81.6 ± 0.7[ab]* | 88.0 ± 0.0[abc]* |
| Distance (m/min) | 70.4 ± 20.0* | 85.4 ± 21.2* | 100.1 ± 15.4[a]* | 82.3 ± 19.6 |
| HSR (m/min) | 6.2 ± 4.9* | 11.7 ± 5.8* | 18.0 ± 4.1[ab]* | 15.3 ± 7.3[a] |
| HSE (number/min) | 0.4 ± 0.3* | 0.7 ± 0.3[a]* | 1.0 ± 0.2[a]* | 0.9 ± 0.3[a] |
| Sprints (number) | 0.1 ± 0.2 | 0.4 ± 0.7 | 3.4 ± 2.8[ab]* | 4.0 ± 4.0[ab] |
| Peak Speed (km/h) | 22.3 ± 3.1 | 24.0 ± 3.5 | 28.4 ± 3.9[ab] | 28.2 ± 3.5[a] |

Mean ± SD; HSR = high-speed running distance, HSE = high-speed efforts, Post-hoc comparisons with groups to the left: [a] significantly different (p<0.05) from U11; [b] from U13; [c] from U15
* significantly different (p<0.05) between training and match

## 4. DISCUSSION

This study is the first to describe the time-motion running demands in junior AF during both training and competition. Running performance demonstrated moderate to very strong relationships (range: 0.408–0.899) with chronological age in this group of players ranging in age from 10.5 to 17.0 years. Relationships were stronger during training than competition suggesting that inherent fitness characteristics are more likely expressed during a structured training environment, as opposed to match conditions where playing position, tactics, level of opposition and the competitive nature of the game may confound this relationship. In a similar recent study in soccer, Buchheit *et al* (2010) demonstrated an increasing trend in match running performance with age in highly trained young players, and when adjusted for age and individual playing time, running performance was found to be position-dependent.

Relationships between running fitness (i.e. 20 m shuttle run and sprint) and running performance in AF were also strongly correlated (range: 0.637–0.930) and in the case of peak speed and HSR exhibited stronger relationships than those for age. Running fitness and age are closely linked in this group of young players with approximately 65% of the variance being explained by age. Other factors such as training derived fitness and biological maturity may further contribute to running performance other than those that might be attributed to age-related increases in size and stature alone. Indeed Mendez-Villanueva *et al.* (2011) recently suggested that the positive effects of age on running speed qualities in their sample of well-trained youth soccer players were more related to biological maturation than to anthropometric characteristics only.

The very strong correlation between aerobic fitness and 20 m sprint in this group of recreational young AF players and between aerobic fitness and HSR and peak speed in a match suggest that running abilities are less specialised in children, and that specialised speed/power or endurance profiles are more likely developed later in adolescence (Falk and Bar-Or 1993; Malina *et al.*, 2004). Children who perform well in sprinting tasks also perform well in endurance activities, and vice versa (Malina *et al.*, 2004). Mendez-Villanueva *et al.* (2011) also observed very strong correlations between acceleration, maximum aerobic running speed, and repeated sprint ability and concluded that running speed was more of a general quality in young soccer players.

Performance in repeated-sprint ability improves during maturation of highly trained youth soccer players, although a plateau occurs from 15 years of age (Mujika *et al.*, 2009). A levelling off was also evident in our data, with speed and endurance running fitness found to be similar in the U15 and U17 age groups yet significantly different from both the U11 and U13 groups. Training and match activity profiles were also similar in the U15 and U17 groups, with the exception of distance and the number of sprints during training. These age groups span mid- and late-puberty and include individuals close to or beyond peak height velocity (Malina, 2003) such that differences related to growth may be less pronounced than those seen between the younger age groups.

Match activity profiles were generally higher than training for most variables, with the exception of the U17 group where training and competition demands were similar. Data from elite senior AF (Dawson *et al.*, 2004) also found differences between training and competition demands, with training being characterised by longer rest periods between high intensity movements, greater number of ball possessions yet less contested and physical pressure and fewer position-specific activities for the more specialised playing positions (e.g. ruckmen, full-forward and full-backs). Brewer *et al.* (2010) compared match activity demands between two playing levels in AF and found that senior elite players had higher movement demands, including 9% more distance covered per minute and 21% more high intensity efforts per minute than sub-elite AF players. When compared to our junior recreational players, differences in distance covered for senior elite and sub-elite were greater by as much as 82% and 66% respectively in the U11 and as little as 28% and 17% in the U15. Comparisons for HSR and sprints are more difficult as running zones were not the same, however, data for HSE suggest that differences are more than 600% in the U11 and 250% in the U15. Distance is known to be a less discriminating variable than HSR variables in football with elite levels of competition demanding that senior players are able to sprint at faster speeds and more often.

In summary, this study found moderate to very strong relationships between age and activity profiles in training and competition and strong to very strong relationships between measures of aerobic running fitness and speed and AF activity profiles. It is suggested that running fitness in junior recreational AF players is less specialised and more general in nature and likely to become more specialised post-puberty and/or with specialised training. Relationships with age and running fitness and AF activity profiles were generally stronger during training than competition, despite match running demands being higher than in training.

## References

Armstrong, N., and Welsman, J., 2005, Essay: Physiology of the child athlete. *The Lancet*, **366**, S44–S45.

Barnsley, R.H. *et al.*, 1992, Family planning: football style. The relative age effect in football. *Int Rev Sociol Sport*, **27**, 77–88.

Brewer, C. *et al.*, 2010, Movement pattern comparisons in elite (AFL) and sub-elite (WAFL) Australian football games using GPS. *J Sci Med Sport*, **13**, 618–623.

Buchheit, M. *et al.*, 2010, Match running performance and fitness in youth soccer. *Int J Sports Med*, **31**, 818–825.

Cobley, S. *et al.*, 2009, Annual age-grouping and athlete development: A meta-analytical review of relative age effects in sport. *Sports Med*, **39**, 235–256.

Coutts, A.J. *et al.*, 2010, Match running performance in elite Australian Rules Football. *J Sci Med Sport*, **13**, 543–548.

Dawson, B. *et al.*, 2004, Comparison of training activities and game demands in the Australian Football League. *J Sci Med Sport*, **7**, 292–301.

Dawson, B. *et al.*, 2004, Player movement patterns and game activities in the Australian Football League. *J Science Med Sport*, **7**, 278–291.

Falk, B. and Bar-Or, O., 1993, Longitudinal changes in peak aerobic and anaerobic mechanical power of circumpubertal boys. *Pediatric Exercise Science*, **5**, 318–331.

Malina, R. 2003, Growth and maturity status of young soccer players. In *Science and Soccer*, London: Routledge, pp. 287–305.

Malina, R. *et al.*, 2004, *Growth, Maturation, and Physical Activity*. 2nd ed. Champaign, IL: Human Kinetics.

Mendez-Villanueva, A. *et al.*, 2010, Is the relationship between sprinting and maximal aerobic speeds in young soccer players affected by maturation? *Pediatric Exercise Science*, **22**, 497–510.

Mendez-Villanueva, A. *et al.*, 2011, Age-related differences in acceleration, maximum running speed, and repeated-sprint performance in young soccer players. *J Sports Sci*, **29**, 477–484.

Mohr, M. *et al.*, 2003, Match performance of high-standard soccer players with special reference to development of fatigue. *J Sports Sci Med*, **21**, 519–528.

Mujika, I. *et al.*, 2009, Age-related differences in repeated-sprint ability in highly trained youth football players. *J Sports Sci*, **27**, 1581–1590.

Nevill, A.M., 1998, Modeling developmental changes in strength and aerobic power in children. *J Appl Physiol*, **84**, 963–970.

Rampinini, E. *et al.*, 2007, Variation in top-level soccer performance. *Int J Sports Med*, **28**, 1018–1024.

Rampinini, E., 2009, Technical performance during soccer matches of the Italian Serie A league: Effect of fatigue and competitive level. *J Sci Med Sport*, **12**, 227–233.

Van Praagh, E. and Dore, E., 2002, Short-term muscle power during growth and maturation. / Puissance musculaire a court-terme pendant la croissance et la maturation. *Sports Med*, **32**, 701–728.

Young, W.B. and Pryor, L., 2007, Relationship between pre-season anthropometric and fitness measures and indicators of playing performance in elite junior Australian Rules football. *J Sci Med Sport*, **10**, 110–118.

# Index